Also by Daniel Gastelu

All About Bioflavonoids

All About Carnitine

All About Sports Nutrition

Avery's Sports Nutrition Almanac

Dynamic Nutrition for Maximum Performance

Performance Nutrition: The Complete Guide

Weight Control, Fitness, and Performance Nutrition

THE COMPLETE NUTRITIONAL SUPPLEMENTS BUYER'S GUIDE

Detailed information on herbal products • Vitamins, minerals, amino acids, metabolites, fatty acids • Which formulas work best for health and longevity • The top nutrients for stamina, weight loss, sleep, joint health, and memory • The top supplements to beat fatigue, headaches, and depression • The top supplements for women's health • Ingredients you should avoid • And much, much more

DANIEL GASTELU, M.S., M.F.S.

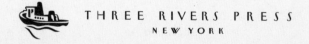

THREE RIVERS PRESS
NEW YORK

Published by Three Rivers Press, New York, New York.
Member of the Crown Publishing Group.

Random House, Inc. New York, Toronto, London, Sydney,
Auckland
www.randomhouse.com

THREE RIVERS PRESS is a registered trademark and the
Three Rivers Press colophon is a trademark of Random
House, Inc.

Printed in the United States of America
Design by Rhea Braunstein

Library of Congress Cataloging-in-Publication Data
Gastelu, Daniel.
The complete nutritional supplements buyer's guide :
detailed information on herbal products . . . /
Daniel Gastelu.—1st pbk. ed.
1. Dietary supplements—Handbooks, manuals, etc. I. Title.
QP141 .G355 2000
613.2´6—dc21
99-59792

ISBN 0-609-80464-2

10 9 8 7 6 5 4 3 2 1
First Edition

IMPORTANT NOTICE

This book is not intended for use as a substitute for consultation with a qualified medical practitioner. If you have symptoms of any illness, it is essential that you see your doctor without delay. You are unique, and your diagnosis and treatment must be individualized for you by your own doctor. This book provides exciting information about nutritional supplements and the ingredients they contain. But no book can replace the personalized care that you need. You are encouraged to work closely with your doctor and other health-care professionals to achieve optimum health.

The author or his agents will not accept responsibility for injury, loss, or damage occasioned to any person acting or refraining to act as a result of material contained in this book, whether or not such injury, loss, or damage is due in any way to any negligent act or omission, breach of duty, or default on the part of the author or his agents.

The brand names included in this book are not intended to endorse products. A product that is included in this book does not imply it is any better than products not included in this book.

A special dedication to
Keith and Tammy

This book is dedicated to the following authors, who have devoted their lives to the promotion of health through education, and have inspired me to write the best book on dietary supplements ever, so that you too can become a champion of health and happiness.

Sal Arria, D.C.

Robert C. Atkins, M.D.

Denise Austin

James F. Balch, M.D.

Phyllis A. Balch, C.N.C.

Kenneth Blum, Ph.D.

Deepak Chopra, M.D.

Alex Duarte, O.D.

H. Winter Griffith, M.D.

Frederick C. Hatfield, Ph.D.

C. Everett Koop, M.D.

Jack La Lanne

Shari Lieberman, Ph.D.

Tony Little

Earl Mindell, Ph.D.

Michael T. Murray, N.D.

Gary Null, Ph.D.

Richard Simmons

Edward A. Taub, M.D.

Varro E. Tyler, Ph.D., Sc.D.

Art Ulene, M.D.

Ben Weider

Joe Weider

Andrew Weil, M.D.

Jonathan Zuess, M.D.

CONTENTS

ACKNOWLEDGMENTS

I am extremely grateful to my family, friends, and colleagues, whose constant support inspired me to be able to make this book an extremely valuable resource for fellow supplement-takers.

I would like to offer my special thanks to the talented team of people at The Crown Publishing Group whose hard work and dedication helped to make this book a reality: Liz Matthews, Peter Guzzardi, Cindy Berman, Carrie Thornton, Tina Constable, and Jennifer Gowins.

Finally, I express my sincere appreciation to President William J. Clinton and the members of the 103rd Congress who had the vision and wisdom to pass the Dietary Supplement, Health, and Education Act; and to the U.S. Food & Drug Administration personnel for their superb work regulating the dietary supplement industry to ensure safe and effective products for the 180 million, and growing, supplement-taking Americans.

PREFACE

Today almost every man, woman, and child consumes dietary supplements, yet this seemingly endless category of products remains a mystery to most. Hence the need for this book.

The contents of this book are based on my vast experience as an industry veteran, scientist, and developer of hundreds of dietary supplement products, combined with direct input from teaching health professionals. I've put all this information together in an easy-to-use format. This is the book you have been waiting for.

In it you will learn:

- What dietary supplements are, and how they are regulated to ensure safety
- How to choose safe and effective formulas that contain the right dosages for your personal needs
- All about the ingredients that medical studies say work best

- The best forms of calcium for protection against osteoporosis
- Guidelines for selecting the best formulas for health and longevity
- All about herbal products, sorting through the facts and misconceptions
- Nutrients for cardiovascular wellness, weight loss, sleep, joint health, and memory
- The best supplements to beat fatigue, headaches, and depression
- The top ten supplements for boosting energy levels
- The best supplements for longevity
- The top eleven supplements for women's health
- The top seventeen supplements for overcoming digestive difficulty
- Ingredients you should avoid
- Special guidelines for selecting supplements for children
- Drug-supplement interactions

- Learn industry secrets, known only to a select few

But this is just the beginning. There's much, much more . . . including a bonus section featuring the Natural-Thin weight loss program.

With this dietary supplement guide you will be truly in charge of your health and well-being. Join the millions of people who are reaping the benefits of taking the right kind of supplements.

This is the only authoritative guide available to the otherwise baffling world of supplements. Reading it will put the power back in your hands. Armed with this new information, you will be able to decode the labels of the thousands of dietary supplement products on the market, and know what the medical research says is best for your health. *So stop what you're doing and read this book before you take or purchase another dietary supplement, to be sure that what you are taking is safe and effective.*

The Complete Nutritional Supplements Buyer's Guide is divided into three parts, making your road to mastering this information as easy as 1-2-3.

Part 1 gives you an insider's view of the process of designing and manufacturing dietary supplements. It goes through the terminology and regulations, which until now were familiar to only a small group of industry experts. The information in these introductory chapters will set the record straight about the safe and effective use of dietary supplements and the numerous benefits taking them has to offer. After reading these chapters, you will also understand the FDA's role in regulating the safety of dietary supplements and the FTC's role in regulating the claims manufacturers make. You will learn why in 1994 Congress passed new rules allowing you, the consumer, access to more ingredients.

Part 2 contains without a doubt the most unique and revealing information ever published about dietary supplements. Within these chapters you will learn just what supplements you need, based on your sex, age, and health goals. You will be privy to information known to only a handful of experts in the world, those who formulate and invent dietary supplements. Part 2 will set the record straight on which formulas are best for you to take. Starting with Chapter 5, you will find special guidelines to help you understand the "why" of the various dietary supplement formulations. After reading this chapter, you will also be able to determine your personal dietary supplement needs. Chapters 6 through 19 are devoted to the best products for specific goals, including healthy cholesterol levels, a strong immune system, weight loss, natural energy, and women's and men's health. These chapters will enable you to fine-tune your wellness program to promote health and extend your life. Amazingly, this can be accomplished with very little effort on your part, and on a tight budget, too. The few seconds a day that are needed to take your supplements can make big improvements in your life.

Part 3 contains an alphabetical listing of the major dietary supplement ingredients on the market today. It includes both common ingredients found in the mass-market brands and uncommon ingredients you may encounter in products sold in health food stores and through direct marketers. Up-to-date medical and scientific information is presented for each ingredient, including common name(s), supplement type, scientific name(s), functions, benefits, best ingredient forms, dosages, cofactors, concerns, and revealing comments. With this information at your fingertips, your decisions about which supplements to take will be sensible and well informed.

The Appendix contains my revolutionary Natural-Thin diet program. This plan includes all the information you will need to be a success at weight loss and weight maintenance. It's the program that lets you eat the delicious foods you love, and includes the top appetite-satisfying foods to help you win the battle of the bulge. The Natural-Thin program has it all, including the best fitness tips and behavioral strategy science has to offer for losing weight and keeping it off. I also include a food guide to help you choose the foods that are best for you and your family.

The information contained within these pages is based on current scientific fact, backed by research findings from thousands of clinical studies as well as the National Institutes of Health, the National Academy of Sciences, the Surgeon General's office, the Council for Responsible Nutrition, the Food and Drug Administration, the U.S. Department of Agriculture, universities, hospitals, the American Heart Association, the American Dietetic Association, and the U.S. Department of Health and Human Services. In addition, a leading natural health products expert, Jonathan Zuess, M.D., took the time to review this information. Peer reviewing of medical and scientific works is regarded as the highest quality standard, and an essential way to further ensure that this information meets the highest academic, industry, and medical standards. The overall goal of this book is to offer you the proven facts on dietary supplements that work best.

On a final note, proper use of the information in this or any health book means working with your health care practitioner to develop a nutrition and dietary supplement program and keeping him or her informed about what supplements you are taking. In this way, your progress will be monitored by a trained health professional, to document your improvements in health and promptly deal with any health issues. It is especially important to work closely with a medical professional if you have an existing health disorder, are on a weight loss program, are involved in strenuous activity, or are pregnant or lactating.

I want you to have fun reading this book. Approach it as if you were reading a novel or magazine—but with this difference: Learning the story of dietary supplements is learning the secrets to optimal health. It is a story you can live for real, and of which you can be the hero.

My personal wish is that you and your loved ones use this valuable information to live a long life filled with health, happiness, and prosperity.

DANIEL GASTELU

INTRODUCTION

Jonathan Zuess, M.D.

You're holding in your hands one of the true fruits of the Information Age. It took a technological revolution in the biosciences to redeem nutritional supplements from their "home remedy" roots of the past decades and put them in their rightful place—the cutting edge of modern medicine. Never before have we had so much information about their effectiveness for preventing and treating illness, not to mention improving overall well-being, mental functioning, athletic performance, and possibly even extending life span. If Bacon was right when he said four hundred years ago, "Knowledge itself is power," then this book represents the power you can take over your own health.

The practice of nutritional medicine is a passion of mine, and I'm glad to see more of this knowledge available for everyone. It's not a simple task to sum up the many thousands of studies on the myriad of different supplements you'll find in health food stores today, but Daniel Gastelu has done it admirably. This book is comprehensive, straightforward, and easy to use. Lay people and health professionals alike will benefit from it—and I mean physicians, too.

THE PRACTICE OF MEDICINE IS CHANGING, WITH NUTRITIONAL PREVENTION BECOMING THE CURE

In the past few years, I've seen some real changes starting to take place within the medical profession. The attitude of most doctors toward supplements is beginning to shift from an unwarranted skepticism born out of ignorance to a willingness to learn more. Courses on herbs and nutritional medicine are becoming popular among physicians, for instance. Staid journals such as *The Archives of Internal Medicine* have devoted entire issues to studies of natural remedies. The National Institutes of Health have just funded two major dietary supplement research centers, one at UCLA and the other at the University of Illinois in Chicago. Nutritional medicine is becoming part of the mainstream.

I've personally received enthusiastic positive feedback when I've given lectures to other doctors on the uses of nutritional medicine. They're interested not only for their patients, but for themselves, too. I have no hesitation in saying that doctors are now among the most dedicated users of supplements. Younger doctors, especially, are taking advantage of supplements for themselves. Like paradigm shifts in other scientific fields, changing of the generations sometimes seems to be required for the field to make progress. Having said that, I also know many older, entirely conventional doctors, who never prescribe supplements to their patients, but who use large numbers of supplements for their own self-care.

Why are these changes occurring? One reason is that medicine itself is becoming more sophisticated. The more we discover about the biochemical basis of illnesses, the more we're appreciating the scientific merit of natural treatments. A good example of this is the use of folate to reduce high homocysteine levels, which we now know to be a risk factor for heart disease.

Our more sophisticated understanding of biochemistry also helps us to address the true underlying causes of illness more effectively than with conventional drugs. For example, I've had two patients who both had severe hypertriglyceridemia, a type of lipid disorder, as well as treatment-resistant bipolar disorder (manic-depression). Their previous doctors had tried essentially every available conventional drug, with little effect. Taking advantage of recent research, I treated them both with high doses of fish oil concentrate. Both patients had marked reductions in their triglyceride levels to near-normal levels, as well as remissions from their bipolar disorders, for the first time in years. The true underlying problem, in both their cases, was probably a severe omega-3 fatty acid deficiency. It took a lot of high-tech science to validate a low-tech supplement.

Probably the most important reason for the changes occurring in the medical profession, though, is that consumers are becoming more educated. For most people, doctors are no longer the main source for medical information. Medical news is featured prominently on television, on-line, and in print media. This book itself is playing a part in the process of change, through educating the public.

An informed public really is important in improving the overall standard of medical care. Let me tell you a story about a certain dietary supplement. It's a true story, and a shocking one, but it is little-known. It definitely proves my point. Be warned: Once you read it, you may become seriously disillusioned about the way the American medical profession has operated in the past, and to some extent, continues to operate.

A TRUE STORY: WHY BECOMING INFORMED IS ESSENTIAL

A certain dietary supplement, whose name I will reveal below, had been available over the counter since the late 1800s and had been claimed to have benefits for a number of conditions. Because it was a simple, natural substance, it was unpatentable. Anyone could make it into tablets and sell it, so its price was always low. As a result, the major pharmaceutical companies, which were only interested in products that could be patented and provide big profits, were not interested in it.

In 1949 an Australian doctor discovered that this supplement was an effective treatment for a certain common, serious, and hard-to-treat illness. Interestingly, the U.S. government removed it from the market that very same year. It was all but forgotten in this country.

European doctors, though, continued to do studies on it, and prescribed it successfully to tens of thousands of patients. Many patients who had been severely ill for years were cured with it. In fact, it's known today that this natural supplement is unquestionably the single most effective treatment that exists for this particular illness. But for around twenty years, from 1950 to 1970, American doctors kept ignoring it. The drug companies had such a powerful financial and political stranglehold over the medical profession in this country, that if a drug

company didn't sell a given product, most doctors simply never heard about it. Europeans published abundant, good-quality scientific research on this supplement. But American doctors ignored it anyway.

During the 1950s and 1960s, the American media would occasionally run a story on the use of this dietary supplement overseas. If a patient read about it and asked their doctor to try it out, they were told something like, "Sorry, there isn't enough evidence to support its use." So some patients, desperate for an effective medicine, would fly to Europe to get a prescription for it.

Finally, because of their patients' demands, a few American doctors reluctantly began prescribing it. They worried that other doctors would consider them quacks. In 1970 the FDA at last approved its use, and American doctors were allowed to catch up with their European peers.

This simple, natural supplement was lithium. It's now considered the first-line treatment for bipolar disorder. Today, the history of the American medical profession's prejudice against it and deliberate ignorance about it are described, even by conventional doctors, as a "black mark" in medical history. It would be nice to think that this story was an isolated incident, an aberration in an otherwise reasonable and unbiased medical system. But unfortunately, a similar story can be told about dozens of other natural supplements. Glucosamine, for example, provides well-proven relief from arthritis and was widely prescribed for years by European doctors, while U.S. doctors ignored it. St. John's wort was already the number one prescription antidepressant in Europe, while U.S. doctors had never heard of it. The same story goes for fish oils, selenium, ginkgo, coenzyme Q_{10}, carnitine, licorice, and dozens of other natural supplements. Today, American doctors are still decades behind their European counterparts when it comes to using natural medicines.

The difference now is that people expect their doctors to know about supplements. And a lot of doctors have gotten tired of admitting that they don't know anything about the subject. So, as I mentioned, they're seeking out information themselves. As a result, people are now becoming partners with their doctors in a way that was rare just a few years ago, researching and applying treatments together.

A NEW PARTNERSHIP— A NEW RESPONSIBILITY

Along with this sharing of information comes a new sharing of responsibility. Supplements can provide tremendous benefits, but no supplement is entirely free of risk. If you don't use them responsibly, heeding the contraindications for their use—such as are listed in this book—and maintaining alertness for adverse effects, not only can you personally be harmed, but you may make it more likely that the FDA will take away the freedom of all the rest of us to use supplements. I want them to continue to be available for everyone.

Can you overdo supplement use? Of course you can. Some people take doses far in excess of those recommended, reasoning that if a little is good, then more must be better. Unfortunately, biology doesn't follow that kind of logic. As is frequently pointed out, anything can be toxic if used in high enough doses—even water or oxygen. The story of lithium, described above, is also a salutary reminder that natural substances are not necessarily less toxic than synthetic ones. When used therapeutically, lithium levels in the blood need to be carefully monitored in order to avoid potentially serious side effects. In this book you'll find invaluable guidelines about how to use supplements safely: who will benefit from them, who should avoid them, how much to take, and how often.

Another way that some people overdo supplement use is by becoming overreliant on them. I remember a patient I treated in the hospital for fluid overload, which was in his case a complication of chronic renal (kidney) failure, and which had very nearly been fatal. He showed me the list of nutritional supplements he was taking, and it was astounding. The list was three pages long, with around thirty different supplements on it, all taken according to a very complicated schedule. He had been using the supplements to treat himself for the symptoms of chronic renal failure, when it was plain and obvious to any doctor that what he needed was regular dialysis. But he didn't trust conventional medicine, he told me. Another patient I know of decided that nutritional supplements could cure her of her diabetes and so stopped taking her insulin. She went into a diabetic coma. Fortunately, she recovered.

Sure, skepticism of the medical profession is warranted at times. But if you go against their advice, you are taking your life into your own hands. In this book, you'll find clearly indicated in many places when medical supervision is called for in the use of supplements.

As a general rule, you should consult a physician for any symptoms that you may be experiencing, and discuss supplements with your doctor before using them. I also advise people using supplements for weight loss, enhanced athletic performance, or prevention of illness to do so under medical supervision.

WHO WILL BENEFIT FROM SUPPLEMENTS?

There are still a few diehards out there saying that our American diet provides all the essential nutrients we need. They're becoming a minority now, though. Most of us recognize that the standard American diet doesn't provide the levels of nutrients necessary for optimal health and longevity. Not only that, but for some Americans, it may not even provide the minimal levels of nutrients necessary for *life*. A colleague of mine at our hospital recently treated a young man who had almost bled to death—requiring massive transfusions—because he had scurvy, which is caused by severe vitamin C deficiency. It turns out that, like many people, this young man was fond of fast food, and he ate a lot of burgers from a certain well-known fast-food chain, which will remain nameless. And, of course, he was not into supplements. Maybe if he'd special-ordered extra slices of tomato on his burgers he would have been okay.

One of the things that makes this book so valuable is that unlike other books on supplements, it includes a discussion of how to eat healthily. Your diet is the bedrock of your health. Eating right should be your first goal. Despite this, to maintain optimal well-being, we often need more of particular nutrients than even a perfectly balanced diet can provide. It makes good sense for all of us to take supplements.

In this book, you'll discover basic nutrient blends tailored for your individual needs, whether you're interested in stress relief, extra energy, increased mental clarity, or in treating a particular illness. You'll find all you need to start reaping benefits today from one of the most significant developments currently taking place in all of science—the revolution in nutritional medicine.

Part 1

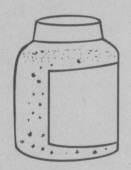

1

Getting Started the Right Way with Dietary Supplements

Dietary supplements are widely available through many retail outlets, from pharmacies to mail order catalogs. They come in many forms—tablets, powders, extracts, drinks, and conventional foods. Almost daily the media report on how dietary supplements can help enhance health, fine-tune the way the body works, improve the body's structure, and cure or prevent diseases.

To many, however, the thousands and thousands of products found on the shelves are still a mystery. They offer an endless variety of ingredients with seemingly incomprehensible names. The good news is that to the trained professionals who make their career designing and manufacturing dietary supplements, the benefits these products have to offer are increasingly well understood. These days the same scientific community that only ten or so years ago was skeptical of dietary supplements now dedicates entire journals to dietary supplements and their beneficial effects on your health and well-being. In January 1999 the National Institutes of Health's Office of Dietary Supplements opened its brand-new scientific database dedicated to dietary supplement research. This database, the International Bibliographic Information on Dietary Supplements (IBIDS), is designed to help both professionals and the public understand and have access to the latest research on dietary supplements. The IBIDS database contains over 350,000 scientific articles on dietary supplement ingredients. Harvard Medical School even teamed up with the Corporate Alliance for Integrative Medicine to conduct studies on dietary supplements. The Corporate Alliance for Integrative Medicine is a group of leading dietary supplement manufacturers and suppliers dedicated to providing the public, the medical profession, and the natural health industry with a more thorough understanding of dietary supplements.

Despite all of the research on supplement ingredients and the regulations that govern the manufacturing of dietary supplements, a huge gap still exists in the public's understanding of what products are safe, what products are effective, and what products people should take on a daily basis to meet their personal needs. For example, it is now well established and accepted that garlic supplements will help maintain healthy cholesterol levels and that for some individuals who have high cholesterol, using garlic supplements each day along with other prescribed therapies can reduce cholesterol levels significantly. Questions such as what type of garlic, how much to take, and how long to continue taking the supplement remain unanswered in many people's minds. These questions, and many more, are answered in this book.

Let me provide a historical perspective on the use of dietary supplements and show exactly how supplements fit in with food and drugs, in order to pave the way toward understanding the many issues associated with dietary supplement products.

The twentieth century was marked by remarkable advances in medical science. In the last fifty years synthetic drugs have been providing miracle cures. But in 1900 natural products—herbal products in particular—were the primary mode of medical treatment, along with a healthy diet, exercise, and a positive outlook. People kept themselves healthy by building a strong foundation to enhance their ability to fight diseases off naturally. As the century progressed, modern medicine developed, but we also created food products that could be stored longer and appealed to our palates but were stripped of vital nutrients and full of artificial ingredients. I find it fascinating that as the twentieth century drew to a close, 42 percent of the adult American population had at some time sought alternative-medicine treatments to help treat their ailments, give them more energy, build stronger bodies, fight off disease, and live a longer life. It says something about the value of following nature's way that in the quest for maximizing well-being we keep returning to time-tested supplements and treatments. By the same token, science supports the notion that with the proper ingredients in your lifestyle you can easily attain a hundred productive and happiness-filled years of life. For example, in a recent study on centenarians, researchers found two interesting things about their biochemistry. When compared to younger adults, fifty years old and above, it was found that the centenarians had higher amounts of antioxidants—vitamins C and E—in their blood. These substances have been proven to protect the body from damage at the cellular level and to enhance cellular function. The researchers also found that the centenarians' insulin system functioned extremely well. Those of you who read health magazines are probably aware that impaired insulin system function is associated with cardiovascular disease and obesity. It can be corrected through lifestyle, diet, and the use of dietary supplements.

HOW ARE DIETARY SUPPLEMENTS REGULATED?

A few years ago, when I was visiting a client in the business of manufacturing and selling dietary supplements, I noticed something curious in the company's lobby display of products from its hundred-year history. Among the vials containing elixirs made of herbs and other natural compounds was one bottle that looked as if it had come from an apothecary shop. As I took a closer look at the label of this slender, tapered bottle with the black cap, I found, to my amazement, that the key ingredients were cocaine, heroin, and morphine. It is hard to believe today that this type of product was sold over the counter in the late 1800s. Of course, such products were likely to cause serious adverse health effects.

The Pure Food and Drug Act was passed in 1906 to deal with unsafe foods, harmful elixirs, and misbranded products. It limited access to products that were potentially harmful and prevented "snake oil" salesmen from peddling their mystery formulas to the public. In 1938 the Food, Drug and Cosmetic Act established specific categories for a food's special dietary use,

and shortly thereafter, in 1941, the Food and Drug Administration (FDA) established regulations governing vitamin and mineral supplements. It was also during this period that the first reference standards for dietary supplement ingredients were established. The minimum daily requirement (MDR) was established, based on the amounts of vitamins and minerals needed to avoid deficiency diseases.

During the 1960s and 1970s, the FDA revised the MDR and gave it a new name: the U.S. recommended daily allowance, or USRDA. During this period the FDA also sought to have various disclaimers printed on the labels of dietary supplements and to limit the amount of vitamins and minerals that could be allowed in dietary supplement products. A series of court battles were initiated by industry and other groups interested in preventing such restrictions, and the FDA's proposals were never implemented. It is important to note that dietary supplements had always been regulated as food products. It's just that amounts and combinations were never regulated—nor are they today, except where there is a known health risk.

In 1976 Congress passed legislation that prohibited the FDA from classifying vitamin and mineral supplements as drugs based solely on the combination or potency of the ingredients (though some dietary supplement ingredients are used as approved drugs). Then in 1990 Congress passed the Nutrition,

Labeling and Education Act (NLEA), which regulated product labeling and allowed supplement manufacturers to make health claims that were based on scientific evidence. For example, a common claim seen today on product labels and in advertising is that calcium helps prevent osteoporosis. NLEA legislation also directed the FDA to replace the current RDA system for essential vitamins and minerals with a new system, recommended daily intake (RDI).

At the request of Congress, during the 1990s government-sponsored studies gathered data on the use of and need for dietary supplements in the American population. The findings showed that among the more than twenty thousand people studied, not a single one was ingesting the full Recommended Daily Allowance (RDA) of ten key vitamins and minerals identified by science as essential to health. It became apparent that different segments of the population, in particular the elderly, were more at risk than others for deficiencies of vitamins and minerals, with potentially major health consequences. For example, while a slow decline in cognitive function in the elderly is commonly observed, research has found that this decline may be prevented and even reversed by increased intake of certain vitamins and other dietary supplements. Also, studies have shown that intake of vitamin-mineral supplements can improve immune system function, which may translate into lifestyle, health, and economic benefits (the

last from cutting the number of sick days per year in half). And researchers found that folic acid supplementation in the earliest stages of pregnancy could help prevent certain birth defects in newborn children.

The findings of this congressional report outlined some exciting research on how vitamins and minerals can help protect against heart disease, cataracts, osteoporosis, and perhaps even many types of cancer. One of the most widely reported findings, known as the Harvard Study, showed that nurses and other health professionals who took at least 100 international units (IU) of vitamin E per day for at least two years lowered their risk of heart disease by 40 percent over those who did not take vitamin E supplements.

Some of the other interesting research findings reported to Congress included the health-enhancing effect of herbs, amino acids, and other dietary supplements. For example:

Echinacea has been reported to boost immune system function and ward off colds and flu.

Ginkgo has been shown to help improve peripheral circulation and enhance memory, particularly in the aged.

Garlic and other herbs have been shown to reduce the risk of cardiovascular disease.

Coenzyme Q_{10}, important in normal fat and energy metabolism, has been shown to help individuals at risk of angina by preventing the accumulation of fatty acids within the heart. Coenzyme Q_{10} has also been shown to have beneficial effects by preventing the breakdown of LDL cholesterol, or "bad" cholesterol, thereby helping prevent arteriosclerosis. Researchers have recently determined that LDL cholesterol, damaged by free radicals, is more likely to contribute to cholesterol deposits forming on the lining of artery walls.

Glucosamine, a naturally occurring substance found in high concentrations in the joints, has been shown to help with joint repair, thus benefiting individuals with osteoarthritis.

As a result of the presentation of all of this research to the members of Congress, as well as from the efforts of millions of individuals petitioning the government to acknowledge the many beneficial effects that dietary supplements could have on the nation's health, in 1994 Congress passed the Dietary Supplement Health and Education Act. Under its new regulations, dietary supplements would still be regulated by the FDA as food products, but as a special category. Some of the act's important provisions include:

- Implementation of improved manufacturing standards to ensure product quality

- Expanding the information available to customers where dietary supplements are sold
- Ensuring access to safe and effective dietary supplement ingredients
- Establishing of the Office of Dietary Supplements at the National Institutes of Health
- Statements about how dietary supplements can benefit your body and health
- Mandating uniform labeling, using the Supplement Facts convention, to make it easier to understand what is contained in a dietary supplement product

One issue of particular interest is maintaining a distinction between the proper use of dietary supplements and the unauthorized use of dietary supplement products as drugs, that is, for the prevention, diagnosis, treatment, or cure of diseases. Many people find this distinction ambiguous, as they are in fact taking vitamins, minerals, herbs, and other dietary supplement products as nutritional therapy, to cure or prevent a disease. The information contained in Chapter 2 defines exactly what dietary supplements are and what they are not. Chapter 3 provides a concise review of what claims manufacturers may legitimately make for dietary supplements, and will explain what's on the labels of the thousands of products found in stores.

GRAPPLING WITH SCIENTIFIC TERMS ON DIETARY SUPPLEMENT LABELS

One obstacle in trying to understand what dietary supplements are and what they do is the scientific terminology found on the labels. Think of it this way: Salt and pepper are two of the oldest and most widely used "dietary supplements"—they are found in every restaurant and every house. But had I started talking about how common sodium chloride and *Piper nigrum* are, you may have found yourself scratching your head in bewilderment. Yet table salt is sodium chloride, and *Piper nigrum* is the scientific name for the plant black pepper is derived from.

Part 3 of this book lists dietary supplement ingredients and information about them in easy-to-understand language. Some scientific terminology is required in order to adequately explain how some ingredients work, but don't let a few words act as a barrier to understanding the rest of the information. Take it one step at a time. You may find that jotting down notes on the different terms used for ingredients may be helpful. In Chapter 5 there is a worksheet intended to help you put together a list of the ingredients, together with dosage ranges, to use when you go shopping for dietary supplements and when you meet with your doctor or other health professional.

DIETARY SUPPLEMENT DOSAGES

Both professionals and lay people alike can get confused by dosages of different dietary supplements. For now, let me note simply that there are primarily two categories of dosage ranges: therapeutic dosage range and nutritional dosage range.

Therapeutic dosage ranges are determined from scientific studies performed in clinical settings, which are primarily designed to measure the effects of a particular dietary supplement ingredient on patients with a disease condition. One example is the use of garlic for lowering cholesterol levels and in some cases blood pressure. For individuals with cholesterol or blood pressure high enough to be classified as a disease, researchers have found that using high dosages of garlic over short periods of time will help lower cholesterol levels and blood pressure. However, when it comes to using high levels of garlic supplementation for very long periods of time in healthy individuals, the benefits (and possible side effects) are unknown, because long-term studies have not been conducted yet (see Part 3 for details on using garlic supplements). Unlike drugs, which are required to undergo several years of safety and effectiveness testing, dietary supplement ingredients, being foods, are already considered safe, so no formal testing is required. Additionally, because there is generally no patent protection for dietary supplement ingredients, there is no industry incentive to bear the costs of long-term studies. So the majority of studies found in the medical and scientific journals are conducted over the short term—a few weeks to a few months. Researchers use high dosages to increase their chances of determining a biological effect during the short study period.

This is where the concept of nutritional dosages comes into the dietary supplement picture. Scientific studies and practitioner experiences indicate that for currently healthy individuals, using lower-than-therapeutic dosages of dietary supplement ingredients will help promote health and well-being in many cases. Let's look at a popular supplement, glucosamine. High dosages of glucosamine, 1,500 to 3,000 mg per day, have been shown to reduce the symptoms of osteoarthritis. The beneficial effects of these therapeutic dosages of glucosamine occur within weeks of beginning to take it and have lasting effects. However, whether or not these high dosages are necessary for healthy individuals is another question. Dosages of 250 to 500 mg a day may be more appropriate for people who are not in a disease state but who want to derive benefits from glucosamine intake, such as building strong ligaments and joints and improving the health of the circulatory system.

When you review the information in Parts 2 and 3, keep in mind these dynamics of dietary supplement dosages.

Why Take Dietary Supplements?

- Supplements supply a measurable amount of nutrients.
- Supplements make up for the poor nutrient content of many foods we eat.
- Supplements ensure that you are getting adequate amounts of the essential nutrients.
- Supplements replace nutrients destroyed in foods by cooking and in the body by smoking, alcohol consumption, drug use, and pollution.
- Most supplements are either calorie- and fat-free or very nearly so.
- People with food allergies can get the nutrients they need with special supplement formulations free of allergens.
- Stress can increase the body's need for certain nutrients, such as the B vitamins, which can be easily obtained from supplements.
- Pregnant women require a reliable supply of all the essential nutrients, including iron, folic acid, calcium, zinc, vitamin D, and protein.
- Lack of sunlight (as in many parts of the Northern Hemisphere during the winter months, and among the elderly who don't get outside much) requires intake of higher amounts of vitamin D.
- The elderly need supplemental nutrition because they often eat less, and because they digest poorly the foods they do eat.

- Supplemental amounts of antioxidants help counter the effects of aging and protect the body from free-radical and other chemical damage.
- Athletes and fitness enthusiasts can use supplements to ensure optimal supplies of nutrients for maximum performance.
- Intake of some nutrients in greater amounts than can normally be supplied from food in the diet (such as vitamin E) have been shown to improve health.
- Dietary supplements can enhance the structure and function of your body.
- Dietary supplements can prevent certain degenerative disease, such as coronary heart disease, diabetes, and osteoporosis.

2

Defining Dietary Supplements

The passage of the Dietary Supplement Health and Education Act (DSHEA) in 1994 introduced a whole new set of criteria and terms that have newly reshaped the identity of supplement products found in health food stores, pharmacies, and supermarkets. Understanding how these regulations determine what a dietary supplement is will certainly help you in your personal quest for nutritional wellness and facilitate proper use of the dietary supplement products available in the marketplace.

The A, B, Cs of Supplement Common Jargon

Unless you are a student majoring in nutrition or a recent graduate, you probably do not understand the differences between the various nutrient values in popular use today. You may not even realize that there are any differences. To aid you in your quest

to improve your nutritional acumen, I have compiled the following list of definitions:

Adequate Intake (AI): A value based on observed or experimentally determined estimates of nutrient intake by a group, or groups, of healthy people. It is used when an RDA cannot be determined.

Amino Acids: Amino acids are a special class of organic molecules that contain nitrogen. Amino acids are linked together to form proteins. Most amino acids come in two forms. The two forms are isomers, mirror images of each other, and are denoted by the letter "D" or "L" placed in front of the name of the amino acid. In general, the L-form is more compatible with human biochemistry and the only form that should be ingested. As a general rule, never use a supplement that contains only the D-form. However, some products will contain a mixture of the D- and L-forms. The only two amino acids whose DL-forms have been observed to have metabolic advantages in humans are phenylalanine and methionine.

Botanical: Refers to ingredients that are of plant origin. A botanical ingredient can be from a whole plant, such as an entire herb or mushroom, or part of a plant, such as seeds, leaves, bark, roots, etc.

Daily Reference Values (DRVs): Food- and supplement-label nutrient values created by the Food and Drug Administration for the macronutrients and two electrolytes. DRVs, based on a reference diet of 2,000 or 2,500 calories, have been assigned to fat, saturated fat, cholesterol, total carbohydrate, fiber, protein, sodium, and potassium. These values, the same as the Reference Daily Intakes (RDIs), are presented on the new nutrition labels as percent Daily Values (DVs).

Daily Values (DVs): A system created by the Food and Drug Administration to help manufacturers present their Reference Daily Intake (RDI) and Daily Reference Value (DRV) information on food and supplement labels. The RDI and DRV values are presented as percent Daily Values—that is, the amount of the nutrient in the product is described as a percentage, with 100 percent being equivalent to the total amount of the nutrient required by a reference individual consuming a 2,000-calorie-per-day diet. The terms Reference Daily Intakes and Daily Reference Values (RDI and DRV) never actually appear on the supplement or nutrition labels.

Estimated Average Requirements (EAR): A nutrient intake value that is estimated to meet the requirement of half the healthy individuals in a group. It is used in the assessment of the prevalence of inadequate intakes within a group, or possibility of inadequacy of an individual.

Estimated Safe and Adequate Daily Dietary Intakes (ESADDIs): A group of nutrient values compiled by the National Research Council that represents safe and adequate intake levels for a number of essential nutrients for which the data were sufficient to estimate a range of requirements but not sufficient enough to assign RDAs.

Metabolites: These are substances that take part in metabolism. Some are produced in the body as part of the metabolic process, while others are derived from food sources. Some are now also available in supplemental form. Even though the body is able to make many of these substances, taking them can improve the structure or function of the body. Some examples of metabolites covered in Part 3 include carnitine, glucosamine, melatonin, and SAMe.

Minerals: These are inorganic nutrients or inorganic-organic complexes that are essential structural components in the body and necessary for many vital metabolic processes, even though they make up only about 4 percent of the body's weight. Every day the body needs minerals such as calcium in large amounts, about 1,200 milligrams or more, while it needs other minerals, such as chromium, in smaller amounts, measured in micrograms.

Recommended Dietary Allowances (RDAs): A database compiled by the National

Research Council that has become the accepted source of nutrient allowances for healthy people. The RDAs serve as the basis for the Reference Daily Intakes (RDIs) and Daily Reference Values (DRVs). The RDAs are presented in a book entitled Recommended Dietary Allowances, first published in 1943; the tenth edition was published in 1989.

Reference Daily Intakes (RDIs): Food- and supplement-label nutrient values created by the Food and Drug Administration to replace its U.S. Recommended Daily Allowances (USRDAs) but still based on the National Research Council's Recommended Dietary Allowances (RDAs). The original mandate, which grew out of a number of proposals, was published in January 1994, and the RDIs completely took the place of the USRDAs by January 1997. Consult table 2.4 for the current vitamins and minerals with assigned RDIs. These values are represented on the new nutrition labels as percent Daily Values (DVs).

Standardized: This term is usually applied to botanical ingredients that are specially prepared to contain an exact amount of one or more of the phytonutrients it contains. For example, ginseng standardized to ginsenosides. By using standardized botanical ingredients, manufacturers can ensure that each product they make will have the same biological activity.

Sustained-released: In a sold dosage dietary supplement, capsule or tablet, the ingredients can be mixed in with a matrix that causes the product to slowly digest over a few hours. These types of products are sometimes referred to as sustained released.

Time-released: In some cases, dietary products are made with small bead-like ingredients. These tiny beads are specially prepared to dissolve in specific areas of the digestive system; thus the term time-released.

Tolerable Upper Intake Level (UL): The highest level of daily nutrient intake that is likely to pose no risks of adverse health effects to almost all individuals in the general population.

U.S. Recommended Daily Allowances (USRDAs): A group of nutrient values created by the Food and Drug Administration to help the manufacturers of processed foods and supplements meet its nutrition-labeling criteria. The values were based on the National Research Council's Recommended Dietary Allowances (RDAs). The FDA took the RDAs, which are the average recommended nutrient intakes for promotion of health, and created the USRDAs, which are the nutrient values used on food and supplement labels. The USRDAs were completely phased out and replaced with the FDA's Reference Daily Intakes (RDIs) by January 1997. However, you may sometimes encounter them still on some products.

Vitamins: These are organic compounds that the body needs for the maintenance of good health and for growth. By convention, the name vitamin is reserved for certain nutrients that the body cannot manufacture and therefore must get from food.

Table 2.1

EXAMPLES OF DIETARY SUPPLEMENT INGREDIENTS, BY DEFINITION TYPE

AMINO ACIDS
L-arginine
L-glutamine
L-leucine
L-lysine
L-phenylalanine
L-valine

BOTANICALS / HERBS
Black cohosh
Garlic
Ginseng
Ginkgo
Echinacea
Feverfew
Gotu kola
Ginger
Hawthorn
St. John's wort
Saw Palmetto
Valerian

Constituents—Botanical
Allicin
Anthocyanidins
Apigenin
Curcuminoids
Eleutherosides
Ginsenosides
Isoflavones
Kavalactones
Ligustilide
Phytosterols

Salicin
Silymarin
Valerenic acid

METABOLITES
Coenzyme Q_{10}
Creatine
DHEA
Glucosamine
Lipoic acid
Melatonin

MINERALS
Calcium
Copper
Iodine
Iron
Magnesium
Manganese
Potassium
Selenium
Zinc

VITAMINS
Choline
Folic acid
Niacin
Pantothenic acid
Vitamin A
Vitamin B_1
Vitamin B_2
Vitamin C
Vitamin E

WHAT IS A DIETARY SUPPLEMENT?

As defined by the letter of the regulations, the term *dietary supplement* means a product (other than tobacco) that is intended to supplement the diet and which contains one or more of the following ingredients: a vitamin, a mineral, an herb or other botanical, an amino acid, a metabolite, a concentrate, an extract, a constituent, any other dietary substance for use by humans to supplement the diet by increasing the total dietary intake, or any combination of these. A dietary supplement must be labeled clearly as a dietary supplement and not claim that it is a conventional food or is to be used as the sole component of a meal.

The Dietary Supplement Health and Education Act defined as dietary supplement ingredients all those ingredients that were available for sale in interstate commerce at the time the act was passed, in 1994. This greatly expanded the number of ingredients that were allowed in dietary supplement products. Before DSHEA, only a limited number of ingredients that were considered to be generally recognized as safe or that were FDA-approved food additives were authorized for use in foods and dietary supplements. (However, note that conventional food products—those with a Nutrition Facts panel on the label—can still include only ingredients that are FDA-approved food additives or generally recognized as safe.)

MAJOR FORMS OF DIETARY SUPPLEMENTS

Dietary supplements come in several major types and forms (also referred to as delivery systems):

Tablets
Capsules
Softgels
Powders
Liquids
Nutrition bars

Tablets

These start out as a blend of powdered nutrients, which are then pressed by machines into the characteristic round or oval solid form. Tablets come in many sizes, but there is an upper limit based on the maximum size that can be safely swallowed. Tablets are also made in chewable forms. The term *caplet* is currently being used to describe tablets that are shaped like capsules. (Originally the caplet was a tamper-proof one-piece capsule with a hard outer layer and loosely bound contents.)

Tablet delivery systems vary. Current manufacturing technology allows tablets to be digested quickly or to provide sustained or timed release of nutrients. These features give tablets an edge over other forms of dietary supplements. Tablets also have a long shelf life, typically over two years. Tablets need to be manufactured properly, so do not assume that all products on the market will digest as expected. If you ever encounter a tablet that passes through your system undigested, switch brands. Products labeled "USP" (which stands for United States Pharmacopeia) are guaranteed to be properly digested. However, this does not mean that brands not made using USP standards will not digest well. Put a tablet of your brand into a glass of vinegar or water to see how long it takes to start dissolving. It should start dissolving within an hour, unless the formulation is sustained-release, in which case it should take a few hours. Note that if the product you are testing is enteric-coated, it probably won't dissolve at all, because it requires special digestive enzymes found in the intestines.

Capsules

Capsules are delivery systems that consist of two hollow halves, into which a powder blend is injected. The two halves are then brought together by a machine to form the capsule. In general, nutrition supplement capsules will be digested quickly. They are not designed with a sustained-release system, and there are very few dietary supplement capsule products that are in timed-release form. Capsules do not offer the advantages that they did decades ago, when tablets dissolved less easily. Capsules offer no real advantage over tablets, and are generally more expensive to make. One advantage is that capsules require a lesser amount of excipients—fillers, binders, and other inactive components (though some are needed to help the powders flow easily through the machines, and for stability).

Softgels

Softgels were developed to hold liquid supplement ingredients such as lecithin, cod liver oil, and vitamin E. They consist of an outer gelatin shell, soft or hard, that is filled with liquid. They are generally quickly digested. Some people prefer gelatin capsules because they find them easier to swallow.

Note that the material used to make capsules and gelatin capsules is, by and large, animal in origin. Only recently have some companies developed vegetarian capsules and softgels. This is important to know if you are a strict vegetarian.

Powders

The most common powder formulations are protein powders, diet powders, energy powders, greens powders, and weight gain powders. Supplement powders are a convenient way to get high-quality nutrition in the exact amounts you need, when you need it. Most people have very busy schedules and cannot find the time to eat the five or six recommended small complete meals per day (twenty minutes devoted to each meal would mean that you spend two hours a day just eating). Powdered nutrition supplements therefore provide a convenient high-density source of nutrition to meet your individual needs.

Liquids

Liquid dietary supplements include protein drinks, carbohydrate drinks, weight gain drinks, herbal extracts, herbal tinctures, liquid vitamins, and minerals. Many of these concoctions are also available in dry form, either as powders or as pills. Athletes are most familiar with the host of carbohydrate drinks and weight gain drinks presently on the market.

Nutrition Bars

Nutrition bars have been around for many years now but are currently becoming popular as more people recognize their quality nutrition content and convenience. These scientifically developed snacks are high in healthy carbohydrates and protein, and low in fat. This is the opposite of what most mass-market candy bars have to offer. Nutrition bars should become part of your daily performance diet. Keep a few with you to serve as between-meal snacks.

Other Forms

Recently Hain Foods introduced a line of canned soups labeled as dietary supplements—for example, chicken soup with echinacea, to be used when you have a cold or the flu. Doubtless dietary supplement manufacturers will be coming up with other new ideas for delivery systems in the future.

LABELING OF DIETARY SUPPLEMENTS VERSUS OTHER PRODUCTS

Dietary supplements must by law have a label clearly stating that it is a dietary supplement, herbal supplement, vitamin supplement, calcium supplement, nutritional supplement, or the like. The Supplement Facts box is another part of the identification system found on labels. This box lists the active ingredients and other ingredients contained in the dietary supplement.

Nevertheless, sometimes food, drugs, homeopathic products, and other types of products on the shelves are confused with dietary supplement products. To clear up the identity of dietary supplements versus other products, the following information provides comparisons and definitions to make your understanding of these products much clearer and to make it easier and safer for you to select and use a supplement.

Table 2.2

UNDERSTANDING THE SUPPLEMENT FACTS INFORMATION PANEL

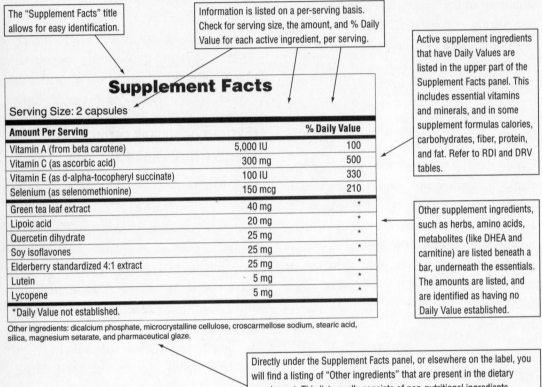

The "Supplement Facts" title allows for easy identification.

Information is listed on a per-serving basis. Check for serving size, the amount, and % Daily Value for each active ingredient, per serving.

Active supplement ingredients that have Daily Values are listed in the upper part of the Supplement Facts panel. This includes essential vitamins and minerals, and in some supplement formulas calories, carbohydrates, fiber, protein, and fat. Refer to RDI and DRV tables.

Supplement Facts

Serving Size: 2 capsules

Amount Per Serving		% Daily Value
Vitamin A (from beta carotene)	5,000 IU	100
Vitamin C (as ascorbic acid)	300 mg	500
Vitamin E (as d-alpha-tocopheryl succinate)	100 IU	330
Selenium (as selenomethionine)	150 mcg	210
Green tea leaf extract	40 mg	*
Lipoic acid	20 mg	*
Quercetin dihydrate	25 mg	*
Soy isoflavones	25 mg	*
Elderberry standardized 4:1 extract	25 mg	*
Lutein	5 mg	*
Lycopene	5 mg	*

*Daily Value not established.

Other ingredients: dicalcium phosphate, microcrystalline cellulose, croscarmellose sodium, stearic acid, silica, magnesium setarate, and pharmaceutical glaze.

Other supplement ingredients, such as herbs, amino acids, metabolites (like DHEA and carnitine) are listed beneath a bar, underneath the essentials. The amounts are listed, and are identified as having no Daily Value established.

Directly under the Supplement Facts panel, or elsewhere on the label, you will find a listing of "Other ingredients" that are present in the dietary supplement. This list usually consists of non-nutritional ingredients (excipients) needed to make the dosage form. It may also contain the source ingredient of the vitamin or minerals, if not listed in the Supplement Facts panel; for example, ascorbic acid, the source of vitamin C.

Miscellaneous:

Botanical ingredients should list the part of the plant used. They can be listed using their common (vernacular) name, as listed in the reference book *Herbs of Commerce.* The scientific names can also appear or be used solely when an herb's common name is not listed in the *Herbs of Commerce.*

Proprietary blends of nonessential nutrients, like botanicals, amino acids, and metabolites, may be listed using the weight for the total blend only. When this is done, components of the blend must be listed in descending order of predominance by weight.

The appearance, size of type, and lines that make up the Supplement Facts panel are all specified by the Food and Drug regulations.

Table 2.3

UNDERSTANDING THE NUTRITION FACTS INFORMATION PANEL

The "Nutrition Facts" title allows for easy identification.

Serving size indicates the amount per serving that contains the nutrition information listed in the Nutrition Facts panel. Also included is the number of servings per container.

Nutrition Facts

Serving Size: 1/2 cup (114 g)
Servings Per Container 4

Amount Per Serving	
Calories 90	Calories from Fat 30

The amount of "calories" is the total number of calories per serving. The amount of calories from fat is also included. In this example, the total number of calories is 90 calories per serving, and of that total number of calories, 30 calories are from the fat content.

	% Daily Value*
Total Fat 3 g	5%
Saturated Fat 0 g	0%
Cholesterol 0 mg	0%
Sodium 240 mg	10%
Potassium 450 mg	13%
Total Carbohydrate 13 g	4%
Dietary Fiber 3 g	12%
Sugars 3 g	
Protein 3 g	

Vitamin A	80%	•	Vitamin C	60%
Calcium	4%	•	Iron	4%

% Daily Value are calculated from the Daily Reference Values (DRVs) and Reference Daily Intakes (RDIs). Refer to those tables to see the 100% Daily Values.

The amount of total fat is listed, in this case 3 g. The amount of saturated fat is also indicated; in this example it is zero. This means that all the fat is unsaturated.

Nutrient ingredient information is listed to help you make healthy food choices and track the intake of key nutrients. This information helps select foods with adequate nutrient content.

The percentages of vitamin A, vitamin C, calcium, and iron are always listed, even if none is contained in the product. Amounts for the other vitamins and minerals with RDI amounts can be listed when present in a product.

*Percent Daily Values are based on a 2,000 calorie diet. Your daily values may be higher or lower depending on your calorie needs:

	Calories:	2,000	2,500
Total Fat	Less than	65 g	80 g
Sat Fat	Less than	20 g	25 g
Cholesterol	Less than	300 mg	300 mg
Sodium	Less than	2,400 mg	2,400 mg
Total Carbohydrate		300 mg	375 mg
Dietary Fiber		25 mg	30 mg

This information states whether the % Daily Value calculations were based on one of the two standard daily diets, 2,000 or 2,500 calories per day. In this example, 2,000 calories per day were used. Also note the sentence: "Your daily values may be higher or lower depending on your calorie needs." This statement is sometimes missing on food labels but underscores the importance of knowing your individual needs.

Calories per gram:
Fat 6 • Carbohydrate 4 • Protein 4

Ingredients (This is where all the ingredients contained in the food are listed.)

This information is optional, and when included, it provides reference information about the 100% Daily Values for the 2,000 and 2,500 calorie reference diets.

This is more reference information about the number of calories in a gram of fat, carbohydrate, or protein. Note that g = grams, and there are about 28 g in an ounce. Also, mg = milligrams, and there are 1,000 mg in 1 g.

Table 2.4

REFERENCE DAILY INTAKES (RDI'S)

These are the set of nutrient standards to be used for calculating % Daily Values on supplement and nutrition labels. There are five different sets of standards, but most Supplement Facts and Nutrition Facts panels are based on the first column on the left: "Adults and Children 4 or more years old." I think it is interesting that the government experts established that these values are supposed to supply adequate essential nutrition for four year olds and adults of all ages. So when you see a % Daily Value of 50 on a supplement label for vitamin E, you know that the serving size contains 50% of 30 IUs, or 15 IUs, by having this chart to refer to.

REFERENCE DAILY INTAKES BY AGE GROUP

Nutrient	Adults and Children 4 or more years old	Children less than 4 years old	Infants	Pregnant Women	Lactating Women
Vitamin A	5,000 IU	2,500 IU	1,500 IU	8,000 IU	8,000 IU
Vitamin C	60 mg	40 mg	35 mg	60 mg	60 mg
Vitamin D	400 IU	400 IU	400 IU	400 IU	400 IU
Vitamin E	30 IU	10 IU	5 IU	30 IU	30 IU
Vitamin K	80 mcg	*	*	*	*
Thiamin	1.5 mg	0.7 mg	0.5 mg	1.7 mg	1.7 mg
Riboflavin	1.7 mg	0.8 mg	0.6 mg	2.0 mg	2.0 mg
Niacin	20 mg	9.0 mg	8.0 mg	20 mg	20 mg
Vitamin B6	2.0 mg	0.7 mg	0.4 mg	2.5 mg	2.5 mg
Folate	400 mcg	200 mcg	100 mcg	800 mcg	800 mcg
Vitamin B12	6 mcg	3 mcg	2 mcg	8 mcg	8 mcg
Biotin	300 mcg	150 mcg	50 mcg	300 mcg	300 mcg
Pantothenic Acid	10 mg	5 mg	3 mg	10 mg	10 mg
Calcium	1,000 mg	800 mg	600 mg	1,300 mg	1,300 mg
Iron	18 mg	10 mg	15 mg	18 mg	18 mg
Phosphorus	1,000 mg	800 mg	500 mg	1,300 mg	1,300 mg
Iodine	150 mcg	70 mcg	45 mcg	150 mcg	150 mcg
Magnesium	400 mg	200 mg	70 mg	450 mg	450 mg
Zinc	15 mg	8 mg	5 mg	15 mg	15 mg
Selenium	70 mcg	*	*	*	*
Copper	2.0 mg	1.0 mg	0.6 mg	2.0 mg	2.0 mg
Manganese	2.0 mg	*	*	*	*
Chromium	120 mcg	*	*	*	*
Molybdenum	75 mcg	*	*	*	*
Chloride	3,400 mg	*	*	*	*

*RDI values have not been established for these age groups.

Table 2.5

DAILY REFERENCE VALUES (DRV'S)

These are the sets of nutrient standards to be used for calculating % Daily Values on the supplement and nutrition labels macronutrients, sodium, and potassium. There are five different sets of standards, but most Supplement Facts and Nutrition Facts panels are based on the first column on the left: "Adults and Children 4 or more years old." Also, only a Daily Reference Value for protein has been established for the other age groups.

DAILY REFERENCE VALUES BY AGE GROUP, BASED ON REFERENCE DIET OF 2,000 CALORIES PER DAY

Nutrient	Adults and Children 4 or more years old	Children less than 4 years old	Infants	Pregnant Women	Lactating Women
Fat	65 g	*	*	*	*
Saturated Fat	20 g	*	*	*	*
Cholesterol	300 mg	*	*	*	*
Total Carbohydrate	300 g	*	*	*	*
Fiber	25 g	*	*	*	*
Sodium	2,400 mg	*	*	*	*
Potassium	3,500 mg	*	*	*	*
Protein	50 g	16 g	14 g	60 g	65 g

*DRV values have not been established for these groups.

DIETARY SUPPLEMENTS VERSUS FOODS

Food products take many forms. One distinction between dietary supplements and food products is that food products list their ingredients and nutrition information in an area of the label designated as the Nutrition Facts box, and do not display a Supplement Facts box. In some cases the manufacturer can choose to label products as either dietary supplement products or as food products, based on the company's marketing objectives. For example, a high-quality nutrient drink product could be sold as a dietary supplement, which would mean the label must identify it as a "dietary supplement" and the Supplement Facts box has to appear on the label. If the manufacturer chooses to identify and sell the product as a dietary supplement, it can only be used to supplement the diet and therefore cannot technically be sold as a meal or meal replacement product. On the other hand, if the manufacturer chooses to identify the product as a food, it would have to bear a Nutrition Facts box on the label, and would most likely be identified in advertising or on the label as a nutritious meal or meal replacement product.

Another point of distinction when selling a dietary supplement versus a food product is that a dietary supplement can make claims of nutritional support as well as the approved health claims. Food products, on the other hand, may *only* bear approved health claims, such as that calcium can help prevent osteoporosis. Chapter 3 will expand on these details. The object of this regulation is to remind consumers that supplements are meant to add to the nutritional value of their diets and not to replace eating a healthy diet.

DIETARY SUPPLEMENTS VERSUS DRUGS

The drug category is probably the category people most often confuse with dietary supplement products, primarily because they are similar in appearance and packaging. Adding to the confusion, some dietary supplements, such as prescription prenatal vitamins and some children's vitamins, are also sold as drugs. But when you look more closely you will notice that over-the-counter drug products have one or more ingredients listed under the heading "Active Ingredients," and are labeled according to the diseases they are intended to treat. In fact, you will soon be seeing over-the-counter drug products conforming to new FDA label standards, which include listing the information in a Drugs Facts box.

The term *drug* can be defined as follows: anything intended for use in the diagnosis, cure, mitigation, treatment, or prevention of disease. When selecting products, there are prescription drug products and nonprescription drug products. There are almost a hundred different categories of nonprescription drug products found on the shelves, used both topically and internally for ailments ranging from acne and colds to insomnia and sunburn. It is estimated that there are over three hundred thousand separate nonprescription drug products currently being marketed, but these products contain only about seven hundred distinct, approved active nonprescription drug ingredients. *The United States Pharmacopeia, Homeopathic Pharmacopoeia of the United States,* and *National Formulary* are official reference texts that list the historical uses of drug ingredients.

The definition of a drug product also includes articles (other than food) intended to affect the structure of the body or any of its functions. This is the part of the definition where there is some overlap with dietary supplement products. Dietary supplement products can make claims relating to their effects on the body's structure or function, which will be discussed in detail in Chapter 3, but they cannot be recommended to diagnose, cure, mitigate, treat, or prevent diseases.

When a manufacturer of a dietary supplement product makes unauthorized drug claims for the product and gets caught, the FDA notifies it that it must stop making the claim. Dietary supplement companies respond by agreeing to cease making the unapproved drug claims, or sometimes by sending letters arguing that the claim they are making is not a drug claim and in fact falls under the function claims allowed under the regulations governing dietary supplements.

It is interesting to follow these interactions between the FDA and manufacturers of supplement products, because sometimes the distinction between dietary supplement products and drugs is not as clear as you may think. In fact, the FDA is currently in the process of clearing up some of the gray areas between dietary supplement claims and drug claims. For example, is saying that a product can reduce inflammation a drug claim or a supplement claim? Does stating that a nutrition product can relieve the symptoms of PMS or menopause make a drug claim or a supplement claim? As of the writing of this book, the FDA contends that these would be considered unapproved drug claims, because inflammation, PMS, and menopause are considered disease conditions. However, many consumers and health professionals argue that these are natural conditions the body experiences, not diseases. As a consumer, when you are confronted with such debate in articles and on television, go with what science supports—which is that the use of dietary supplement products as well as drug products can relieve these common conditions.

DIETARY SUPPLEMENTS VERSUS HOMEOPATHIC PRODUCTS

Homeopathic remedies officially are classified as drugs. Many are sold over the counter for use in treating diseases and afflictions that are considered not to be serious or life-threatening, or that will cure themselves without the use of any drug intervention. The use of homeopathic products as prescription drugs is permitted only when products have official approval from the Food and Drug Administration; homeopathic physicians often use prescription homeopathic drug products for the treatment of serious disease conditions under their direct supervision. Homeopathic products typically contain ingredients similar to those in dietary supplements, such as herbs, which adds to the confusion when trying to determine what's on the shelves. When in doubt, ask an employee working in the store. Herbal supplements and homeopathic herbal products are *not* the same thing.

Homeopathy is a medical approach that was developed in the 1700s, before the development of modern drugs, by Samuel Hahnemann, a German physician and chemist. The remedies used to make homeopathic products come from many sources, including minerals, botanicals, and animals, and are based on the concept of like curing like, with additional consideration given to the specific personality and medical history of the person being treated. Homeopathic remedies contain ingredients that stimulate the body to produce symptoms similar to the ailment the practitioner is trying to cure. Practitioners of homeopathy believe, contrary to our modern medical therapeutic approach, that a substance's strength and effectiveness is increased the more it is diluted. Consequently, dilutions as low as one part of active ingredient per million parts of water are common in homeopathic remedies. In fact, today's homeopathic remedies are so dilute that many do not contain one molecule of the healing substance that the preparation started with. It is the belief of the homeopathic practitioner that during the dilution process, the active substance leaves an imprint or healing essence that is enough to stimulate the body to heal itself.

In the early 1900s, when drug laws were formalized, homeopathic physicians were more common, which is one reason why homeopathy was accepted and written into the FDA regulations for drug therapies. Today the FDA tolerates homeopathic products because there is no real concern over their safety. This is because such products are very dilute and because over-the-counter products are used only for conditions that would go away even if left untreated. While there are over two thousand homeopathic remedies identified in the official pharmacopeia, a homeopathic drug that claims to treat a serious disease such as cancer must be sold by prescription and can be used only if it has the proper approvals.

In the late 1980s I teamed up with a manufacturer of homeopathic products to test how some of these products would work on healthy people who are undergoing athletic training. I tested formulas for pain and for energy and did not find any measurable significant improvements. But I did not test their effectiveness for sick people, which is the primary use for homeopathic remedies. A 1997 *Lancet* study that reviewed 186 clinical trials of homeopathic products found that only 89 of those studies had been conducted according to accepted standards for medical research. After analyzing those 89 studies, however, the article's authors determined that in many cases homeopathic therapies were effective and safe for the treatment of many self-limiting disorders such as allergies, dermatological problems, intestinal problems, musculoskeletal complaints, neurological problems, and obstetrical and gynecological problems. In my own experience, it seems that about 30 to 50 percent of people using homeopathic products for conditions such as headaches, PMS, menopause, allergies, and arthritis experience positive results.

In Europe, homeopathic products are usually taken along with drugs and supplements in a holistic healing approach. Millions of Americans are also using holistic approaches to improve their health. As the medical community continues to study various holistic therapies and track their results, we will learn more and more about which combinations work best for particular conditions.

The following table lists some of the disorders that the researchers found homeopathic remedies were most effective with:

Allergic asthma	Premenstrual
Pollinosis	syndrome (PMS)
Skin lesions	Cystitis
Dermatoses	Cough
Gastritis	Otitis media
Irritable bowel	Rheumatoid
Sprains	arthritis
Haemarthrosis	Fibrositis
Cramps	Myalgia
Dental	Postoperative ileus
neuralgia	Tooth extraction
Migraine	Bruises
Seasickness	Obesity

DIETARY SUPPLEMENTS VERSUS NUTRACEUTICALS

Recently scientists and medical researchers have been conducting research on the beneficial effects that foods have on health. Almost every day you encounter reports in newspapers, in magazines, and on television of how a food product or food ingredient—soy, for example—can have beneficial effects on health or is associated with reducing the risks of certain cancers. This category of foods has been termed *nutraceuticals*.

Nutraceuticals are foods that do more than just provide good nutrition—they have specific disease-prevention or -curing benefits. This idea of foods that heal is not new, and can be traced back to early Greek civilization. In fact, the "father of modern medicine," Hippocrates, is thought to have said, "Let food be your medicine, and let medicine be your food." For those of you who have suffered ailments related to a poor diet, such as cardiovascular disease or diabetes, you know firsthand how proper diet can heal these conditions. So doesn't it make sense to routinely eat a healing diet to prevent diseases and live a long life?

The research on how food can prevent disease is so compelling that the Food and Drug Administration has allowed a series of health claims for foods and dietary supplements, which is discussed further in Chapter 3. As more and more research establishes a food's or supplement's beneficial effects on health, submissions can be made to the FDA to have new health claims approved to be used on those products.

Since it may take decades to accumulate enough scientific studies to support approval of new health claims, you as a consumer must be discerning in your selection of foods to help enhance your health and well-being. A word of caution: While diet is extremely important in maintaining health and preventing certain diseases from occurring, if you are suffering from a serious health condition, always work with a doctor or other health professional to make sure you are using every possible mode of treatment—

drugs, dietary supplements, foods, meditation, and so on—that has been shown to be effective in healing your condition. Contrary to some popular beliefs, there are no real miracle cures for diseases. There are natural cures and drug cures that are backed by science, and an occasional new breakthrough is discovered. When it comes to serious or life-threatening illness, use all the best types of medicine that modern science and alternative approaches have to offer.

DIETARY SUPPLEMENTS VERSUS PHYTOMEDICINES

The World Health Organization estimates that about 80 percent of the world's population relies on herbal medicines for the management and treatment of many diseases. However, in the United States there is no separate category for botanical medicines. In order for a phytomedicine to be sold for use as a drug, it must be approved by the FDA under existing procedures for over-the-counter or prescription drugs. (Botanical ingredients may be found in homeopathic products, but these products are not the same as phytomedicines.)

Phytomedicinal products are very popular in Asia and in European countries, and can often be found for sale in the United States, mostly in ethnic communities, such as Chinese herbal medicines sold in traditional Chinese pharmacies. Botanical products are allowed to be sold as dietary supplements only if they have no therapeutic or curative drug claims associated with their sale.

One of the most common botanical supplements is echinacea, used to help reduce the symptoms of the flu and the common cold. Echinacea, like many of the products sold on the market as dietary supplements, is often sold under claims that it "supports immune function" or "helps stimulate proper immune function." These are allowable claims, as they relate to the product's effect on one of the body's functions. However, marketers of dietary supplements sometimes expand these claims on echinacea products, suggesting that they be used specifically during cold season. The FDA considers this a drug claim, and usually warns the companies to change the wording so as not to imply that echinacea cures colds (which are a disease condition).

Botanical products are available in the United States in a variety of forms. You can purchase dried plant parts, to be prepared as a tea. Then there are a range of manufactured products, which include herbal powders ground up and put in capsules or compressed into tablets. Liquid forms of botanical supplements are also common, and are available in water-, glycerin-, or alcohol-based preparations (or combinations of these). Liquid concentrates are also made into softgels.

Herbs are technically nonwoody plants. However, as you read the labels of herbal supplements and become more aware of the ingredients, you will notice that the labels may list bark, leaves, roots, and berries of woody plants. One of the most common botanical products on the market is ginkgo, made from the leaves of the ginkgo tree.

Many familiar over-the-counter products also use botanically derived ingredients. For example, if you read the label for Ex-Lax Natural, you will see sennosides listed as an active ingredient. Sennosides are derived from a plant called senna, and the company has gone through the official process to have their naturally derived products categorized as laxatives.

As time passes, undoubtedly we will see more and more over-the-counter drug products that include botanical ingredients. However, the more desirable path would be for the Food and Drug Administration to officially create a separate category for phytomedicines, following the models already established in other countries such as Germany, Japan, China, France, and Italy.

If you use botanical products, be aware that they are not always standardized and are not always produced in accordance with accepted drug product manufacturing procedures. This means that you may not be getting the proper dosages that the scientific studies have shown will help with your particular ailment. When using botanical products to treat a disease condition, it is well advised that you do so only under the supervision of a trained naturopathic doctor or other health practitioner who is experienced in using nutrition and herbal products to treat disease conditions. Do not substitute herbal medicines for conventional medicines when treating serious health conditions such as cardiovascular disease, cancer, arthritis, diabetes, and others. While there is research that shows natural products will help in the prevention, cure, and treatment of many of these disorders, be sure to use them in concert with your physician.

MORE INSIGHTS ON NUTRITIONAL USES VERSUS THERAPEUTIC USES OF DIETARY SUPPLEMENTS

When using the information in Part 3, which lists numerous dietary supplement ingredients and the dosages found to be effective to help promote health and well-being, it is important to distinguish between therapeutic uses and nutritional uses of these dietary supplements. For example, many medical studies used a daily dosage of 120 to 180 mg of standardized *Ginkgo biloba* leaf extracts. Using these therapeutic dosages has been shown to produce beneficial effects, such as curing peripheral circulatory insufficiencies and improving memory in people with various dementias. While millions of people worldwide are using these high therapeutic dosages daily as a dietary supplement, smaller dosages can be equally effective in stimulating or maintaining the proper structure and function of the circulatory system over longer periods of time. As more research on dietary supplements is conducted, the lower and upper ranges of beneficial dosages will continue to be better defined. For the purposes of this guide, I chose to provide nutritional dosages, and therapeutic dosages when appropriate, to enable you to use dietary supplements to your best advantage. The next chapter will begin to discuss the many advantages that dietary supplements have to offer in your quest for improved health.

3

Special Claims for Dietary Supplements: Understanding What's on the Labels

One of the most significant impacts of the Dietary Supplement Health and Education Act is that it authorizes manufacturers of dietary supplements to make certain types of claims about their products. Broadly speaking, there are two categories of claims now allowed on dietary supplement products. These claims are referred to as "statements of nutritional support" and "health claims."

Statements of nutritional support include (1) claims of benefit related to a classic nutrient-deficiency disease, (2) description of the role of a nutrient or dietary ingredient intended to affect the structure or function of the body, (3) characterization of the documented mechanism by which the ingredient acts to maintain structure or function, and (4) description of general improvements in well-being related to consumption of the ingredient.

The other type of claims, health claims, are special types of claims allowed in food labeling. Health claims are based on a relationship between the particular food or food ingredient and the prevention of a disease or health-related condition. In order for health claims to be made, manufacturers must submit to the FDA substantial scientific studies that then undergo an official review process. The experts decide if the scientific evidence supports the health claim and can be included in the product labeling.

Many dietary supplement products tiptoe around the boundaries imposed by these regulations. Some of these include such claims as "supports heart health," "supports a healthy prostate," and "improves well-being." When a statement of nutritional support is used on the label or on promotional literature sold with the product, a disclaimer must be listed that states the following: "This product has not been evaluated by the Food and Drug Administration. This product is not intended to diagnose, treat, cure, or prevent any disease." This disclaimer is required as part of a compromise made to get the FDA to permit structure/function claims and other claims of nutritional support on dietary supplement labels. While it may seem cumbersome, it is intended as a safeguard for consumers.

Yet much information is found in books and the media concerning how ingredients found in dietary supplements can indeed help cure or prevent diseases. For example, scientific studies have clearly demonstrated that glucosamine will help in the treatment of osteoarthritis. Millions of people take glucosamine-containing supplements for this very reason. However, until someone makes a formal submission to the FDA, with all the existing research, to get this drug claim approved, marketers must craft their claims to meet the dietary supplement structure/functions claims criteria. Thus they use wording such as "strengthens your joints," "promotes joint health," and "helps nourish cartilage and cushion your joints." (If you are interested in joint health, see Chapter 11 for guidelines.)

In my experience, the Food and Drug Administration does not evaluate whether or not a claim of nutrition support is a valid one. They only determine whether the manufacturer's statement falls into the dietary supplement claim category or the drug claim category. The manufacturer must have the proper scientific evidence on file in case it is ever required by a government agency to substantiate the claims it is making on its products and in its advertising. So while the FDA's policy of allowing only certain claims for dietary supplement products is designed to protect the consumer from unwarranted claims, it provides no help in sorting through the thousands of scientific studies that report on how dietary supplement ingredients can also help with disease conditions.

This chapter is dedicated to educating you on the various aspects of claims of nutritional support that you will encounter when purchasing dietary supplements. It will also discuss the approved health claims. You will find guidelines on the type of wording to look for to detect whether or not a manufacturer is making an unauthorized drug claim. (Keep in mind that many dietary supplement ingredients have been shown in clinical studies to effectively treat diseases, alone or in conjunction with drug therapy. Parts 2 and 3 will provide information on the ingredients that have good scientific support, which will enable you to work with health care professionals to better treat your condition.) Finally, I will review the ins and outs of the scientific studies and the criteria used to qualify them as acceptable for substantiating claims of nutritional support. This will give you important insights on the quality and quantity of research that does exist on the benefits of dietary supplement products, and will make you realize that information in magazine or newspaper articles and on TV is not considered substantiation. Only high-quality scientific studies that have been reviewed by other scientists and whose results can be reproduced in subsequent studies by different researchers are considered valid. This is the standard that I maintain when including claims about ingredients in this book.

STATEMENTS CLAIMING A BENEFIT RELATED TO CLASSIC NUTRIENT-DEFICIENCY DISEASE

If a manufacturer claims that its product can help someone avoid or treat a disease caused by a lack of a specific nutrient, such as a vitamin or mineral, it must also disclose the prevalence of that disease in the United States. For example, while it is true that vitamin C supplements can help prevent scurvy, scurvy is not a common deficiency disease in the United States. The thinking behind this is that people should not be misled into thinking that if they did not take the supplement product, they would develop a deficiency condition. While it is important to have adequate essential vitamin and mineral intake, most companies are not currently using these types of claims on dietary supplement products, because those diseases are rare.

STATEMENTS DESCRIBING THE ROLE OF A NUTRIENT OR DIETARY INGREDIENT INTENDED TO AFFECT STRUCTURE OR FUNCTION IN HUMANS

The claims that you will mostly encounter on dietary supplement labels fall under the heading of structure or function claims. These types of claims prescribe how an ingredient in a dietary supplement product, or perhaps its entire formula, works to benefit the structure or function of your body. The wording of such claims is becoming something of an art, because scientists and marketers working together need to make sure that they craft the statements in such a way as not to make unapproved drug claims. Words commonly used in such claims include *stimulate, maintain, support, regulate,* and *promote.* Following are some examples of structure/function claims that have been submitted to the FDA for their review and comment. Reviewing these examples will help you develop an understanding of how dietary supplement ingredients can affect the structure and function of the body, such as calcium improving bone structure, and bilberry promoting good eye function.

> Scientific studies have shown that regular consumption of carotenes helps maintain a strong, healthy immune system.
>
> Phytochemicals are a key to good health.
>
> Good for antioxidant and cellular health.

Research shows that antioxidants help fight free-radical damage caused by environmental factors and other toxic insults.

CoQ_{10} [coenzyme Q_{10}] is a nutrient that supports heart function and promotes energy production in cells.

Supports immune system function.

Alpha-lipoic acid helps maintain the function of the cardiovascular system and acts as a protective antioxidant.

Supports healthy heart function as the body ages.

Helps support cardiovascular function and a healthy circulatory system.

Helps the walls of arteries, capillaries, and veins stay flexible and strong.

Nourishment for a healthy heart.

Helps maintain healthy blood cholesterol levels.

Nutritional support for healthy heart function.

For cardiovascular health.

Promotes normal blood clotting.

Nutritionally supports healthy vein function.

Aids digestion naturally.

Nutritionally supports normal digestive processes.

Support for healthy digestive system.

Acidophilus organisms help maintain a healthy digestive tract.

Promotes good health.

Nutritionally supports normal energy production processes.

Supports endurance and stamina.

Promotes energy and mental clarity.

Helps maintain physical performance.

Rich in energizing nutrients.

Supports normal joint function and lubrication.

Promotes healthy joints and cartilage.

Nutritional formula for optimal bone formation.

Vitamin D is necessary for healthy teeth and bones and enhances calcium absorption.

For strong bones and teeth.

Nutritional support for connective tissue.

Promotes relaxation.

Supports normal memory function and reduces absentmindedness.

Positive mood enhancer.

Nutritional support for mental function.

Nourishment for your nervous system.

Shown to have relaxing effects and sleep-promoting action.

Supports natural sleep [or normal sleep patterns].

Ginkgo supplements benefit memory, mental clarity, and alertness.

Naturally relaxing dietary supplements.

Promotes a calm, healthy attitude.

Nutritionally supports feelings of well-being.

Supports the eye's ability to focus at a distance.

Bilberry has been proven to support healthy eye function and help enhance night vision.

Enhances visual health.

Supports healthy vision function.

Vitamin A is necessary for new cell growth and healthy tissues and is essential for vision in dim light.

Supports healthy liver function.

Traditional herb for kidney function.

Helps promote urinary tract health.

Nutritional support to help maintain a healthy prostate.

Nutritional support for the male reproductive system.

Herbal support for women.

Required for reproductive function.

Helps replace those nutrients lost during the menstrual cycle.

Nutritional support for women's health.

Nutritional support for healthy estrogen function.

Promotes women's health and well-being.

As you can see, the structure/function claims are quite diversified.

When a company starts to market products with claims of nutritional support and submits a notification to the Food and Drug Administration, the people reviewing the claims at the FDA determine if the claims are allowable under the rules discussed above. The following list includes some actual examples of the purported claims of nutritional support that the FDA determined were really drug claims. In such cases the agency sent out a letter to the manufacturer advising it to change the claim or be subject to fines or other penalties. If you compare this list to the list of permitted structure/function claims, above, you will quickly pick up on why the FDA considered these to be drug claims.

Promotes cold sore relief.

Decreases risk of heart disease.

Lowers cholesterol.

Inhibits hemoglobin and blocks the growth and nourishment of malignant tumors.

For nutritional support during the cold season.

Resistance to viruses may be enhanced.

Eating a diet high in tomatoes and foods rich in tomato extract has been related to a lower risk of prostate and other cancers.

For relief of symptoms of cold, flu, and sore throats.

Promotes healing.

Reduces the pain and stiffness associated with arthritis.

Decreases the effects of alcohol intoxication.

Alleviates constipation.

I find it remarkable that people with scientific and medical degrees submitted such obvious drug claims to the FDA. However, some of the claims, such as "lowers cholesterol," are less clearly drug claims, especially when you consider that the claim "maintains healthy cholesterol levels" is seen widely on many garlic supplements and other products purported to help promote circulatory system wellness. The people at the FDA argue that claiming a dietary supplement product "lowers cholesterol" implies that it will cure the disease conditions hypercholesterolemia and hyperlipidemia (which in fact it may) and may mislead unsuspecting consumers, even though it would carry a disclaimer saying that the FDA has not evaluated the product. On the other hand, "maintains healthy cholesterol levels" is an allowable structure/function claim because it limits and restricts the claims to a healthy state. The situation is quite confusing, and during the writing of this book, the FDA and the public were again grappling with some of these gray-area issues.

In 1998 the Food and Drug Administration proposed some new regulations on structure/function claims made for dietary supplements. These regulations were intended to better define what would be considered allowable claims and to make the claims more informative, reliable, and uniform. Perhaps a more straightforward approach in the future will enable you as a consumer to better understand how a given product can help you maintain health. In the meantime, use the information in this book to gain a clear understanding of the different ingredients, the amounts that are safe and effective, and the type of benefits you can expect from using various dietary supplement products.

CLAIMS CHARACTERIZING DOCUMENTED MECHANISMS BY WHICH A NUTRIENT OR DIETARY INGREDIENT ACTS TO MAINTAIN STRUCTURE OR FUNCTION

Claims of this type are sometimes mixed in with the other types of structure/function claims listed above, but can get more descriptive and specific about how a specific dietary supplement ingredient works inside the body. For example, the statement that the herb valerian "helps promote restful sleep" is a valid structure/function claim (see Chapter 15 if you want a perfect night's sleep). Taking the claim a step further would describe the physiological mechanism through which valerian's chemical ingredients promote more restful sleep: "Valerenic acid stimulates the release and uptake of the calming neurotransmitter GABA, which results in relaxation and promotion of restful sleep."

As you can imagine, using technical structure and function claims like this one would make reading dietary supplement labels like reading biochemistry textbooks. For this reason most manufacturers spare you the scientific details on the labels, but you may encounter biochemical jargon in brochures and articles. As a regulatory matter, promotional literature for dietary supplement products is considered to be an extension of the label, and the claims in promotional literature are subject to the limitations of the Dietary Supplement Health and Education Act. The publications or reprints cannot be false or misleading, they must be displayed in an area with other publications and literature, and they must contain a balanced view of the subject matter. So when you read an article on how taking ginkgo or Acetyl-L-carnitine can help treat Alzheimer's disease, don't expect to see the same claims in brochures or on the labels; instead you will see "improves brain wellness," "improves memory," or the like.

STATEMENTS DESCRIBING GENERAL WELL-BEING FROM CONSUMPTION OF A NUTRIENT OR DIETARY INGREDIENT

Stating that a product or product ingredients will enhance your well-being is a sort of catchall that avoids the problem of substantiating more specific claims but lets the consumer know what the product may do.

HEALTH CLAIMS ALLOWED FOR DIETARY SUPPLEMENT PRODUCTS

As part of the 1990 Nutrition Labeling and Education Act, the FDA authorized certain health claims, and made provisions for companies to get more health claims approved. These health claims show a relationship between consumption of a nutrient or other substances in foods and a disease or health-related condition. The intended purpose of health claims is to provide consumers with information on healthful eating patterns that may help reduce the risk of cancer, heart disease, osteoporosis, high blood pressure, dental cavities, or certain birth defects. In order to get a health claim approved, scientific studies must be submitted to the Food and Drug Administration.

The current approved health claims (as of May 1999) for dietary supplements and conventional foods include the following:

Calcium supplementation can prevent osteoporosis.

Soluble fiber from whole oats and psyllium can reduce the risk of coronary heart disease.

Use of sugar-free gum containing sugar alcohols (such as sorbitol, mannitol, and xylitol) can prevent tooth decay.

Folate supplements can prevent neural tube defects.

Some health claims are allowed to be made only for food products, that is, products with a Nutrition Facts panel, not dietary supplement products. These include the following:

Diets low in sodium will help lower blood pressure and related risks in many people.

Low-fat diets reduce the risk of some types of cancer, such as cancers of the breast, colon, and prostate.

Diets low in saturated fat and cholesterol decrease the risk of coronary heart disease.

Diets low in fat and rich in fiber-containing grain products, fruits, and vegetables may reduce the risk of some types of cancer.

Diets low in saturated fat and cholesterol and rich in fruits, vegetables, and grain products that contain fiber, particularly soluble fiber, will reduce the risk of coronary heart disease.

Diets low in fat and rich in fruits and vegetables will reduce the risk of some cancers.

As more scientific research accumulates supporting the role of particular foods or nutrients in their prevention of diseases, new health claims will certainly be added to these lists.

SCIENTIFIC SUBSTANTIATION

One of the primary requirements for making claims of nutritional support on dietary supplement labels, or for submitting a petition to the FDA for approval of new health claims, is that the claims must be substantiated by significant scientific agreement and evidence. In the case of nutritional support claims for dietary supplements, the companies making claims of nutritional support must maintain files backing up these claims at their place of business. However, at this point in time none of the legislation sets out a specific definition of what exactly constitutes adequate substantiation.

The kind and amount of evidence needed to support a claim will depend upon the statement of nutritional support being made. For example, evidence of how a vitamin or a mineral is related to a classic nutrient deficiency disease is well known. On the other hand, some structure/function claims require well-controlled clinical studies as evidence. The gold standard of scientific studies is those published in peer-reviewed scientific journals with high credibility.

In the arena of scientific research, submitting your study to a journal that has independent scientists review the material is considered the preferred way of verifying that the research results are well founded. This level of peer scrutiny is required because no researcher is perfect, and complex issues that may arise when conducting scientific studies can sometimes be overlooked. However, other types of studies that are not reported in peer-reviewed journals may also be considered valid evidence in support of a structure/function claim. It is best to look at the total body of knowledge when determining whether or not a structure/function claim is truthful and not misleading.

Scientific research can include a wide range of activities. *In vitro* studies involve research conducted in test tubes, outside of living organisms. In vitro studies are useful when scientists are trying to figure out specific aspects of the biochemistry of a particular compound. Researchers use in vitro studies to help sort out details of processes that are observed in living systems.

Another type of study is called *ex vivo*. These studies use parts of animals or humans experimentally outside the body and subject them to various tests. Ex vivo tests commonly use living cells in a laboratory setting to measure the effects of a drug or dietary supplement ingredient.

In vivo studies are conducted in living systems. These include experimental studies using animals (to measure toxicity, for example) and experimental studies on humans (usually called clinical studies). Well-conducted clinical studies must exist to verify the effects of a dietary supplement in order to support claims for nutritional support. But just because scientific studies have not been conducted yet does not mean that a dietary supplement ingredient should automatically be judged ineffective. Some ingredients have a history of use that demonstrates their effectiveness. For example, it is well known what effects you can expect from drinking a glass or two of prune juice. But, there are few well-controlled clinical studies to verify prune juice's laxative effects.

When selecting information to include in this book, I adhered to the highest standards of scientific evidence. While there are some instances, in particular with herbal products, where legitimate traditional uses are also recognized as adequate evidence, I have been conservative about including such evidence, because I would rather err on the side of safety than stretch weak evidence. There are many legitimate claims for nutrients that you can be comfortable relying on. You don't need to experiment with ingredients.

THE FEDERAL TRADE COMMISSION'S ROLE IN REGULATING DIETARY SUPPLEMENT CLAIMS

While the FDA's responsibility is the regulation of claims on product labeling, which includes packaging, inserts, and other promotional materials distributed at the point of sale, the Federal Trade Commission, on the other hand, has primary responsibility for regulating claims in advertising, including print and broadcast ads, catalogs and similar direct marketing materials, and infomercials. In 1998 the FTC published specific advertising guidelines for the marketing of dietary supplement products, in response to all of the new claims that the Dietary Supplement Health and Education Act made possible.

These guidelines point out that as a general rule, well-controlled human clinical studies are the most reliable form of evidence. To underscore this point, I would like to share with you a glimpse into a court proceeding concerning a matter between the FTC and a dietary supplement company during 1994–1996. The company was marketing a dietary supplement that contained calcium in the form of a chemical compound called hydroxyapatite. The FTC challenged several advertising claims made about the product and its effects on the body. This was an interesting case, because most companies usually settle with the FTC on advertising issues rather than go to court. In this case, the company thought its claims well substantiated and decided to defend itself.

The FTC hired scientific experts on calcium, and the marketer of the calcium product hired its own experts as well. Many scientific studies, articles, editorials, and abstracts were offered as evidence in support of advertising claims. After the experts reviewed over a hundred scientific studies and other supportive materials, the judge ruled that only well-designed and controlled clinical studies would be considered as evidence. Other scientific studies, review articles, and abstracts were considered substantiation for the findings of such clinical studies. All articles in magazines, chapters in books, and other secondary literature were not accepted as qualified evidence at all.

After a very lengthy and expensive court proceeding, the court rendered the following decisions on the several advertising claims:

1. Builds bone or increases bone thickness (substantiated)

2. Restores lost bone greater than the amount of bone lost (not substantiated)

3. Halts or prevents bone loss or bone thinning (substantiated)

4. Restores bone strength (not substantiated)

5. Halts, prevents, or treats osteoporosis (substantiated)

6. Reduces or eliminates pain associated with bone ailments (not substantiated)

7. Is superior to and is more effective than other forms of calcium in the prevention or treatment of bone ailment (not substantiated)

8. Is more bioavailable, more absorbable, and more effectively utilized by the body than other forms of calcium (not substantiated)

The outcome of this case sends the message to marketers of dietary supplements that they had better make sure they are making advertising claims based on scientific fact, not guesses. It is interesting to realize that during and after this case, the company was never restricted from selling the calcium supplement; all it had to do, in the end, was change unsubstantiated advertising claims. It is also interesting to note that now there is good scientific evidence to support the claim that taking calcium supplements can restore lost bone in many cases.

SAFETY OF DIETARY SUPPLEMENTS

As discussed earlier, the passage of the Dietary Supplement Health and Education Act permitted dietary supplements to include all ingredients that were currently available in interstate commerce when the act was passed, in 1994. To the delight of the dietary supplement marketers, this provision covered a significant number of ingredients that the FDA was at the time battling to exclude from the market: metabolites, amino acids, and all of the herbal products. In other words, until proven otherwise, all ingredients in dietary supplements were considered safe. The burden was put on the FDA to declare a dietary supplement ingredient as being not safe and an imminent hazard to public health or safety. Any dietary supplement ingredient introduced after 1994 would have to be submitted to the FDA with supportive scientific research to prove its safety. However, if a dietary supplement contains ingredients that are already present in the food supply, are used for food, or have a history of use as dietary supplement ingredients, it is automatically approved for use.

The issue of whether dietary supplement products, especially botanical supplements, are safe has received substantial coverage on television and in the print media, with some justification (though the media's coverage of most issues concerning dietary supplements is frequently very superficial and usually flawed). Some herbal products are safe when used properly but can pose potential health risks if used improperly. The catch is that, unlike drugs, the regulations for dietary supplements generally do not provide for the establishment of approved dosages, instructions, warnings, and use guidelines. This is left up to the manufacturers. Fortunately, most manufacturers take a responsible approach to formulating their products and include only ingredients that are safe when taken according to package instructions. If the FDA becomes aware of the rare supplement that contains hazardous ingredients or ingredients that should not be taken in the amounts recommended, the agency responds very quickly to correct the situation and recall the problematic product. The information in Parts 2 and 3 will help you determine whether the supplements you are taking now (or are considering taking) are safe and effective for you and your family. It is also important to consult with your doctor or other health professional to ensure that the diet you are following and the supplements you are taking will provide beneficial results.

When taking supplements, you must keep in mind three things: the ingredients, the dosage, and the duration of use. There may be occasions when you need to take high dosages of an ingredient for short periods of time. On the other hand, most dietary supplements you take will contain effective ingredients in amounts that are safe for long-term use. The information contained in Part 2 will help you understand what science and history have shown to be the optimal diet and supplement program for achieving ultimate health.

What about supplement ingredients that should be avoided? First let's put things in perspective. Safety issues concerning supplements are usually blown out of proportion by the media. There are many more times the number of reports of adverse health events from taking drugs and eating conventional food than from supplements. The track record for dietary supplements is extremely safe. However, there are instances where irresponsible companies put unsafe ingredients in their products, or contaminated raw materials get into products, or otherwise safe products are misused by customers. Another area of health concern deals with supplement-drug interactions. The following information will provide you with some recent examples of reported adverse effects of supplement or supplement-like products; although, keep in mind that even essential nutrients (vitamins and minerals) can be harmful if not used properly.

In recent years, the FDA has been confronted with removing certain products from the market, products that were essentially dangerous, unapproved drugs, sometimes sold as dietary supplements. These products included the following ingredients: gamma hydroxybutyric acid (GHB); gamma butyrolactone (GBL); and 1,4 butanediol (BD). Products containing these ingredients have been associated with dangerous side effects; avoid them. They are sold for their alleged benefits for body building, weight loss, and sleep aids.

Examples of misused products that the FDA reports can result in illness or injuries include: chaparral, comfrey, slimming/dieter's tea, ephedra, germander, lobelia, magnolia-stephania preparation, willow bark, wormwood, vitamin A (in dosages of 25,000 or more IUs per day), vitamin B_6 (in doses above 100 mg a day), niacin (in slow-released dosages of 500 mg or more a day, or immediate-release dosages of 750 mg or more a day), selenium (in dosages of about 800 mcg to 1,000 mcg a day), germanium, and L-tryptophan (most likely from a contaminant).

Drug interactions are an increasing concern as more people with illnesses are turning to using supplements as complementary or alternative treatments to the drugs they are taking. Part 3 entries offer information on commonly encountered drug-supplement concerns. Recently, a study conducted by The National Institutes of Health showed that use of St. John's wort substantially decreased the plasma concentrations of the drug indinavir; in other words, it reduced the drug's effectiveness.

Refer to Parts 2 and 3 for detailed information on choosing and using safe and effective supplements for your specific needs. You can also visit the FDA's Web site found at http://www.fda.gov/.

4

To Supplement Right, First Eat Right

My quest for nutritional truth started when I was a fourteen-year-old wrestler confronted with having to maintain an unnaturally low body weight for my age. It soon became apparent to me that the practices of the day used for "making weight," such as starving, taking laxatives, and sweating off pounds, were not healthy, and in fact were dangerous. So I began to read every book I could get my hands on about nutrition and weight loss. After looking through dozens of books, I came to the conclusion that the field of weight loss and weight maintenance was filled with inconsistencies and confusion. So many diets on the market made no nutritional sense. How could this be?

When I entered college and became a scientist, I was exposed to a whole new world of nutrition information in hundreds of scientific journals containing thousands of articles published each year. After several years of reading and conducting research of my own on how food affects health, performance, and body composition, a unified nutrition model began to develop in my mind. During this time I developed a scientific model to understand why some diets around the world were reported to benefit health, while those of most industrialized nations were reported to adversely affect health.

My Natural-Thin plan is the result of evaluating and testing a massive body of scientific knowledge and nutritional wisdom that accumulated over many years. It is based not on opinion but on scientific conclusions. The Natural-Thin approach includes eating foods with nutraceutical value. Why wait until you develop a diet-related life-threatening illness, such as diabetes, coronary heart disease, obesity, or cancer, before beginning to eat the right way? Start by following this simple rule: Include in your diet foods that will benefit your health, and exclude or minimize foods that will not.

The Natural-Thin approach includes proper diet, healthy lifestyle behaviors, and dietary supplements. I cannot stress too strongly that exercise, along with diet, is the foundation of super health; supplements alone will not put you in peak condition. Mental wellness is also a key component. The Natural-Thin approach is a result of my multidisciplinary training and interests, which include various fields of science as well as philosophy and spirituality.

Start your quest for nutritional excellence by realizing that achieving optimal health in the twenty-first century is not as easy as you may believe. You are surrounded by low-quality foods that tempt you to eat them and are easily overconsumed. Each day you are conditioned by advertisements to believe that snack foods are something that the human race cannot live without, even though they were only invented in this century. Your cultural eating values are deeply ingrained, and they have a huge impact on your daily eating patterns.

For the past hundred thousand years, our species, *Homo sapiens,* has thrived by eating natural, wholesome foods, rich in essential life-giving nutrients. Today, however, it is a different story. In our industrialized society, we are confronted with many highly refined foods that are sparse in nutrients and may be filled with chemicals. The food in our supermarkets is quite different from what was available to our grandparents. Back then, animals and fish were raised in a far less polluted environment and fed fewer hormones. Fruits and vegetables were grown with fewer chemicals and in richer soils. Grains were less refined and so more nutrient-rich as well as higher in fiber. Then in the 1940s, technology began to dominate food production, altering the way foods are grown and processed and giving them a longer shelf life. Modern technology has created a more reliable food supply, but along the way we've lost a lot—and gained a potent dose of potentially harmful chemicals. Don't take my word for it—look at the ingredient lists and Nutrition Facts panels of the foods in your house, and see how hard it is to find foods high in fiber and rich in essential vitamins and minerals, not to mention foods free of artificial ingredients and unhealthful fats. It's no wonder that as we begin a new century millions of people are buying more foods from natural food stores and seeking alternative approaches to keep the body healthy.

As a result of this technology-based food supply, millions of people develop diet-related diseases each year, such as diabetes, coronary heart disease, obesity, high blood pressure, and cancer. In addition, we tend to live a less active, higher-stress lifestyle than our ancestors, and we eat more out of habit than out of need. To illustrate this point in my lectures, I call this new "sub-species" *Homo sapiens technoramus,* because technology is the environmental force behind its emergence. By contrast, *Homo sapiens* lives more of a tribal life. They eat wholesome, healthy foods, high in nutrition and low in added chemicals. The diet of *Homo sapiens* contains very little (if any) refined sugars, added salt, refined flours, or high-fat animal products; its diet is low in total fat, high in fiber, lean meats, vegetables, and fruit. *Homo sapiens* also is moderately active and avoids a high-stress lifestyle. *Homo sapiens* also eats purposefully; that is, thinking before eating and not overeating.

Here are some things to consider to see if you have become, or on the verge of becoming a *Homo sapiens technoramus*:

1. Do you think about what you eat and when you eat it, or do you eat unconsciously, out of habit?
2. Do you have a potentially diet-related condition such as diabetes, cardiovascular disease, cancer, dental caries, macular degeneration, obesity, gastrointestinal problems, cirrhosis, arthritis, or osteoporosis?
3. Do you rely solely on drugs to manage your diet-related disease?

Answering yes to questions 1 and/or 2 means that you need to become aware of how your eating habits may be putting your health at risk. If you answered yes to all three questions, you may be on the verge of evolving into a *Homo sapiens technoramus*, and need to make significant changes in your eating and lifestyle habits to correct your state of health. Don't be too hard on yourself; you still have time to make changes. For some people making the changes will be easy, and for others it might be very difficult. If you are having trouble, reach out for the support of your family and friends, and seek the advice of a health professional. Eating is a skill, and mastering any skill takes work and dedication.

NUTRITIONAL REVELATIONS

The following list includes the main nutritional problems in most people's diets. The information in the remainder of this chapter, and in Appendix A, where full details of the Natural-Thin program can be found, will help you correct these nutritional inadequacies.

Most American diets are:
Too high in total fat
Too high in saturated fat
Too high in cholesterol
Too high in sodium
Too high in sugar
Too high in processed foods
Too high in empty-calorie foods
Too high in snack foods
Too high in junk foods
Too high in refined flours
Too high in total calories
Too low in potassium
Too low in calcium
Too low in magnesium

Too low in antioxidants

Too low in other essential vitamins and minerals

Too low in alpha-linolenic acid

Too low in the heart-healthy fatty acids eicosapentaenoic acid (EPA) and docosahexaenoic acid (DHA)

Too low in protein

Too low in fiber

Too low in fluid (water)

GOAL SETTING: GETTING THE RESULTS YOU WANT

Establishing your health goals is as important as setting goals in other aspects of your life. Psychologists estimate that it takes at least three weeks to make or break habits and implement new lifestyle changes, so be patient. Knowing how to apply psychology to work for you, not against you, is part of the Natural-Thin approach. (To help with your quest for nutrition excellence, see the worksheet in the Appendix.)

NUTRITION OVERVIEW

The following information will provide the basics of nutrition; the full Natural-Thin plan, in the Appendix, provides detailed eating and lifestyle strategies.

When we think of food, most of us relate what we eat to the "food group" approach we learned in school: fruit and vegetables, meat and fish, dairy, and breads and grains. The old food groups have recently been revised into the new food pyramid, and basing a diet on this can be useful. However, while a meal consisting of steak, potatoes with butter, broccoli, salad, and soda may contain most of the essential nutrients you need, such a meal is likely to contain too many calories, too much fat, too much sugar, and too much salt. You must begin to think of food as the stuff that supplies the nutrition you need for optimal health, and know which foods should be avoided or limited in your diet.

During the 1990s, the U.S. Department of Agriculture devised the Food Guide Pyramid to help consumers implement healthy eating habits. The Food Guide Pyramid is not meant to be perfect, and, in fact, it is not. It does try to imprint a mental image in our minds of the foods we should focus on eating more of, and those we should eat less of.

The USDA Food Guide Pyramid recommends the following foods be eaten each day:

8 to 11 servings of grain products, such as bread, cereal, rice, and pasta

3 to 5 servings of vegetables

2 to 4 servings of fruit

2 to 3 servings of meat, poultry, fish, dry beans, eggs, or nuts

2 to 3 servings of milk, yogurt, and cheese

Use fats, oils, and sweets sparingly

It's interesting to note that other food guide pyramids have been established, such as the Mediterranean Diet Pyramid and Asian Diet Pyramid. These pyramids are similar in that they recommend similar servings of grain foods, fruits, and vegetables, but recommend getting more protein from plant foods and eating less dairy and red meats. However you choose to eat, make sure that you maintain a high intake of nonstarchy vegetables and spread your daily caloric intake out over several smaller meals/snacks each day. Overeating even the healthiest foods can cause obesity and other health problems.

Macronutrients are those nutrients needed in large amounts. These include protein, carbohydrates, lipids (fats and oils), and water. These nutrients play a variety of metabolic roles: Carbohydrates and fats supply energy, protein provides the building blocks of body tissues such as muscle, and water is an essential macronutrient that the body needs all day long (and the physically active need more of it).

Oxygen is also very important for the proper functioning of each cell. Not normally thought of as a nutrient in the traditional sense, it is the most essential one; you can survive only a few minutes without it. There are ways to ensure that you get a good supply of the oxygen you need. The first is being physically fit. When the body is fit, it can take in and use oxygen more efficiently. You can also strive to maintain and improve your cardiovascular health by eating foods and taking dietary supplements that help improve circulation and the health of your blood components. This will result in better blood flow, delivering nutrients and oxygen more efficiently to the cells and clearing unwanted waste products. A healthy circulatory system is the foundation of a healthy metabolism. Anyone who has experienced a circulation problem or knows someone who has been afflicted with one is aware of how it can impair health.

Micronutrients are nutrients required in smaller amounts, particularly vitamins, minerals, metabolic cofactors, and phytochemicals. Micronutrients play very essential roles in health, growth, development, resistance to the problems of aging, and mental wellness. They generally function as cofactors in many biochemical reactions and may also be involved in protecting our bodies from damage caused by chemicals. Micronutrients can also be critical to the body's structure, such as calcium and magnesium in bone, and iron in hemoglobin.

The Five Nutrient Categories, Their Physiologic Functions, and Good Sources

Protein: Builds and repairs body tissue. Occurs in large amounts in egg whites, fish, seafood, low-fat dairy, soy products, and lean meats (turkey, chicken, fish, beef, and lamb).

Carbohydrates: Provide energy for the body. Found in whole grains, pasta, potatoes, beans, cereals.

Fat: Is a necessary part of every cell, carries fat-soluble vitamins, provides energy. Most beneficial types are flaxseed oil, soy oil, walnut oil, fish oil, corn oil, lecithin.

Vitamins/Minerals: Regulate body processes, serve as metabolic cofactors. Present in all foods—fruits, vegetables, dairy, fish, meats—and dietary supplements.

Water: Important for the many chemical reactions in the body, prevents dehydration. Good sources are low-cal beverages and certain foods as well as plain water.

WHY DO YOU NEED TO EAT?

We have been conditioned from watching television commercials to think of eating as an event or celebration. We are also conditioned to think about eating those foods we see the most in TV commercials and print advertisements. These foods may smell and taste great, but they might not be the healthiest choices. First and foremost, you need to eat for growth, development, and promotion of good health, not for pleasure or to satisfy hunger. Your diet provides you with the nutrients you need for energy and to build and repair the body. However, if you eat too much food, the excess is stored as fat. If not enough of the right nutrients are obtained from the diet, your health may suffer. Your body needs a daily supply of carbohydrates, protein, small amounts of essential fatty acids, essential vitamins and minerals, botanical health factors, and water to thrive.

FOOD AND SUPPLEMENTS

The nutrients you need each day are best supplied from eating healthy foods. Whole foods—foods served the way nature made them—tend to provide higher-quality nutrition than processed foods. Although most foods contain both macronutrients and micronutrients, research has shown that the quantity of many micronutrients, particularly minerals, can vary even in foods of the same type. Additionally, micronutrients, especially certain vitamins, are commonly destroyed in the cooking process.

Nutrition research continues to confirm that we can benefit from extra amounts of some nutrients, such as vitamin E and vitamin C. However, it would be impractical to get these extra quantities from food, because this would mean overeating. This is where dietary supplements come in. In addition to supplying you with a pure, high-quality nutrient source, supplements are specially blended to have the exact amounts of nutrients needed to meet your specific nutrition requirements. Supplements are a great way of getting the highly bioavailable nutrients you need, when you need them.

MEAL TIMING

I have found that spreading your food intake over five or six meals per day (including snacks) is more effective than lumping your food intake into three large meals daily. The reason is very simple. Your body can assimilate only a fixed number of calories per meal; this number depends on your body size, activity level, and metabolism. Eating smaller, more frequent meals also helps maintain blood sugar at a steady level, which promotes greater energy, a higher degree of mental alertness, and better appetite control.

For example, a 140-pound adult woman may need 1,600 calories a day to meet daily energy requirements. Most breakfasts and lunches need to be only 250 to 400 calories each, with the balance of the calories being eaten at dinner and spread over snacks. If you eat too much at one meal, the excess calories usually end up getting converted to fat; the valuable proteins and other nutrients are wasted, and so is your money. Similarly, a 170-pound adult man may require 2,700 calories a day to meet daily energy requirements. This would be best accomplished by spreading out this intake over five or six meals and snacks. My Natural-Thin nutrition program focuses on providing you with the nutrition you need while minimizing excess calories, fat, and sodium.

ABOUT THE MACRONUTRIENTS

As previously mentioned, the primary macronutrients are protein, carbohydrates, lipids, and water. As you can imagine, there are many types of foods and supplements that can be used to supply these macronutrients. Additionally, there is much diversity within each macronutrient category. For example, there are many types of carbohydrates, including simple and complex. Proteins also come in many types.

Carbohydrates

On a calories-per-day basis, carbohydrates will be the most plentiful part of your diet. It is generally recommended that carbohydrates make up 50 to 55 percent of your daily calories. Most food sources of carbohydrates are very low in fat. Carbohydrates are generally grouped into three categories: monosaccharides, disaccharides, and polysaccharides.

Monosaccharides are simple sugar molecules. These include glucose and fructose (the most common), galactose, mannose, sorbitol, and mannitol. These simple sugars tend to cause a fast rise and fall in blood sugar levels, which can create surges in hunger and sharp drops in energy level. It seems that because simple sugars get into the bloodstream more quickly, they can be converted to fat more easily than other carbohydrates.

Disaccharides are carbohydrates made of two monosaccharides bound together. Some common disaccharides include sucrose (also called table sugar), maltose, and lactose. Intake of disaccharides should also be minimized, for the same reasons we limit monosaccharides.

The *polysaccharides,* or complex carbohydrates, include starch, dextrin, maltodextrin, and cellulose. Starch, dextrin, and maltodextrin are very large molecules consisting of chains of glucose. Because they are larger, they take longer to digest than simple sugars, and so provide a sustained supply of glucose to the bloodstream. Steady blood glucose levels, in turn, control your appetite and prevent steep declines in your energy level.

Carbohydrates in your diet are important sources of energy in themselves, and studies have determined that fat burns better in the presence of carbohydrates as well. Glucose is also the main energy source for the brain, which is why diets that restrict carbohydrates may not be healthy. Another use for glucose is as a building block for connective tissues. Glucose is made into glucosamine, which is one of the chemicals used to make connective tissue. I bring up this point because of the increasing popularity of very-low-carbohydrate diets. While reducing carbohydrate intake may help jump-start your diet, keep in mind that consuming too few carbohydrates may cause connective tissues to break down, and may

result in long-term structural damage to your body.

Fiber (cellulose, hemicellulose, lignin, gums, mucilages, pectins) is also an important carbohydrate. It seems that the presence of fiber in the intestines helps the digestion process of other nutrients and also plays an important role in the release of nutrients into the body by improving digestion. Virtually all vegetables and fruit contain fiber, however, some are better sources than others. Plants like celery and broccoli that are stalky and low calorie tend to be a good source of fiber, as do most beans, whole-grain breads and cereals, apples, figs, oranges, and almonds. Increasing the amount of fiber you take in helps reduce the amount of fat absorbed into the body, and thus plays a part in maintaining healthy levels of triglycerides and cholesterol. Studies have concluded that some soluble fibers, like those from oats and psyllium seed husk, can help reduce cholesterol levels and reduce the risk of coronary heart disease. Fiber also creates a full feeling and satisfies your appetite.

Good carbohydrate sources such as grains, breads, pasta, and potatoes have received unwarranted bad press over the years as foods that contribute to obesity. In fact, a closer look by nutritionists reveals that the real problem is the heavy sauces and high-fat spreads that usually accompany these foods, as well as overeating. These foods should be a regular part of your daily diet, but make sure you choose whole grains and minimally processed products whenever possible.

Protein

Daily intake of protein is essential. Protein, which is made up of subunits called amino acids, comes in many types and is used to build and restore body tissues; it is also essential to all the body's chemical processes. Under certain circumstances proteins are also used for energy, mainly during exercise.

Maintaining a moderate intake of protein, based on your body size and level of activity, is essential for optimal performance and muscle growth. However, like carbohydrates, proteins can also be converted to fat if your total daily caloric intake is too high. Since protein-rich foods and amino acid supplements tend to be the most expensive items in your diet, overeating them will stress your budget, too. The by-products of protein breakdown are ammonia and uric acid, and excessive protein consumption can cause an unhealthy rise in the levels of these chemicals, putting strain on your kidneys.

Proteins occur in animal and plant food sources and in dietary supplement products. Animal foods contain complete protein— that is, they contain all the amino acids the human body cannot make for itself—but animal foods may also be high in saturated fat and cholesterol. The best choices include egg whites and moderate amounts of whole eggs, low-fat dairy products, chicken, turkey, shellfish, and fish. Always trim visible fat from your meats, choose leaner cuts, and remove the skin from poultry to reduce total fat intake.

Depending on your level of activity, protein should be about 15 to 20 percent of your total daily caloric intake, and can be as high as 35 percent for competitive strength athletes. Also, some people who have trouble losing weight because they are insulin-resistant, may respond to a temporary diet that is higher in protein, and lower in carbohydrates and calories.

To understand what is meant by the term insulin resistance, you must know what insulin does in the body. Insulin is a hormone that stimulates your body's cells to take up glucose, fatty acids, and other nutrients. In some people, their cells become unresponsive to insulin, thereby causing the body to produce even more. Eventually individuals with cells that are unresponsive to insulin overproduce insulin. People with this condition typically have one or more symptoms, including blood lipid disorders, obesity, and hypertension. People with insulin resistance and high insulin blood levels are at risk for developing cardiovascular disease. One thing is certain, eating right, physical activity, and maintaining proper body weight can reverse insulin resistance in most people.

Lipids (Fats & Oils)

Lipids are the group of macronutrients which include fats, oils, and cholesterol. Some lipids have recently gotten a bad reputation for causing coronary heart disease, certain cancers, and other health disorders when eaten in large amounts. But lipids are an essential part of our diet because they serve as carriers for lipid-soluble vitamins (A, D, E, and K) and are a source of essential fatty acids, which are used to manufacture many biomolecules and are essential in maintaining the structure and function of cell membranes. You need a certain amount of lipids in your diet for good health. Like carbohydrates and proteins, though, some types of lipids are healthier than others.

Fats and oils are the most concentrated source of energy found in the diet. By weight, fats and oils have more than twice as many calories as carbohydrates and proteins.

Fats and oils are the primary source of dietary lipids, making up about 99 percent of all lipids ingested. Animal fats and palm and coconut oils are high in saturated fatty acids (the bad fatty acids), and fish and most vegetable oils are high in unsaturated fatty acids (the good fatty acids). Some good sources of essential fatty acids include fish oils, nuts, flax oil, pumpkin seed oil, walnut oil, soy oil, safflower oil, sunflower oil, corn oil, sesame seed oil, and lecithin. Oil from cold-water fish is especially high in the heart-healthy essential fatty acids EPA and DHA. Conversely, a high intake of saturated fat is associated with a higher risk of heart disease, certain cancers, and obesity.

Total dietary fat intake should be kept under 30 percent of your total daily calories, and lower percentages are recommended by many nutritionists—20 to 25 percent of total daily calories. Saturated fatty acids should account for under 10 percent of daily caloric intake, and the intake of cholesterol should be less than 300 mg. Remember, fat makes you fat.

Water

Water is not often thought of as a nutrient, but it is very essential to health and survival. Without it you will last only a few days. Water makes up a major part of your body weight and is present in every living cell. Water is obtained by drinking fluids and eating foods with a high water content. Drinking eight 8-ounce glasses of water each day is highly recommended. However, for active people water intake can be double this amount.

MICRONUTRIENTS

The main micronutrients include vitamins, minerals, and vitaminlike nutrients. Roughly twenty-six have been identified as essential for human health, and more will probably be identified in the future. One or another micronutrient is involved in every biochemical process. For example, it was recently determined that the trace mineral chromium is an essential cofactor for insulin function; insulin is the key hormone that regulates blood glucose and helps transfer it into the body's cells. It also promotes the uptake of amino acids in muscle tissue. However, if chromium levels are low, the insulin cannot work efficiently, and the nutrients circulating in your bloodstream will go back to the liver and be converted to fat.

The chromium story is one of many in which micronutrients play important roles. The major micronutrients include vitamins A, D, E, K, C, thiamin, riboflavin, folate, B_{12}, biotin, and pantothenic acid, as well as minerals such as calcium, phosphorus, magnesium, iron, zinc, iodine, selenium, copper, manganese, chromium, and molybdenum.

It is becoming easy to see how dietary supplements can make an important contribution to even the healthiest eating plan. You will discover a treasure trove of information about the benefits and uses of these micronutrients, and more than 200 other dietary supplement ingredients, in Parts 2 and 3.

Part 2

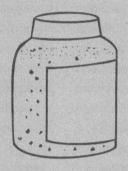

5

Perfecting Your Dietary Supplement Program for Optimal Results

The chapters in Part 1 provided you with important background and insights into the regulations and science that shape the dietary supplement products found in the marketplace. This chapter is aimed at providing you with guidelines for understanding and developing a personalized nutrition supplement program for your own particular health and wellness goals. To assist you in this endeavor, I devised a simple three-factor-approach to serve as the basis for understanding the different dietary supplement products you will encounter. Next I present guidelines for the most essential supplement ingredients to look for, and dosage ranges found to be safe and effective for daily use. This will enable you to ensure adequate intake of the most essential nutrients. These are most important for optimal health and longevity, such as vitamins, minerals, and antioxidants.

The chapters that follow this one address special supplement topics. For example, you

may have a concern about promoting cardiovascular health, or you may want to improve your memory. If you are an adult male, you may be interested in knowing which supplements to take for prostate health and function. If you are a woman going through menopause or approaching it, you may be interested in taking a supplement to help with the symptoms. There is a separate chapter on losing weight, and the Appendix outlines my Natural-Thin program.

You are well aware from your reading in Part 1 how the Dietary Supplement Health and Education Act and other regulations dictate what types of ingredients are allowed in dietary supplement products and what kind of claims can be made about how such products will benefit you. But no set of regulations is perfect. One element missing from the dietary supplement regulations is oversight of the amounts and combinations of ingredients in supplements. There are also no standards for who is doing the formulating, which means that unqualified people could be dreaming up supplement concoctions. While most manufacturers are responsible and sell only safe and effective ingredients in safe and effective dosages, the guidelines provided here and in Part 3 will help you to make sure that you are taking supplements in the most appropriate way.

In the 1940s only a few nutrients were considered essential to human life. As time went on, more and more essential vitamins and minerals were discovered, and supplement companies regularly updated their formulas to include these new ingredients. During the 1970s, 1980s, and 1990s, progressive nutrition researchers and product developers began to look beyond the essential functions of vitamins and minerals to discoveries being made about other beneficial effects nutrients have on the body. For example, many of the essential vitamins and minerals, in particular the water-soluble vitamins such as vitamin C and the B vitamins, have additional beneficial effects when taken in amounts greater than the RDI.

One of the tools scientists have used to find out more about how nutrients can benefit us is epidemiological research. In this type of research, investigators look at the distribution of health problems among a large group of people and try to ascertain which factors are important in determining who stays well and who will develop diseases. In this case, researchers examine the link between health statistics and diet. For example, scientists have learned from studying Asian populations compared to other groups that there is a connection between increased consumption of foods made from soy and reduced risk from heart disease. Further research on this topic has been so convincing that the FDA approved a new health claim that diets high in soy will reduce your risk of cardiovascular disease. Another epidemiological discovery made in Japan established a relationship between high consumption of green tea and a reduced risk of developing gastrointestinal cancer. Moreover, in some populations consuming large amounts of green tea—several glasses a day—a reduced risk of all types of disease was observed. These sorts of discoveries will continue to inspire dietary supplement formulators to extract the biologically active ingredients of foods that have been determined to be beneficial to health, and include them in dietary supplement products on the shelves. However, until high-quality clinical studies establish the health-enhancing effects of supplements based on these foods, you should continue to eat and drink the actual foods and beverages discovered to have the health-promoting effects.

Another important category of scientific research deals with the therapeutic uses of dietary supplement products. This is one of the most extensively researched areas, which includes looking at how different dietary supplement ingredients can be used successfully in support of drugs in the treatment or prevention of disease. Results from these kinds of studies are the ones you hear most about in the media. As you know from Part 1, while there may be valid roles for dietary supplements in disease treatment and prevention, these are considered drug uses, and manufacturers are prohibited from making such claims about products sold as dietary supplements. But the reality is that a significant proportion of people—as many as 40 percent or more of dietary supplement takers—are in fact using supplements to help cure, prevent, or manage a particular illness.

The important thing to remember, when and if you use dietary supplements for management of a particular disease, is to let your doctor know you are doing so, and do not ever treat any serious illness nutritionally without the supervision of your doctor. If your doctor is not open to using nutritional therapies along with modern medical therapies, then find a doctor who is. There are many medical doctors who understand the benefits of using certain dietary supplements in support of drug therapies. There are also other highly qualified and licensed health professionals, such as naturopathic doctors, acupuncturists, herbalists, and clinical nutritionists, who are well versed in the proper use of nutrition and dietary sup-

plements as part of disease prevention, curing, and management.

Supplements have changed over the years not just because of scientific research but because we have developed new approaches to health. For example, traditional mass-market multivitamin-mineral products, designed to be taken once daily, are an artifact of the antiquated RDA approach established sixty years ago. More and more you will see, especially in health food stores but also on supermarket and drugstore shelves, that many new products consist of a broad range of ingredients. Sophisticated supplements are so packed with ingredients that the daily dosage requires four or more tablets, softgels, and/or capsules. These products are designed using the optimal daily nutrition philosophy, which got its start in the late 1970s and early 1980s and is flourishing as we move into the twenty-first century.

While many authors have written books about optimal nutrition and supplement programs, it was *Life Extension*, by Dirk Pearson and Sandy Shaw, that made a nationwide impact in the early 1980s. Dr. Pearson and Dr. Shaw focused on optimal nutrition and showed people how dietary supplements can be used for improving memory, skin health, longevity, cardiovascular health, and so on. As science continues to yield new discoveries revealing the relationship between nutrients and function and structure of the human body, more and more new dietary supplement formulations and products will continue to appear on the shelves.

The more scientists look at our modern diets, the more they discover that the population is deficient in many essential vitamins and minerals, and could benefit greatly from certain dietary supplement ingredients. The story of vitamin E serves as testimony to this point. Medical research continues to conclude that taking vitamin E supplements, in amounts greater than the RDI, will help reduce the risk of cardiovascular disease in men and women by more than 35 percent. This means that if a hundred people who were at risk for developing cardiovascular disease simply took a vitamin E supplement each day, thirty-five of these people would not develop a disease condition. Knowing this, how could you not take vitamin E supplements? The research on vitamin E is only the tip of the iceberg. There is excellent research on how many other supplement ingredients will benefit your health as well.

QUALITY OF DIETARY SUPPLEMENTS

Most people—health professionals and consumers alike—don't know how to tell if a product is high-quality, safe, and effective. In working with over a hundred supplement companies, I have found that a range of product quality exists in the marketplace. As a general rule, larger companies, which usually make their own products, are more likely to do a much better job on quality control. They have more resources and more qualified personnel. However, this does not mean that a small company cannot make a quality product. Some of the highest-quality products are made by smaller, family-owned supplement companies.

The first feature of a quality product is that the ingredients are contained in the product in their prescribed dosages. When making vitamin and mineral products, this is easy, because there are many reliable raw material suppliers and time-tested manufacturing methods. With botanical products it is more difficult to exactly meet the label claim, due to problems inherent in processing natural materials. When choosing supplement products, you should be aware that about 60 percent of the companies that market dietary supplement products have contract manufacturers making the products for them. Look at the labels for the following statements: "distributed by" and "manufactured by." When you see "manufactured by," this clearly indicates that the company makes the product. But if it states "distributed by," chances are good that the company does not make the product itself.

Other quality factors include the digestibility of the product—how well its contents will dissolve in your gastrointestinal system to be absorbed into your body. While many manufacturers follow different approaches for this, some manufacturers follow the USP (United States Pharmacopeia) standard. This is indicated by "USP" on the label next to the names of certain ingredients.

The United States Pharmacopeia is an independent organization established in the 1800s to set strict manufacturing standards for drug products. More recently, standards were established for vitamins, minerals, amino acids, and some botanical dietary supplement ingredients. In order to declare that a product meets USP standards, the manufacturer has to undertake rigorous quality control and quality assurance analyses to ensure product purity, potency, disintegration, and dissolution. The USP purity specifications establish standards for ingredients, which in turn ensure that the raw materials being used to manufacture dietary supplement products will be pure and uncontaminated. USP standards for potency ensure that a particular vitamin, mineral, or other dietary supplement ingredient will be present in the product in the amount declared on the label. As a general rule of thumb, there is usually a plus or minus 10 percent range allowed for ingredients. For example, if 10 mg of an ingredient is listed on the label, this means that legally it could contain a range from 9 to 11 mg. The need for a lower limit is obvious. Establishing an upper limit is equally important, since many ingredients, if taken in excessive amounts for long periods of time, may cause harmful side effects. Ensuring that the amount of an ingredient is as close as possible to what is declared on the label is extremely important.

The next USP requirement is referred to as disintegration—how fast a tablet or capsule will break up into smaller pieces upon ingestion. Unless disintegration tests are done, there is no way to be sure if a product will be completely digested. When a product declares it conforms to USP standards, this indicates that disintegration testing was performed, and that the product's digestibility has been confirmed. However, please note that companies choosing not to follow the USP standards can use other methods to confirm that their products will be properly digested. If you are taking a brand you like and it does not indicate it follows USP requirements, give the manufacturer a call to make sure that it is performing some type of disintegration testing. First ask if its facility follows "good manufacturing practices," and if they are certified by an independent organization. Good manufacturing practices are a set of rules and procedures established by the FDA that manufacturers must follow to ensure that products contain the ingredients stated on the label and are free from contaminants. Then ask how it determines that the products it makes have the ingredients it claims are supposed to be in them. Ask if a "certificate of analysis" is available for the product you are interested in; this is prepared when analysis verifies that the product contains the ingredients it should. It is best to see if the company has its products periodically tested by an independent laboratory. The company should be willing to provide you with some documentation to verify that its product contains the ingredients listed on the labels, that it was produced using good manufacturing practices, and that it will be digested properly.

Disintegration testing only confirms that the tablet will break apart; it does not confirm that the ingredients completely dissolved and are available to be absorbed into the body. This is what dissolution testing is for. Meeting the USP standard for dissolution requires a sophisticated analysis. However, as with the previous USP requirement, just because a company does not perform dissolution testing does not mean that the product will not dissolve. Another point about dissolution testing: It does not guarantee that the nutrients will be fully absorbed. I hope that in the future supplement manufacturers will take steps to verify that after their product is ingested it is fully absorbed and causes a rise in blood levels of the active ingredient(s). This type of testing is not currently required for supplement products, and I am sure that companies taking the lead on verifying the bioavailability of their supplements will attract consumers over brands that do not.

There is a final quality point to consider: expiration dates. Expiration dates on dietary supplement products are useful, but do not have exactly the same meaning as they do on drug products, for which they were originally developed. If a drug product is used after the expiration date, the drug may be only partially active or perhaps totally inactive. If you are suffering from a disease, using a drug product past its expiration date could have adverse effects on your health. Using a dietary supplement product after its expiration date may result in reduced nutritional potency. Over an extended period of time this could lead to nutritional deficiency of essential vitamins and minerals. Some products can become harmful past their expiration date, liquid products and powdered drink mixes in particular. When a product declares an expiration date, the company is required to perform shelf stability testing, which ensures that the declared amount of a dietary supplement ingredient has been shown to hold its potency until that specific expiration date. Some companies that don't have the ability to determine expiration dates exactly will use rules of thumb to estimate a "best used by" date. Some companies, especially herbal product marketers, don't put any dates on them at all. One of the main results expected to emerge from the FDA's pending regulations on good manufacturing procedures for supplements will be to exactly define an expiration date system specifically for these products.

SUMMARY OF MAJOR MANUFACTURERS AND BRANDS
OF QUALITY DIETARY SUPPLEMENT PRODUCTS

If your brand is not included in this table, it does not mean that it is not a quality product. I included only the companies and brands I am currently familiar with. Therefore, exclusion from this list is incidental. Use the information in this chapter and give the company a call to question them about what steps they take to ensure a quality product.

Manufacturer	Brand(s)	Manufacturer	Brand(s)
Abbott Laboratories, Ross	Optilets	East Earth Herbs	Jade Chinese Herbals
American Home Products,		Enzymatic Therapy	Enzymatic Therapy
Whitehall-Robins, Lederle	Caltrate	PhytoPharmica	Remifemin
	Centrum	General Nutrition Company	Basic Nutrition
	Ferro-Sequels		Challenge
	Ocuvite		Energia
	Protegra		Fitness Systems
	Stresstab		Ginseng Gold
AmeriFIT	AmeriFIT		GNC
Amway	Nutrilite		Harvest of Nature
Avon Products	Avon Life Supplements		Herbal Plus
Bayer	Bugs Bunny		Nature's Fingerprint
	Fergon		Ultra Mega
	Flintstones	Genisoy Soy Protein Products	Genisoy
	One-A-Day	Herbalife International	Herbalife
BeautiControl Cosmetics	Within Beauty	IVC Industries	Fields of Nature
Bodyonics	Bodyonics Longevity AgeErasers		Synergy Plus
Pharmaton Natural Health Products	Ginkgoba	J. R. Carlson Laboratories	Carlson
	Ginsana	Leiner Health Products	Your Life
	Movana	Mary Kay Cosmetics	Daily Benefits
	Venastat	Nature's Way Products	Nature's Way
	Vitasana	Nabisco, Knox	Knox NutraJoint
Bristol-Meyers Squibb,		Natrol	Natrol
Mead Johnson Nutritionals	Theragran	NBTY	American Health
	Poly-Vi-Sol		Good'N Natural
	Tri-Vi-Sol		Puritan's Pride
Celestial Seasonings	Celestial Seasonings Herbs	Nu Skin	Interior Design Nutritionals
Chattem, Sunsource Health Products	Garlique	Otsuka Pharmaceutical	Nature Made
	Harmonex	Perrigo	OneSource
	Insomnia Relief	Rexall Sundown	Rexall
	Melatonex		Sundown
	Propalmex		Thompson
	Rejuvenex	Shaklee	Shaklee
Ciba Consumer Pharmaceuticals	SlowFE	SmithKline Beecham	Feosol
	Sunkist Vitamin C		Geritol
Country Life Vitamins	Biochem		Tums
	Country Life	Pharmacia & Upjohn	Os-Cal 500

SUMMARY OF MAJOR MANUFACTURERS AND BRANDS
OF QUALITY DIETARY SUPPLEMENT PRODUCTS

Manufacturer	Brand(s)	Manufacturer	Brand(s)
Solgar Laboratories	Solgar	Goldshield Healthcare	Acumen
Twin Laboratories	Nature's Herbs		Centural
	TwinLab		Fortify
Weider Nutrition	Excel		Memoloba
	Great American Nutrition		Natural Care
	Schiff		Pessicalm
	Weider		Vitaboost
Windmill Consumer Products	DietWorks		Vitaguard
	Foods Plus	Wal-Mart	Spring Valley
	HerbScience		
	NutritionWorks		
	Rx Interactives		
	Windmill		

GUIDELINES FOR SELECTING YOUR DAILY SUPPLEMENT ESSENTIALS

Now that you have a feel for some of the quality issues related to the supplement formulas on the shelves, it is time to consider what vitamins and minerals, and in what dosages, you should be seeking for your core dietary supplement program. To help you with this decision-making process, I have prepared a series of reference tables that integrate my own research and experience making dietary supplement products with the findings of numerous scientific studies and guidelines published by government and independent dietary supplement organizations.

The table on pp. 66–69 provides guidelines for what are considered the most essential nutrients, such as vitamins and

minerals, for daily use by healthy adults. When you are reviewing the table, keep in mind that in most cases the RDI values listed in Table 2.4 are considered the minimum intake of a nutrient, for purposes of survival, and is not intended to promote optimal health. So the dosage ranges I recommend here may be higher than the RDI. I specify ranges rather than one specific figure because smaller or less active individuals will not need as much of a given nutrient as larger or active individuals do. Most people will be taking supplements containing amounts somewhere in the middle of the range.

To further assist in your optimal health supplement efforts, I included blank columns for you to use to keep track of your personal total daily supplement intakes from all of the different dietary supplement

Table 5.1

EXAMPLES OF WHERE TO PURCHASE NUTRITIONAL SUPPLEMENT PRODUCTS

Mass Market Stores: Grocery stores, pharmacies, Wal-Mart

Health Food Stores: General nutrition centers, local health food stores

Mail-Order Nutrition Companies: Goldshield Healthcare

Television Shopping Networks: HSN, QVC

Health Practitioners: Nutritionists, herbalists, doctors

Direct Sales (Multilevel Marketing) Companies: Amway, Avon, Golden Pride International, Herbalife, Mary Kay, NuSkin, Rexall Showcase International, Shaklee

formulas you may be taking. This will help you make sure that you are not overdoing any ingredient that may have adverse effects over the long term. This will become important when you are increasing your daily intake of certain nutrients for special reasons, described in the chapters that follow. Take the time to read the detailed information in Part 3 on each ingredient to ensure proper use.

First use the table to assess your current supplement program, or to purchase a comprehensive vitamin-mineral formula. Then check to make sure your supplements have the essential antioxidants, in particular vitamin C, vitamin E, and beta-carotene. Then select other supplement products to fill in the essential nutrient gaps. Multiple supplements are best taken with meals, unless otherwise directed. This is especially true for minerals, such as calcium, and for the B vitamins. Also, consider taking your supplements in divided dosages two or three times

per day for better assimilation. (Note that some supplements, such as valerian for sleep, may need to be taken at certain times of the day, and on an empty stomach.) If you are not accustomed to taking these amounts of nutrients and feel that you are taking in too much too soon, then begin with half the suggested amounts, and work your way up to the full dosage over a few months. Your body may need time to adjust to the increased nutrient intake.

When it comes to benefiting from your essential nutrient supplement program, consistency is the key. So take your supplements on a regular basis for best results, even times when you may feel like swallowing only a few tablets per day. However, taking supplements is not like taking drugs (unless you are using supplements as part of a medically supervised therapy program). You want to try to take them at the same times every day, but if you skip a dosage or a day or two, just resume your program as soon as you can. You don't have to be concerned about catching up. Finally, realize that you will not find one dietary supplement product containing all of the ingredients in the suggested daily intake ranges. You will have to select two or more products to meet your optimum supplement program goals. I have listed some supplement brands as examples to assist you in your quest for super health. However, I reached a point where the product list I was developing started to become too long and confusing. Therefore, you should rely more upon using the guidelines to evaluate the product you are currently taking, or products sold where you like to shop. Once you start taking a close look at the products you are taking then at the ones on the shelves, it will quickly become apparent how you need to modify your supplement program.

Supplement Facts™ Buyer's Guide Information

In Chapters 5 through 19, you will find a table with the general heading of SUPPLEMENT FACTS™ Buyer's Guide. Each table contains a listing of supplement ingredients, safe and effective daily supplement dosage ranges, comments, and a space for your personal daily supplement intake notes. The criteria for selecting a supplement ingredient in these tables was that it had to have a history of safe and effective use, and have clinical research studies to prove a benefit. With this information, you can evaluate the supplement products

you are taking, or plan to take. I encourage you to also read the entries in Part 3, which include details on the documented proper use of these supplement ingredients.

I also included some product examples that meet the general guidelines. The best approach is for you to use the information to evaluate the brands that you are taking or plan to take. Choose products that are readily available to you.

Follow these simple steps to construct your winning supplement program.

- Thoroughly review the information in this book.
- Use the SUPPLEMENT FACTS™ Buyer's Guide tables to make notes on supplement ingredients and dosages you plan on taking.
- If a medical condition exists, consult your doctor.
- Once you have completed your SUPPLEMENT FACTS™ Buyer's Guide tables, then it's time to go shopping.
- Make a copy of the SUPPLEMENT FACTS™ Buyer's Guide tables and take them to the store with you. Use them to select the products that meet the safe and effective criteria.
- Ask a store employee for help in selecting your supplements. They can assist in choosing products that have the ingredients you want, as well as determine the most economical brands to purchase.
- Give the supplement selection process adequate time and consideration. The

time spent on selecting supplement products with effective ingredients and dosages at a reasonable price is your ultimate goal.

- Every month, reevaluate your supplement program needs and make the necessary adjustments to the products you purchase.
- Keep in mind that your supplement program will probably include two or more different products to meet your needs. Look for one of the comprehensive multivitamin/mineral products to use as your core program. Then select additional products to fill in the gaps.
- It is best to consult a health professional to verify the adequacy of your diet and the supplements you have selected.
- The Final Step is to live a long, healthy, and happy life.

The following lists some brand examples of multivitamin and multimineral formulas. To achieve your optimum daily dietary supplement intake, you will most likely have to purchase two or more products. Although the mega-multiformulas, which are loaded with the essentials and more, may have all you need. Use the list and shop around for products to act as your core supplement program. Then you can add other supplements as needed for special concerns and conditions, as discussed in other Part 2 chapters. Here are some supplement product examples to start with.

Vitamin/Mineral Formulas

Caltrate
Centrum
Comprehensive Formula Men Stage I
Comprehensive Formula Women Stage II
Futurebiotics Hi Energy Multi For Men
Geritol Complete
GNC Maximum Nutrition System
GNC Men's MegaMen
GNC Woman's 50 Plus VitaPak
GNC Women's Maximum Nutrition
   System
Goldshield Central
Goldshield Central Gold
Goldshield Super Multivitamins and
   Minerals
Isotek Multi Vitamin/Mineral Drink
LifePak
Natrol Liquid Multi-Vitamin
   Supplement
Natrol My Favorite Multiple
Nature's Code Men over 50 Formula
Nature's Code Men's Formula
Nature's Code Women's Formula
Nature's Code Women over 50 Formula
Nutrilite
NutritionWorks Maximum Female
Nutrition Works Maximum Male
One-A-Day
Protegra
Stresstab
Tree of Life Super Multivitamin and
   Mineral Dietary Supplement
Twinlab Dualtabs
Vitamin Health Centers OmegaPak
   Nutrient Support System

Supplement Facts™

Buyer's Guide for Super Health and Well-Being—Supplement Products for Your Daily Essential Nutrient Supplement Program

These supplement ingredient ranges are for both men and women. Refer to the men's and women's chapters for gender-specific supplement recommendations. In general, the lower amounts specified in the Effective Daily Supplement Dosage Range are for smaller, less active individuals. The upper range is for larger, more active people. Individual requirements may vary, and you can adjust your supplement intake accordingly.

Nutrient	Safe and Effective Daily Supplement Dosage Range	Comments	Your Personal Daily Supplement Intake Notes Section
The Vitamins: The following guidelines will help you determine if your supplements have safe and effective dosages of vitamins. Note that it is typical for supplements to contain high amounts of the water-soluble vitamins, in particular the B vitamins and C.			
Vitamin A (from acetate and palmitate)	1,000 IU to 10,000 IU	Because vitamin A from acetate and palmitate has the potential to build up in your body and cause side effects, most people should stay in this range. Women who are pregnant should keep under 2,500 IU per day. If you want to increase your vitamin A intake, take supplements with pro-vitamin A, beta-carotene	
Beta-carotene (as vitamin A activity)	2,500 IU to 40,000 IU	Choose supplements containing beta-carotene as the source of vitamin A for best results. Also, the new trend is to include mixed carotenoids; alpha-carotene and lycopene (see Beta-Carotene, Carotenoids, and Vitamin A Part 3 entries)	
Lutein	5 mg to 60 mg	This "new" carotenoid has recently been linked to improving vision, circulatory system health, and immune system function	
Lycopene	2 mg to 40 mg	This is another carotenoid that recent research has determined beneficial health effects. As with other antioxidants, an adequate intake of lycopene is associated with a lower chance of developing degenerative diseases	
Vitamin D	200 IU to 1,000 IU	Take higher levels of vitamin D (600 IU to 800 IU) as you get older, if you do not spend much time exposed to the sun; exposure to sunlight stimulates natural vitamin D production in your body	
Vitamin E	100 IU to 1,000 IU	The most recent research indicates that a daily intake of vitamin E between 200 IU and 800 IU is ideal	
Vitamin K	20 mcg to 160 mcg	Vitamin K intake has been related to bone health, as well as its role in blood clotting	
Vitamin C	60 mg to 2,000 mg	The most recent research confirms that higher amounts of vitamin C intake are needed to produce results. Consistent intake of 1,000 mg per day has been shown to improve immunity and reduce risk of infectious diseases	
Vitamin B$_1$ Thiamin	1.5 mg to 90 mg	The B vitamins are essential for normal growth, development, and reproduction. They are active in many metabolic reactions. Most of the B vitamins are consumed in supplements in many times the RDI values. Take higher amounts of thiamin if you are under stress, 35 mg or higher	
Vitamin B$_2$ Riboflavin	1.7 mg to 100 mg	Taker higher amounts of B$_2$ if you are under stress, 35 mg or higher	

Nutrient	Safe and Effective Daily Supplement Dosage Range	Comments	Your Personal Daily Supplement Intake Notes Section
Vitamin B_3 (niacin)	10 mg to 100 mg	Higher doses (50 mg or more) of vitamin B_3, as nicotinic acid may cause a temporary skin flushing response. Choose products with niacinimide if you are sensitive to this	
Vitamin B_5 Pantothenic acid	10 mg to 100 mg	Take higher amounts of B_5 if you are under stress, 50 mg or higher	
Vitamin B_6	2 mg to 50 mg	Take high amounts when under stress, 40 mg or higher. Also, take 100 mg per day to help overcome carpal tunnel syndrome under doctor supervision	
Folate	200 mcg to 1,000 mcg	Maintain adequate supplement intake of folate, helps reduce heart disease. Also, important for pregnant women to take 800 mcg per day	
Vitamin B_{12}	6 mcg to 200 mcg	B_{12} has developed a reputation for increasing energy levels and improving cardiovascular health. B_{12} is very safe and sometimes taken in very high amounts to help restore energy, 1,000 mcg or higher	
Biotin	200 mcg to 400 mcg	Maintain adequate supplement intake for optimum health	

The Minerals: Essential minerals are vital to good health. Most minerals should not be taken in excessive amounts. The following will help you select supplements with safe and effective dosage ranges.

Calcium	500 mg to 1,500 mg	Most women should take a supplement containing 800 mg to 1,200 of calcium each day	
Phosphorus	20 mg to 800 mg	Most supplements don't contain phosphorus because it is abundant in the diet	
Magnesium	80 mg to 400 mg	Women should take a magnesium supplement containing 200 mg to 400 mg per day	
Iron	4 mg to 30 mg	Pregnant women may need to increase iron intake up to 60 mg per day, check with your doctor	
Zinc	5 mg to 35 mg	During cold season, zinc intake may be increased higher than 35 mg per day. Take zinc lozenges to ward off upper respiratory infections	
Iodine	30 mcg to 300 mcg	Do not exceed 300 mcg per day of iodine intake from supplements for long periods of time	
Selenium	20 mcg to 300 mcg	Selenium is important in supporting the body's natural anti-oxidant systems. Most studies indicate that 200 mcg from supplements is ideal	
Copper	0.5 mg to 10 mg	Maintain moderate copper intake	
Manganese	0.5 mg to 10 mg	Maintain moderate manganese intake	
Chromium	60 mcg to 300 mcg	During periods of weight loss, higher intake of chromium may be indicated, up to 600 mcg per day	
Molybdenum	25 mcg to 150 mcg	Maintain moderate molybdenum intake	
Sodium	none or less than 200 mg	Sodium is not usually contained in supplements, because it is abundant in the diet and most people want to reduce sodium in their diets	
Chloride	none or less than 200 mg	Chloride is not usually contained in supplements, because it is abundant in the diet	

Nutrient	Safe and Effective Daily Supplement Dosage Range	Comments	Your Personal Daily Supplement Intake Notes Section
Potassium	20 mg to 400 mg	Adequate potassium intake is usually adequate from food, but it does occur in some supplement formulas, tablets, and powdered drinks to ensure adequate intake in active people and the elderly	
Boron	0.5 mg to 6 mg	Boron is especially important for people concerned about bone health	
Choline	20 mg to 400 mg	This new essential vitamin is sometimes taken in very high amounts for short periods of time during weight loss, over 500 mg per day	

Additional Supplement Ingredients: The following supplement ingredients can provide you with additional health benefits, beyond the conventional essential vitamins and minerals. These include added antioxidant protection, improved metabolic function, digestive system health, circulatory system health, and prevention of degenerative diseases.

Nutrient	Safe and Effective Daily Supplement Dosage Range	Comments	Your Personal Daily Supplement Intake Notes Section
Inositol	20 mg to 400 mg	Maintain moderate supplement intake	
Bioflavonoids	60 mg to 600 mg	Bioflavonoids are usually present in multinutrient supplement formulas from different types, principally rutin and quercitin	
Lipoic acid	5 mg to 30 mg	This is a new anti-aging antioxidant found in some multi-nutrient supplements, in super-antioxidant formulas, or taken as a separate product. Higher amounts are also well tolerated	
Coenzyme Q_{10}	10 mg to 60 mg	Important for circulatory system health. Also, higher amounts taken for heart health, over 120 mg per day	
Grape seed extract (50% to 85% pro-anthocyanidins)	25 mg to 150 mg	Very important for circulatory system health. Powerful anti-oxidants	
Green tea extract (35% to 50% polyphenols)	30 mg to 300 mg	For digestive system health and protection against degenerative diseases. Powerful antioxidant	
Ginkgo biloba extract (25% ginkgo flavoglyco-sides, 6% lactones)	15 mg to 60 mg	In addition to its role in improving memory and circulation, ginkgo is added to formulas for its antioxidant benefits. Higher amounts are indicated to treat specific circulatory system problems and improve mental function, 80 mg to 140 mg	
Cysteine or N-acetylcysteine	250 mg to 500 mg	Helps form glutathione, an important antioxidant and detoxifying compound made in the body	

The Fatty Acids: While most diets are too high in fat, many adults benefit from taking supplements containing these health-promoting fatty acids. The top fatty acid sources used in supplements include fish oils, evening primrose oil, hemp oil, black currant oil, borage oil, pumpkin seed oil, and flaxseed oil.

Nutrient	Safe and Effective Daily Supplement Dosage Range	Comments	Your Personal Daily Supplement Intake Notes Section
EPA	50 mg to 250 mg	EPA is also safe to take in higher amounts	
DHA	50 mg to 250 mg	DHA is also safe to take in higher amounts	
Alpha-linolenic acid	500 mg to 4,000 mg	Alpha-linolenic acid is safe at higher amounts	
Linoleic acid	200 mg to 6,000 mg	Optional, only take if you are on a low-calorie/low-fat diet. Linoleic acid is present in all of the plant oils and is usually adequate from food intake	
GLA (gamma linolenic Acid)	40 mg to 300 mg	GLA is safe to take higher amount, which is typically required for individuals using GLA for pain control	

Nutrient	Safe and Effective Daily Supplement Dosage Range	Comments	Your Personal Daily Supplement Intake Notes Section
The Probiotics: The beneficial effects of maintaining a dominant population of beneficial intestinal microflora are well established. Take a mega-multinutrient that includes probiotics, or a separate probiotic formula. See Chapter 8 for additional information.			
Lactobacillus and bifidobacterium	2 to 10 billion cells	Increase probiotic intake when taking antibiotics, or after bouts of diarrhea	
Miscellaneous: Some multinutrient formulas will contain a variety of other supplement ingredients. These other ingredients are usually added in small amounts, or qualitatively in the ingredient list. They usually include fruit and vegetable extracts, and digestive enzymes. The trace minerals nickel and tin are common ingredients in mass market multinutrient formulas.			

IU = International Units, *mg* = milligrams, *mcg* = micrograms (also abbreviated µg)

Note: Refer to the specific entries in Part 3 for details on these nutrients and special concerns. Guidelines for other nutrients not included in this table, such as amino acids, botanicals, and metabolites, are covered under the different topics in subsequent Part 2 chapters, and in Part 3 under their individual listings.

Vitamin Health Centers OptiPak 2000

Windmill Hi-Potency Multivitamin and Mineral

Your Life Daily Pak Essentials

Your Life Daily Pak Maximum

Daily Health Herbal/Combination Formulas

Goldshield Super Antio High Strength Antioxidant Formulation

Herbal Advantage

Ricola HerbalHealth Antioxidant Formula

Solgar Advanced Proanthocyanidin Complex

Fatty Acid Formulas

Efamol Essential Fatty Acids

Goldshield Cardio Plus Omega 3 Pure Fish Oil

Goldshield Essential Fatty Acids Plus

Health from the Sun EFA's

Health from the Sun Flax Liquid Gold

Windmill Natural Lecithin

When selecting and choosing supplements to meet your dietary requirements, keep a few points in mind. First of all, nutritionists have determined that no matter how well you eat, many dietary needs cannot be adequately filled by food alone. Dietary supplements meet a real need; they don't just give you expensive urine (although you will observe that when you start ingesting higher intake of nutrients, you will excrete them at a higher rate). Your body consists of trillions of cells, with thousands of biochemical reactions happening each day. Taking supplemental amounts of essential nutrients ensures that each of the cells in your body will be properly nourished. For those of you who are on a limited budget, shop in supermarkets and drug chains, or buy through discount mail order catalogs or over the Internet. If you are really into taking supplements, you may even want to think about getting involved in direct sales and making a business out of it, so that you can take the supplements you want and make money in the process. (There are several direct sales companies in the list on page 63.)

Individuals have different nutrient requirements. Smaller or less active people will need smaller amounts than larger or more active people. People who are under stress or going through a period of disease during cold season, for example, may want to take more vitamin C and B vitamins, and echinacea to strengthen their immune system.

Keep in mind that your dietary supplement program may be a little bit more dynamic than just taking the same pills each day. Once you get your core program perfected and become familiar with the other benefits that supplements have to offer, you may decide to add supplements for short periods, depending on emotional, physical, and seasonal factors. Do your best to take your core supplements on a consistent basis. But, if you find that you can't or don't like to take your supplements every day, then do the best you can; it's better to take supplements a few days a week than not at all. Whatever your personal strategy is, remember that consistency is a vital factor.

Exercise and stress management are important, too; try to find the time to do them each day. However, you have to eat every day, so eat purposefully, making healthy food choices. Before you put something in your mouth, ask yourself if it is going to improve your health or not. Will it load up your bloodstream with fats, or will it load it up with healthy nutrients that reduce cholesterol levels and make your circulatory system healthy? Take supplements that you know are going to benefit your health and well-being. You will live a longer and happier life as a result of developing these new habits and skills.

ABOUT ANTIOXIDANTS

Longevity researchers continue to confirm the health-promoting power of antioxidants. As I mentioned earlier, a recent study found that people who lived to be a hundred years old had higher blood levels of antioxidants such as vitamins E and C than unhealthy younger adults. Antioxidant nutrients reduce damage to the body's cells from both naturally occurring and introduced chemicals. Specifically, antioxidant compounds have the ability to neutralize free radicals, a group of compounds that are unstable and need to react with other substances in the body. This reaction results in damage to molecules, such as DNA, as well as to structures of the body, such as cell walls, the circulatory system, and nerves. These free-radical reactions continue to occur throughout life and are thought to be responsible for some of the conditions associated with aging. Researchers from the University of California have concluded that you need extra amounts of the antioxidants vitamins E and C and beta-carotene for their antiaging effects to have maximum impact.

Some of the more popular new antioxidants include botanical substances such as the bioflavonoids and polyphenols, lipoic acid, and botanical extracts such as green tea leaf, bilberry fruit, ginkgo, and grape seed extracts. During the past twenty years we have gained much understanding of how herbal compounds function as antioxidants in the body. We also have learned that there are seven major kinds of free radicals: hydrogen peroxide, hydroxyl radical, organic or fatty acid hydroperoxide, oxidized protein, polyunsaturated fatty acid radical, singlet oxygen, and superoxide anion radical. It takes a variety of vitamin and herbal antioxidants to combat these different types of free radicals.

Additionally, certain antioxidants appear to exhibit free-radical scavenging activity that is specific to different parts of the body. For example, vitamin E's antioxidant activity is especially beneficial to the circulatory system and skin. Some other site-specific antioxidant herbs include turmeric (for the liver), bilberry (eyes), soy isoflavones (breast tissue), and lycopene (prostate). As researchers continue to examine the beneficial effects of antioxidants, they suggest that taking a number of different types of antioxidants will enable you to best protect the whole body and all of its complex systems and tissues. Research continues, so keep on the lookout for additional announcements about antioxidants. Make your goal to be healthy at one hundred years old. That is the true gold medal of life, and it is an award that each one of us has the ability to earn.

A NOTE ON SUPPLEMENTING WITH MACRONUTRIENTS

In addition to dietary supplements that include essential vitamins and minerals, you may also find it beneficial to include a fiber supplement, protein supplement, or energy drink containing carbohydrates. There are lots of good protein supplements, which are among the most widely used, on the market these days. People looking to enhance cardiovascular health and get a low-fat protein source with beneficial fiber should give powdered beverages containing soy protein a try. Protein supplements containing whey, casein, and egg white are good choices, too; their protein is considered very high-quality.

When using protein supplements, remember they do add calories to your diet (most contain between 80 and 160 calories per serving), so keep track of these calories just as you would with other foods. Protein supplements can be taken with meals or between meals as a nutritious snack. A lot of people like to take them to work or on trips as a portable meal or snack, but you don't need to pay extra money for single-serving pouches; purchase a large container of your favorite supplement when it is on sale, and make your own single-serving sizes by scooping a serving into a plastic bag. This will save you a small fortune in the long run.

Carbohydrate supplement products can provide an energy boost, and may be especially useful for those of you who are into fitness and athletics. These products usually include other nutrients, such as electrolytes and B vitamins. Again, keep in mind that they contain calories; check the label.

Essential fatty acids (EFAs) are available as single-ingredient supplements or as part of a multinutrient product. Keep in mind that EFA-containing oils, such as flaxseed oil and evening primrose oil, are high in calories, with about 130 per tablespoon. While taking essential fatty acid supplements can promote health benefits, you must make extra sure to reduce your fat intake from other food sources, especially when preparing meals. There is no extra benefit to taking EFAs if you are overeating other types of fat in your diet. As a rule of thumb, you should be keeping your total daily fat intake under 30 percent of total calories, and in most cases you should stay between 20 and 25 percent of total daily calories from fat.

Finally, remember to drink plenty of pure water: eight glasses per day, or more as needed.

The following chapters present information on how to supplement for special health concerns. In addition to your core dietary supplement program, you may need to take other types of supplements aimed at enhancing, for example, your cardiovascular system, your immune system, your energy, your memory, your digestive system, or your skeletal system. The rise in the use of botanical products during the past few years is a result of people attempting to take control of improving their health status before they fall victim to degenerative diseases. One of the fastest-growing supplement product categories is aimed at protecting and revitalizing joint function, such as with glucosamine. Use of supplement products for improving circulation is another biggie, as more and more people realize that if you don't have good circulation, your body systems, tissues, and organs are vulnerable to slow degradation.

To help you increase your success when dealing with special health issues, Chapters 6 through 19 present information on using supplements for a variety of health concerns. Here is a reference table to guide your way to super health and longevity:

6

Cardiovascular System Health Dietary Supplements

One of the inside secrets for maintaining optimal health is a healthy cardiovascular system. If you focus your eating, supplement program, and lifestyle around maintaining a healthy cardiovascular system, everything else will start falling into place. You will feel more energetic, and your body weight will normalize. When most people think of cardiovascular health, the supplement that most often comes to mind is vitamin E, because of widespread media coverage of recent research proving that taking vitamin E reduces your risk of developing coronary heart disease. While vitamin E is essential to cardiovascular health, you will also find a variety of dietary supplement products on the shelves that contain a single ingredient or multiple ingredients that promote cardiovascular health and wellness.

Cardiovascular system problems and diseases are very preventable and treatable with good nutrition, exercise, and supplements. Adding supplements can give you an extra advantage in avoiding such problems as congestive heart failure, in which the heart is unable to pump sufficient blood to meet the needs of the body; angina pectoris, discomfort in the chest that results from poor blood supply to the heart; hypertension, which can be due in part to poor circulation; arteriosclerosis; and high blood lipid levels.

Some dietary supplement products are designed to provide health benefits for specific aspects of the cardiovascular system. For example, some products, such as the herb hawthorn, coenzyme Q_{10}, carnitine, and the mineral magnesium are targeted at the heart. While these ingredients may also have other benefits, this is a typical ingredient profile of a supplement designed to promote heart health.

Some dietary supplement products focus on maintaining healthy blood lipid characteristics. Garlic is one of the more popular of these for its cholesterol-lowering properties. Other ingredients that can have beneficial cardiovascular effects include ginkgo, niacin, arginine, beta-sitosterol, guggul, and a variety of healthy fatty acids, and oils rich in these healthy fatty acids, such as linoleic acid, linolenic acid, DHA, EPA, and GLA, and flaxseed oil and evening primrose oil (EPO), among others.

In addition to reducing cholesterol and triglycerides, scientists have recently detected another coronary heart disease risk factor: homocysteine, a naturally occurring compound. We now know that certain B vitamins—folic acid, vitamin B_6, and vitamin B_{12}—are associated with reducing and managing homocysteine levels. Keeping homocysteine levels low will help you maintain a healthy cardiovascular system.

The box on page 77 includes a list of the primary dietary supplement ingredients to look for if you're concerned about the health of your cardiovascular system. Make sure you are also following a healthy diet and lifestyle, as prescribed in the Natural-Thin program in Appendix A. If you have a special circulatory system health concern, consider increasing the amounts of certain vitamins and minerals or including other supplements in your daily program, as listed on page 76. But remember, in order for supplements (or drugs, for that matter) to be effective, you must eat right and engage in a program of regular exercise.

Tips for Maintaining a Healthy Cardiovascular System

Eat more nonstarchy vegetables.

Eat two or three servings of fruit per day, especially grapes and grape juice.

Eat more fish, especially tuna, salmon, cod, and halibut.

Learn to love broccoli, green beans, and other fat-free, low-sodium, high-fiber vegetables, which also contain protein and energetic carbohydrates (two to three pounds a day should be your goal, which is only 325 to 400 total calories).

Use healthy oils such as flaxseed oil, pumpkin seed oil, evening primrose oil, and extravirgin olive oil (but watch the calories oil adds).

Reduce total fat consumption.

Reduce cholesterol consumption.

Reduce saturated fat consumption.

Reduce trans-fatty acid consumption, i.e., margarines, shortening, refined oils, anything "dehydrogenated," and deep-fried foods.

Reduce sugar intake.

Choose lean meats.

Eat more whole foods; reduce your intake of processed foods.

Reduce sodium intake.

Increase potassium intake.

Eat more fiber, 35 or more g per day.

Eat more beans.

Eat more egg whites.

Eat more soy products—tofu, soy protein drinks, soy flour, miso, tempeh, soy milk.

Eat more whole oats.

Eat more low-fat whole-grain breads, rice, and pasta.

Eat whole baked or boiled white or sweet potatoes, instead of fried potatoes.

Eat more poultry and seafood.

Get moving with regular exercise or other physical activity.

Keep a positive outlook on life.

Relax several times per day.

Keep your body flexible.

Maintain normal body weight.

Don't use tobacco products.

Avoid alcohol products, or limit their use as directed by your doctor.

Drink plenty of pure water.

Open your heart—to others, and to your own feelings (of Dean Ornish's "Open Your Heart Program")

When you have a cardiovascular disease, don't use multivitamins and mineral tablets that contain iron. This mineral is a pro-oxidant, and in excess, accelerates atherosclerosis. Most people with atherosclerotic heart disease have an overload of iron in their bodies. Look for iron-free supplements, which are widely available. Work closely with your doctor to ensure an adequate dietary intake of iron.

Products

Cholestaid

Country Life Omega-3

Ginkoba

Goldshield Cardio Plus Omega 3 Pure Fish Oil

Goldshield Natural Care Garlic

Health from the Sun the Total EFA

Herbscience Garlic

Herbscience Hawthorn

Kal Max EPA

Medicine Shoppe Coenzyme Q_{10}

Medicine Shoppe Ginkgo Biloba Extract

Medicine Shoppe Grape Seed Extract

Medicine Shoppe Hawthorn Berry Extract

Medicine Shoppe Odorless Garlic Extract

Natrol Hawthorn Berry

Nature Made Garlic

Nature's Herbs Grape Seed Powder

Solgar Grape Seed Extract

Solgar L-Carnitine

Solgar Mega-Max EPA

Spring Valley Vitamin E

Sundown Garlic

Sundown Hawthorn

Sunsource Garlique

Tree of Life CoQ_{10}

Tree of Life Flaxseed Oil

Tree of Life Hawthorn

Tree of Life Odorless Garlic

Tree of Life Omega-3

Tree of Life Vitamin E

TruNature Ginkgo

Twinlab Carnifuel

Twinlab Dale Alexander Omega-3 Fish
   Oil Concentrate

Twinlab L-Carnitine

Windmill Coenzyme Q_{10}

Your Life Cardio Complex

Your Life Circulatory and Heart Body
   Benefits

Your Life Hawthorn Concentrate

Your Life L-Carnitine

Your Life Natural Fish Oil Concentrate

Supplement Facts™

Buyer's Guide for Healthy Cardiovascular System Supplement Products

The following is your personal checklist of supplement ingredients that are known to promote cardiovascular system health. Consult your doctor for safe, adequate treatment of cardiovascular disorders. The high amounts are for short-term use only. Consult Part 3 for details on the proper use of these ingredients.

Supplement Ingredient	Safe and Effective Daily Supplement Dosage Range	Comments	Your Personal Daily Supplement Intake Notes Section
Special Cardiovascular Antioxidants and Circulatory System Health Nutrients: Maintaining adequate intake of antioxidants and antioxidant cofactors is essential to promoting cardiovascular system health and function. As may be required, consider including these nutrients in the amounts specified below. You may need to include one or more additional products in your daily supplement program, as determined by your doctor.			
Vitamin E	400 IU to 1,000 IU	Antioxidant, reduces risk of cardiovascular diseases	
Beta-carotene	20,000 IU to 60,000 IU	Antioxidant, reduces risk of cardiovascular diseases	
Vitamin C	500 mg to 3,000 mg	Antioxidant	
Selenium	150 mcg to 300 mcg	Antioxidant factor	
Coenzyme Q_{10}	60 mg to 180 mg	Antioxidant for circulatory system health and heart health. Definitely take if you are on statin drugs, which deplete coenzyme Q_{10} in your body	
Lipoic acid	30 mg to 90 mg	Antioxidant	
Green tea extract (35% to 50% polyphenols)	100 mg to 300 mg	Antioxidant	
Grape seed extract (50% to 85% proanthocyanidins)	50 mg to 150 mg	Antioxidant, blood thinner, strengthens capillaries	
Ginkgo biloba extract (25% ginkgo flavoglycosides, 6% lactones)	80 mg to 140 mg	Antioxidant, promotes healthy circulation, normalizes blood pressure, blood thinner	
Bilberry extract (25% anthocyanidins)	60 mg to 240 mg	Antioxidant, promotes circulatory system function	
Gotu kola extract (8% to 10% triterpenes or asiaticosides)	50 mg to 150 mg	Improves circulation, strengthens capillaries	

Supplement Ingredient	Safe and Effective Daily Supplement Dosage Range	Comments	Your Personal Daily Supplement Intake Notes Section
Soy isoflavones	25 mg to 60 mg	Antioxidant	
Ginger (4% gingerols)	100 mg to 300 mg	Antioxidant	
EPA	500 mg to 2 g	Circulation	
DHA	500 mg to 2 g	Circulation	
Linolenic acid	2 g to 4 g	Promotes circulatory system health	
Soy protein	15 g to 25 g	Promotes cardiovascular system health. Eat more soy-protein-containing foods and supplements	

Vitamins for Reducing Homocysteine Levels: High homocysteine levels can contribute to damaging your circulatory system and promote atherosclerosis. Make sure you are maintaining these levels of intake.

Folic acid	400 mcg to 1,200 mcg	Reduces homocysteine levels	
Vitamin B$_6$	30 mg to 50 mg	Reduces homocysteine levels. Use higher amounts under doctor supervision	
Vitamin B$_{12}$	100 mcg to 500 mcg	Reduces homocysteine levels	

Blood Lipid Normalizing Factors: Take supplements containing these ingredients when confronted with the need to reduce your cholesterol or fatty acid blood levels. Consider the following.

Garlic extract (0.6% to 1% allicin)	600 mg to 1,200 mg	Start by taking a garlic supplement. Promotes normal blood lipids and blood pressure. Garlic has added benefits in improving cardiovascular system health	
Red yeast rice (0.4% statins, lovastatin)	1,200 mg to 2,400 mg	If your cholesterol levels are still not coming down after using garlic for three or more months, try including red yeast rice. Reduces cholesterol production in the liver and blood levels, works like the statin drugs. Use only for short periods of time	
Guggul (2.5% guggulsterones)	500 mg to 1 g	Normalizes blood lipids	
Beta sitosterol	1 g to 3 g	Blocks cholesterol absorption in the intestines	
Psyllium fiber	1.5 g to 3 g	Reduces cholesterol absorption. Include psyllium fiber supplement immediately in your cholesterol-lowering program	
Niacin (nicotinic acid)	80 mg to 300 mg	Reduces cholesterol levels. Levels over 2 g may be prescribed by your doctor, but beware that side effects can occur	
Chromium	200 mcg to 600 mcg	Helps normalize blood lipid levels	

Ingredients for Blood Pressure and Heart Health: In addition to the circulatory system health nutrients listed above, the additional supplement intake of the following nutrients may be warranted for individuals with heart health problems.

L-taurine	500 mg to 2 g	Blood pressure regulation and antioxidant	
L-arginine	500 mg to 2 g	Promotes circulation by stimulating nitric oxide in blood	
Potassium	99 mg to 600 mg	Promotes regular blood pressure	
L-carnitine	1 g to 3 g	Increases heart function, reduces angina, ischemia	
Hawthorn extract (5% vitexin)	150 mg to 300 mg	Dilates peripheral and heart blood vessels. Use if you have congestive heart conditions and decreased cardiac output	

7

Children's Dietary Supplement Concerns

Nutritionists have recently refocused their attention on the adequacy (or inadequacy) of children's diets. Their research has triggered some definite concerns about nutrient deficiencies in children of all ages. A recent article published in the medical journal *Lancet* reported that infants given diets enriched with the omega-3 fatty acid DHA (docosahexaenoic acid) displayed greater problem-solving ability when compared to infants drinking standard formulas, which were lower in this fatty acid. Other studies report inadequate protein content in children's diets, as well as insufficient intake of certain key minerals such as calcium and zinc.

A common problem is getting children to eat enough vegetables and fruits. Proper intake of fruits and vegetables is very important because these foods contain many essential nutrients, including antioxidants, which help protect the body's cells from damage.

In 1998 Barbara Dennison, M.D., issued a report on her research concerning fruit and vegetable intake in young children, which appeared in the *Journal of the American College of Nutrition.* Her purpose was to determine from a sample of healthy children if they were indeed eating the recommended number of servings per day of fruits and vegetables. By interviewing parents and 223 children in two age groups, two and five years old, Dr. Dennison found that these preschool-age children consumed on average approximately 80 percent of the recommended fruit servings per day, but only 25 percent of the recommended vegetable servings. Dr. Dennison also reported that low intake of fruits and vegetables was associated with inadequate intake of vitamin A, vitamin C, and dietary fiber. These children typically had diets that were too high in total fat and saturated fat. Also, the lower the children's fruit and vegetable intake, the lower their fiber intake. This indicates that for children fruit and vegetables are a major source of dietary fiber, and that many are not getting a significant amount of fiber from the cereals and grains they eat, perhaps because they are highly processed. Dr. Dennison concludes that identification and correction of poor eating habits at an early age is critical to developing lifelong good eating habits. One way to ensure that fruit and vegetables are always available is to keep a supply of fruits and vegetables in the freezer, to supplement the fresh variety. Warehouse stores often sell fresh fruit in bulk as well.

A final word on fruit and vegetables: Fruit juices tend to be very popular with children, but it is always a good idea to dilute them, because they are high in natural sugars, which could contribute to your child's "sweet tooth" and to dental health problems in the long term.

Supplement companies have created a new category of dietary supplements for kids, some of which even include sugar-free fruit and vegetable juice extracts. Starting a good antioxidant protection program at an early age means living a healthier life, reducing the risks of degenerative disease as an adult, and increasing life span. After love, the best gift you can give children is the gift of health.

You should never give children megadoses of any dietary supplements. Stick to the simple formulas that supply the essential nutrients, as indicated in the table in this chapter. You can explore using some of the other supplements, but check with your doctor before starting. Always remember that a supplement does not replace a good, balanced diet, and always encourage your child to eat the proper amounts of the right foods.

For active children, children playing sports, and children entering adolescence, I find that a protein supplement can be very beneficial. It is well established that children need a higher intake of protein for proper growth and development. One way to ensure that your kids get adequate protein is to provide them with a low-fat, nutritious protein drink (sold in powdered form). There are several brands developed for kids that contain one or more high-quality protein sources, such as whey, soy, casein, or egg white. For younger children, start with a serving per day; this supplies 8 to 14 g of protein. For older children, age twelve and up, this should be increased to 15 to 25 g of additional protein per day. This can also take the form of protein supplement bars available on the market, particularly in health food stores. If your child needs to increase total caloric intake as well, then choose a protein supplement that contains 100 or more calories from carbohydrates, per serving. Also look for products that contain fiber; 2 to 6 grams of fiber per serving is ideal.

Whenever you suspect any type of medical condition or growth failure in your child, make sure to consult your doctor immediately. Work with your doctor to seek the advice of a trained clinical nutritionist. If you choose to use dietary supplements for therapeutic reasons, do so only under the guidance of a licensed health professional, and never in place of traditional drug therapies, unless directed by your doctor.

The use of fluoride-containing supplements to promote dental health has been a topic of debate for many years. Such fluoride supplements are considered drugs and need to be prescribed by a doctor. Fluoride supplements may contain other nutrients as well, especially some of the essential vitamins and minerals. Make sure to check the completeness of these formulas, because they typically come up short in one or more essential nutrients—often calcium, magnesium, zinc, vitamin C, or vitamin E. In my experience, it is better to ask your doctor to prescribe a product that contains only fluoride. This gives you flexibility to choose a high-quality multinutrient dietary supplement.

In 1994 the American Dietetic Association (ADA) published a position paper concerning fluoride and its role in dental health. The association concluded that using fluoride products, such as fluoride toothpaste, fluoride-containing mouth rinses, and fluoride treatments in the dental office, as well as consuming fluoride in water, food sources, and dietary supplements, does reduce the risk of dental decay. Fluoride also helps promote enamel remineralization throughout life. Based on this and other research findings, I support the use of a fluoride supplement for children.

For your convenience, the table on page 82 includes the Reference Daily Intakes, for adults and children four years and older. I find it remarkable that the government has established only one set of RDIs for such a wide age range (there are separate RDIs for children younger than four years old, and for infants). It is important to work closely with your health care practitioner to ensure that the diet you are serving your kids is adequately balanced. You need to be on the conservative side about supplements, because most of the research on dietary supplements has involved only adults. This means the details concerning daily intakes and long-term health effects (both beneficial and harmful) of the essential nutrients are less well established for children. Again, do not give children megadoses of supplements. The daily effective supplement dosage ranges listed in the table will help you purchase products that are safe and effective for children from four to early adolescence. For older teenagers, use the guidelines for adults in Chapter 5.

Tips for Maintaining a Healthy Eating Plan for Your Children

Follow the same healthy eating guidelines as for adults.

Ensure adequate intake of calcium and other essential vitamins and minerals.

Supplement Facts™

Buyer's Guide for Children's Supplement Products—
Daily Essential Nutrient Supplement Program

These supplement ingredient ranges are suitable for children over eight years old and preteens. Keep track of your child's total daily supplement intake from all sources, including tablets, capsules, softgels, powdered drinks, and health bars.

Nutrient	Reference Daily Intake for Adults and Children Four Years or Older	Safe and Effective Daily Supplement Dosage Range	Comments on Selected Nutrients	Your Personal Daily Supplement Intake Notes Section
The Vitamins: As a general comment, research studies continue to determine that most children's diets are deficient in several essential nutrients. When studies are performed to determine the benefits of children taking nutrition supplements, these studies always show some type of improvement in growth, health, or intelligence.				
Vitamin A (from acetate and palmitate)	5,000 IU	1,000 IU to 5,000 IU	Higher vitamin A intake may be prescribed for children with lung disorders and acne	
Beta-carotene (as vitamin A activity)	none established	2,500 IU to 15,000 IU	Also look for products containing lycopene	
Vitamin D	400 IU	100 IU to 400 IU		
Vitamin E	30 IU	60 IU to 200 IU		
Vitamin K	80 mcg	20 mcg to 80 mcg		
Vitamin C	60 mg	60 mg to 500 mg	Higher amounts may be taken for short periods during illness	
Vitamin B_1	1.5 mg	1.5 mg to 15 mg	The B vitamins are very safe. Some health food children's formulas may contain amounts higher than these ranges	
Vitamin B_2	1.7 mg	1.7 mg to 15 mg		
Vitamin B_3 (niacin)	20 mg	5 mg to 20 mg		
Vitamin B_6	2 mg	2 mg to 15 mg		
Folate	400 mcg	200 mcg to 400 mcg		
Vitamin B_{12}	6 mcg	6 mcg to 60 mcg		
Biotin	300 mcg	20 mcg to 300 mcg		
Pantothenic acid	10 mg	2 mg to 20 mg		
The Minerals: The minerals have many functions in the body and are essential for normal growth and development. Look for supplements containing all or most of these essential minerals, in particular, calcium, magnesium, and zinc.				
Calcium	1,000 mg	250 mg to 1,000 mg		
Phosphorus	1,000 mg	20 mg to 400 mg		
Magnesium	400 mg	50 mg to 300 mg		
Iron	18 mg	4 mg to 18 mg		
Zinc	15 mg	5 mg to 15 mg		
Iodine	150 mcg	30 mcg to 150 mcg		
Selenium	70 mcg	20 mcg to 70 mcg		
Copper	2 mg	0.5 mg to 2 mg		
Manganese	2 mg	0.5 mg to 6 mg		
Chromium	120 mcg	60 mcg to 120 mcg		
Molybdenum	75 mcg	25 mcg to 75 mcg		

Nutrient	Reference Daily Intake for Adults and Children Four Years or Older	Safe and Effective Daily Supplement Dosage Range	Comments on Selected Nutrients	Your Personal Daily Supplement Intake Notes Section
Sodium	3,400 mg	none or less than 100 mg per serving	Not usually in supplements	
Chloride	3,400 mg	none or less than 100 mg per serving	Not usually in supplements	
Potassium	3,500 mg	20 mg to 100 mg	Not usually in supplements	
Choline		20 mg to 200 mg		
Inositol		20 mg to 200 mg		
Bioflavonoids		20 mg to 500 mg	Look for supplements with citrus bioflavonoids, like rutin	
Lutein		5 mg to 40 mg	Good for healthy vision	

The Fatty Acids: Studies show that children can benefit in many ways from regular intake of these health-promoting fatty acids, in particular, improvements in dry skin, circulatory system health, and improvements in intelligence. The top fatty acid sources used in supplements include fish oils, evening primrose oil, hemp oil, black currant oil, borage oil, pumpkin seed oil, and flaxseed oil. Most health food stores have plant oil products in containers, which gives you flexibility to add to your children's food.

Nutrient				
EPA		30 mg to 150 mg	Great for peak intelligence	
DHA		30 mg to 150 mg	Great for peak intelligence	
Linolenic acid		500 mg to 2,000 mg		
Linoleic acid		200 mg to 2,000 mg		
GLA (gamma linolenic Acid)		40 mg to 100 mg	GLA is optional due to the high cost but is highly recommended for children with dry skin problems	

The Probiotics: The beneficial effects of maintaining a dominant population of beneficial intestinal microflora are well established. Take a mega-multinutrient that includes probiotics, or a separate probiotic formula. See Chapter 8 for additional information.

Nutrient				
Lactobacillus and bifidobacterium		1 to 4 billion cells	Especially useful for children who have irregular bowel movements and consume a lot of sweets	

Protein and Fiber: The most recent studies reveal that many children do not get enough protein and fiber in their diets. If your child is experiencing slow growth or is very active, consider including a protein shake into their daily nutrition program. If your child does not eat several servings of fruits, vegetables, or grains, then consider using a fiber supplement. Fiber supplements can also help overweight children who eat a lot of junk food control their appetite.

Nutrient				
Protein supplements	50 g	8 g to 24 g	If your child does not eat right, include a high-protein supplement drink or nutrition bar into his/her daily diet. Protein supplements are very beneficial for athletic children	
Fiber	25 g	5 g to 16 g	If your child does not eat enough of dietary fiber from food, include a fiber supplement into his/her daily nutrition program. Fiber supplements can be very useful to help children who overeat gain control over their appetite. Also, visit a health food store and purchase snack foods that contain 2 or more grams of fiber per serving	

Miscellaneous: Some multinutrient formulas will contain a variety of other supplement ingredients. These other ingredients are usually added in small amounts, or qualitatively in the ingredients list. They usually include fruit and vegetable extracts and digestive enzymes. I prefer that you choose products that do not include too many of these extra ingredients, due to the fact that the history of use of these exotic ingredients in scientific studies, and in products, has been with adults. The fruit and juice extracts should not be a problem. But children's products with digestive enzymes, bee products, medicinal herbs, and metabolites should be avoided or minimized.

Ensure adequate intake of protein, carbohydrates, fiber, and essential fatty acids.

Recent research has proven that EPA and DHA intake will improve your child's mental development. Fish and flaxseed oil are rich sources of these important fatty acids, as is linoleic acid as well (but most well-balanced diets usually contain plenty of linoleic acid).

Kids should drink more water and diluted fruit juice, and less soda and other soft drinks.

Kids should eat plenty of fresh or frozen vegetables.

Kids should eat two to four servings of fruit per day.

Use healthy nutrition bars (from the health food store) for snacks; they are a good source of protein and essential vitamins and minerals. Choose brands with essential fatty acids and lower sugar content, with 2 to 5 g of fiber per bar.

Start imprinting good eating and fitness habits in your children. Teach them to eat during designated meal and snack times. Don't let them get in the habit of eating in front of the television, or eating freely all day and night long.

Products

Bugs Bunny

Chewy Bears and Friends

Flintstones Complete

GNC Kids (full line of all sorts of supplements for children)

GNC Teens (full line of all sorts of supplements for teens)

Goldshield Centural Children

Health from the Sun Flax Liquid Gold

Natrol A Kid's Companion

Nature's Plus Animal Parade

One-A-Day Kids Complete

Popeye Multi-vitamins Great Tasting Chewables

Popeye Multi-vitamins with Extra C Great Tasting Chewables

Spring Valley Children's Chewables

Twinlabs Animal Friends Chewable

I recommend that you read the following books, which will cover a variety of contemporary issues concerning children's health:

Armstrong, Thomas. *The Myth of the ADD Child.* New York: Penguin Books, 1995.

Institute of Medicine. *Nutrition During Pregnancy: Weight Gain, Nutrient Supplements.* Washington, D.C.: National Academy Press, 1990.

Kushi, Aveline. *Raising Healthy Kids.* Garden City Park: Avery Publishing Group, 1998.

Zand, Janet, Rachel Walton, and Bob Rountree. *Smart Medicine for a Healthier Child.* Garden City Park: Avery Publishing Group, 1994.

8

Digestion Wellness Dietary Supplements

Among the best-selling prescription and over-the-counter drugs are those aimed at treating stomach and intestinal problems. Peptic ulcers, constipation, diarrhea, gastroesophageal reflux, gastritis, intestinal gas, and indigestion are among the most common complaints. Health practitioners attribute this pandemic of gastrointestinal disorders to eating too little fiber and too much sugar and processed foods, topped off by an unhealthy daily dose of chemicals.

In the realm of dietary supplements, there is a range of products for the promotion of digestive health. Some are designed for colon health, such as fiber products and probiotics. Others are for people with gastrointestinal irritation problems; here there is a host of formulas that can be effective, but keep in mind that whenever you experience pain in your gastrointestinal system, make sure to seek immediate supervision from a doctor, because if a serious condition is left untreated, severe health prob-

lems may develop. Dietary supplements can be used in concert with medical treatment or for prevention of problems.

One of the common ingredients you will find in gastrointestinal supplement products is *Aloe vera* gel. It is famous for its soothing and restorative action on the stomach and intestinal linings, and for healing the skin as well. But if you are in the market for a soothing product, look closely at the labels to make sure that the product contains only aloe leaf gel if you are looking for soothing action. If you are looking for a gastrointestinal stimulating action, then take products containing whole leaf aloe; the skin of aloe leaves contains aloin, a bitter substance with mild laxative properties (see Part 3 for details).

You will also commonly see ginger and licorice root in digestive health dietary supplements. They help restore balance, aid the function of your gastrointestinal lining, and promote gastrointestinal secretions.

Another interesting and increasingly popular category of digestive health products is digestive enzymes, taken with meals. The most common ones include papain, bromelain, protease, lactase, amylase, cellulase, and lipase. As people get older, their bodies secrete fewer digestive enzymes, which leads to food not being digested properly. Using digestive enzymes can assist your body in promoting more complete digestion of the foods you eat. Some food allergists believe that inadequate digestion may result in the absorption of large molecules of food compounds into the bloodstream; they suspect the immune system then attacks these molecules, leading to food allergies. Many naturopathic doctors use digestive enzyme supplements to help control food allergies, with good success. However, even the most high-quality enzymes cannot help if you are not eating healthy foods and if you do not adequately chew your foods so they liquefy in your mouth. This may mean taking two or three times longer to eat, but you will be rewarded with a better-functioning digestive system.

Another type of digestive wellness supplement is the probiotics. These include *Lactobacillus acidophilus* and *Bifidobacteria bifidus,* microorganisms that benefit the intestinal tract. Probiotic supplements are an easy way to reestablish the beneficial bacterial populations in your intestines and crowd out the bad bacteria that can produce unhealthy waste products. You will also encounter probiotic formulas containing FOS (fructooligosaccharides). FOS is actually a starchlike compound made of chains of fructose molecules (regular starch consists of chains of glucose molecules). FOS is mostly indigestible by humans. However, the friendly bacteria occupying the intestines can digest FOS; in fact, FOS is the preferred carbohydrate food for these beneficial intestinal bacteria. In fact, studies examining intake of FOS and sugar show that the higher the amount of refined sugars in the diet, the lower the amount of beneficial bacteria and the higher the amount of bad bacteria. People who have never taken probiotics and FOS supplements will experience beneficial effects only after a few weeks. Many health-minded people take probiotic supplements before, during, and after they travel, to avoid travelers' diarrhea. It is interesting to note that whole foods, especially fruits and vegetables, contain FOS, while processed foods do not (and are often high in refined sugar). It's no wonder that so many people are having trouble with their digestive systems. Refer to the table on page 87 for guidelines on selecting digestive health dietary supplements.

Tips for Promoting Digestive System Wellness

Start by using common sense: Don't eat foods that upset your digestive system. Your body is telling you that the food is causing an imbalance or damage.

Supplement Facts™

Buyer's Guide for Digestive System Wellness Supplement Products

The following supplements have been found to be useful in promoting gastrointestinal wellness. If you have a known digestive system medical problem or suspect you have one, consult your doctor for proper medical treatment.

Supplement Ingredient	Safe and Effective Daily Supplement Dosage Range	Comments	Your Personal Daily Supplement Intake Notes Section
Digestive Enzymes: Digestive enzymes are becoming a common ingredient to adult multinutrient formulations. The logic of digestive enzymes is that it is believed that as people get older, their body does not produce adequate digestive enzymes. If you have problems digesting your meals, try taking a digestive enzyme–containing supplement. But keep in mind that some of your digestive system problems may be caused by the foods you eat or an underlying medical condition. Always take digestive enzymes with meals. Refer to Digestive Enzyme entry in Part 3 for more information on these enzymes.			
Papain	5 mg to 30 mg	Don't use if you have an inflammatory GI disease, including gastritis or peptic ulcer disease	
Bromelain	5 mg to 30 mg	Don't use if you have an inflammatory GI disease, including gastritis or peptic ulcer disease	
Protease	5 mg to 30 mg	Don't use if you have an inflammatory GI disease, including gastritis or peptic ulcer disease	
Amylase	5 mg to 30 mg		
Lactase	5 mg to 30 mg		
Cellulase	5 mg to 30 mg		
Lipase	5 mg to 30 mg		
Probiotics Supplements: If you are not taking probiotic-containing supplements as part of your daily supplement program, current research on maintaining digestive system health supports the recommendation of including one in your daily supplement program. Always take probiotics after bouts of gastrointestinal distress and when taking antibiotic drugs to help restore and maintain your body's population of beneficial intestinal microflora.			
Lactobacillus acidophilus	1 to 10 billion cells	Take a single species probiotic formula or multispecies formula. But make sure they include *L. acidophilus* and/or *B. bifidus*	
Bifidobacteria bifidus	1 to 10 billion cells		
FOS-Inulin (prebiotics)	500 mg to 2 g	Take FOS-containing supplements with or without probiotics. Taking 1 or more g per day of FOS will in itself cause your beneficial intestinal microflora to grow	
Soothing Supplements: To help restore and maintain the health and function of the gastrointestinal tract lining. Include these supplements if you are experiencing mild irritation, or as supportive natural therapy along with conventional medical treatment for inflammatory disorders of the GI tract.			
Aloe vera gel (40:1 or 200:1 concentrate)	250 mg to 750 mg	Take aloe vera gel in solid dosage forms, or try one of the liquid concentrate drinks	
Ginger (4% ginerols)	20 mg to 120 mg	Use standardized supplements or teas	
Licorice (2% to 4% glycyrrhizin)	20 mg to 120 mg	Use standardized supplements or teas	

Supplement Ingredient	Safe and Effective Daily Supplement Dosage Range	Comments	Your Personal Daily Supplement Intake Notes Section
Chamomile (1.2% to 2% apigenin)	250 mg to 1,000 mg	Use standardized supplements or teas	
Fiber	5 g to 15 g	Look for powdered drink supplements containing one or more of the beneficial fibers: psyllium, guar gum, oat bran, apple pectin	
L-glutamine	500 mg to 2 g	Use L-glutamine supplements as part of your digestive system healing program	
Natural Laxatives:			
Cascara sagrada (7% to 30% total hydroxyanthracene)	40 mg to 160 mg	Use botanical laxatives with the same caution as using laxative drugs. Only use as directed on the product labels. Consult a doctor if constipation persists for more than 48 hours. Cascara works more gently than OTC drugs and is reported to have a restorative and soothing effect on the GI tract	

Relax before you eat, and take your time. Chew your foods well, until you can easily swallow them. The more you chew your foods, the easier they will be to digest more completely.

Maintain adequate fiber intake, 25 g or more per day. Fiber promotes proper digestive system function. It also reduces the amount of cholesterol and fats absorbed into your body.

Use probiotic and FOS supplements to restore your beneficial gastrointestinal bacteria. Reduce sugar intake, which feeds the bad bacteria.

Drink some stomach-soothing teas, such as peppermint or chamomile.

Don't wait until you develop a serious gastrointestinal problem; seek immediate medical attention if problems persist for more than two or three days.

If you are experiencing minor gastrointestinal problems, give yourself two to four months to rebuild your digestive system health by combining a good diet with digestive system wellness supplements and proper medical treatment.

Avoid drinking alcoholic beverages and other beverages that are filled with chemicals and sugar.

Start drinking more water, aloe gel drinks, and herbal teas to soothe and heal your digestive system.

Products

American Health Chewable Acidophilus with Bifidus

Bifa-15

Country Life Daily Fiber

Dr. Shari Lieberman's for Women Only Aloe Essence Aloe Drink

GNC Natural Brand Acidophilus Plus

GNC Natural Brand Colon Guard

Herbscience Aloe Vera with Yucca

Herbscience Cascara Sagrada with
    Psyllium Seed

Nutrition Now Pro-Biotic Acidophilus

Rainbow Light Everyday Fiber

Spring Valley Acidophilus

Sundown Cascara

Sundown Ginger

Sundown Licorice

Tree of Life Aloe Vera

Tree of Life Cleansing Blend

Tree of Life Digestive Enzyme Blend

Tree of Life Full Spectrum Enzyme
    Complex

Tree of Life Ginger

9

Energy-Promoting Dietary Supplements

Energy—it's what we all want. People of all walks of life around the world are looking to boost their energy levels each day. The fact that most of the world starts off each day with caffeinated beverages such as coffee, tea, or guarana is testimony to this desire. Out of all the supplement categories, energy-promoting products represent one of the largest. But it's also one of the most confusing.

Dietary supplements positioned as energy products fall into several different categories: those that stimulate the nervous system, those that help optimize the metabolism (the way the body turns food into energy), those that contain special concentrated energy sources, and those that actually work at the cellular level to help the body's complex energy-producing biochemical systems function at their best.

The most basic way to boost energy levels is to maintain a proper diet, which includes eating several snacks and meals per day and ensuring an adequate intake of the essential vitamins and minerals and other daily nutrients discussed in Chapter 5. In particular, the B vitamins, as well as copper and magnesium, are involved in all energy-producing metabolic pathways in the body. Iron is an important mineral needed to help make sure that the body's oxygen-carrying hemoglobin is functioning properly. Trace minerals such as chromium are important because they help the body to turn these nutrients into usable energy.

Fatigue Medical Alert

Be advised that persistent or unusual bouts of fatigue warrant a medical evaluation. Many people who experience persistent fatigue can have serious medical conditions, which can only be properly diagnosed by a medical doctor. Medical conditions typically associated with persistent fatigue include depression, borderline hypothyroid function, insomnia, poor sleeping habits (i.e., irregular sleeping hours), chronic fatigue syndrome, or you may find out that you have a normal amount of energy but are trying to do too much. So, consult your doctor if feelings of fatigue persist.

When it comes to improving overall metabolism above and beyond what your dietary supplement and nutrition program will accomplish, consider including ginseng and other energizing botanical supplements in your daily program. Ginseng, one of the biggest botanicals in the United States, is known as an adaptogenic supplement. Adaptogens have a general effect on improving the way the body functions, helping the body become more resistant to fatigue, boosting mental alertness, and increasing the body's capacity to do work. Note that most experts recommend using ginseng and other adaptogenic botanicals in on/off cycles of three months on and two to three weeks off. It is believed by cycling the body will not become unresponsive to the adaptogenic effects. However, note that long-term use of ginseng taken in the recommended dosages has been shown to be safe. And don't expect results to come too fast. This is one area where I find a lot of people who try to push too hard to boost their energy levels end up burning themselves out in the long run. There are practical limitations to what your body can do, and you need to balance your peaks of energy with periods of daily relaxation and rest. Several times each day, do some deep-breathing exercises and stretching. Also, a program of moderate regular exercise helps with stress management as well as with building up your strength and energy levels. These are all key components of a holistic vitalizing lifestyle. You need to allow some time to get your metabolism working correctly, but you will be surprised at how quickly your energy increases.

When all is said and done, however, there are times in our lives when we need more energy, in particular mental energy, to get through the day or perform better at work. Supplements for mental energy usually contain botanicals such as guarana, yerba mate, gotu kola, and the controversial ephedra. These herbs contain either caffeine or, in the case of ephedra, the drug ephedrine, both of which stimulate mental alertness. As with all central nervous system stimulants, after a few days their effects seem to become reduced. If you overdo these products, you will usually be worse off than before you began to use them. Refer to the table on page 93, which summarizes some of these points and lists the more common dietary supplements useful for restoring and maintaining vibrant energy.

If you are very active, you know that eating properly is extremely important for maintaining the high energy level you need to perform well. For sustained physical activity, the body needs to be well hydrated, and for prolonged exercise (over an hour), it needs a good supply of carbohydrates. This is why most athletes drink carbohydrate-containing beverages before, sometimes during, and immediately after exercise and competitions. One particular supplement attracting a lot of attention recently among athletes has been creatine. Creatine helps replenish energy-producing compounds in the body used primarily for short-duration, intensive bursts of power, like in powerlifting or football. More than twenty clinical studies conducted between 1994 and 1999 have concluded that creatine supplements will improve performance for strength athletes, but they are not useful for endurance athletes such as long-distance runners.

BEATING CHRONIC FATIGUE SYNDROME

During the 1990s researchers discovered some interesting insights concerning the nutritional treatment of chronic fatigue syndrome. Dr. Audrius Plioplys and Dr. Sigia Plioplys have been studying ways of treating this problem for many years. They found that some cases of chronic fatigue syndrome may be due in part to dysfunctional energy production at the cellular level. Each cell in your body contains mitochondria, specialized parts that produce most of the cell's energy and which are aptly referred to as the cell's powerhouse. The Plioplyses have discovered that in some people with chronic fatigue syndrome, the mitochondria do not operate as they should.

They theorized that carnitine supplements—carnitine helps with energy production by shuttling high-energy-yielding fatty acids into the cell's mitochondria—would help the mitochondria start working correctly. To test their hypothesis, they examined thirty-five chronic fatigue syndrome patients and determined that they indeed had low blood serum levels of carnitine. They then gave these patients 1 g of carnitine three times a day during the eight-week study period. The researchers measured significant improvement in their patients' energy levels after only four weeks, with additional improvements through to the end of the study period. The results of this research are very encouraging for people suffering from this disorder. However, remember that chronic fatigue syndrome may also have a psychological component. So if you are currently suffering from chronic fatigue syndrome, you may want to bring the results of this study to your doctor's attention, and start taking carnitine supplements under medical supervision. Look for improvements in four to eight weeks if dysfunctional mitochondria is the cause of your problem.

Products

Country Life Octa-Cosanol
Dr. Shari Lieberman's For Women Only
  Maximum Ginseng with Royal Jelly
Ginsana
GNC Ginseng Gold
Goldshield Co-Enzyme Q10
Goldshield Creatine with Dextrose
Goldshield Korean Ginseng
Goldshield Ginseng

Supplement Facts™

Buyer's Guide for Energy-Enhancing Supplement Products

The following supplement ingredients have been found to be safe and effective for increasing physical and mental energy, reducing feelings of fatigue, and improving performance.

Supplement Ingredient	Safe and Effective Daily Supplement Dosage Range	Comments	Your Personal Daily Supplement Intake Notes Section
Botanical Adaptogens: If your energy levels are sagging, then first try an adaptogen product for three months to promote balance and restore vitality. Note that when taking an adaptogen, during the first few weeks you may actually feel less energetic. This is a temporary condition, which will pass, due to the rebalancing action of the adaptogenic herbs. Use one or more of the following botanical adaptogens at a time.			
Ginseng (5% to 14% ginsenosides)	200 mg to 1,000 mg	Take for up to 3 months at a time. I recommend ginseng be taken in the A.M. only for most people (those with adrenal insufficiency may need it in the P.M. too)	
Eleuthero (0.8% eleutherosides)	200 mg to 1,000 mg	Take for up to 3 months at a time	
Arctic root (standardized to rosavin)	50 mg to 300 mg	Take for up to 3 months at a time	
Schisandra (1% schisandrins)	40 mg to 200 mg	Take for up to 3 months at a time	
Energizing Metabolites: Along with taking your botanical adaptogens, you can start taking the following supplements as well, which will help improve your energy production at the cellular level.			
Octacosanol	1 mg to 2 mg	Helps stimulate cellular energy and also improves physical reaction time	
L-carnitine	500 mg to 2 g	Start by taking a minimum of 1 g per day for 3 months. Also improves athletic performance	
Coenzyme Q_{10}	60 mg to 120 mg	CoQ_{10} also improves endurance	
Additional Energy Supplements:			
Energy drinks	2 to 3 servings	If your energy is lagging, make sure you are getting the carbohydrates you need. Ingest a 120 to 220 calorie-per-serving high-carbohydrate energy drink before, during, and after exercise	
Botanical stimulants: Guarana and yerba mate	Consult product labels for suggested use	Use botanical stimulants on an optional basis and only use periodically. If overused, they can burn you out	
Creatine	20 g, for 2 to 4 days, followed by 5 to 10 g per day	Use creatine to boost your strength and power if you are a serious strength athlete	

Goldshield Ginseng
Goldshield Vitaboost
Herbscience Ginseng
Hi-Ener-G, Windmill
Medicine Shoppe Korean Ginseng
  Extract
Nature Made Ginseng

Sundown Ginseng
Tree of Life Energy Blend
Tree of Life Ginseng
Tree of Life Siberian Ginseng
Your Life L-carnitine
Your Life Q_{10}

10

Immune System–Stimulating Dietary Supplements

While eating right and taking the proper vitamin and mineral dietary supplements are important for maintaining a properly functioning immune system (and remember that a poor diet, with too much fat, alcohol, sugar, and empty calories, can reduce your immunity), there will be some times during the year when you can benefit from boosting your immune system function—times when you are exposed to a higher amount of infectious agents, such as bacteria and viruses, or times when you may be working too hard or are emotionally stressed. These conditions can contribute to weakening your immune system, which is often followed by illness setting in. You know best what times of the year or what conditions can precede catching a cold or the flu, which means you can do some planning and take preventative measures to strengthen your immunity. One of the most popular practices in recent years has been to take an immune-stimulating product—vita-min A, beta-carotene, vitamin C, zinc, copper, glutamine, lysine, and echinacea.

When fighting off upper respiratory infections such as colds or flu, one of the most beneficial herbs, shown in scientific studies to help shorten the duration of the illness and reduce the severity of its symptoms, is the herb echinacea. Echinacea needs to be taken in high amounts, however, as indicated in the table on page 96 and as discussed on page 171 in Part 3, and should be used as supportive therapy along with any other drug or nutritional therapies. Studies have shown that taking echinacea before upper respiratory infections hit will reduce the number of times you get sick and the duration of illness if you do get sick. Even if you already have an upper respiratory infection, it's not too late to take echinacea, because studies also show that if you start taking it as soon as illness sets in, it will help shorten the duration of the illness and alleviate the symptoms.

Supplement Facts™

Buyer's Guide for Immune System–Stimulating Supplement Products

Take these supplements on a periodic basis when you want to promote/stimulate immune system function. Great for cold and flu season, or when you're overworked.

Supplement Ingredient	Safe and Effective Daily Supplement Dosage Range	Comments	Your Personal Daily Supplement Intake Notes Section
First start by increasing your antioxidant intake, which improves immune system function and helps fight infections. For upper respiratory infections, take zinc lozenges. Concerning botanicals, start immediately taking echinacea.			
Extra vitamin C	1,000 mg to 3,000 mg	Increase your total daily vitamin C supplement intake to within this range	
Extra vitamin E	600 mg to 1,200 mg	Increase your total daily vitamin E supplement intake to within this range	
Extra vitamin A and beta-carotene	10,000 IU to 30,000 IU	Increase your total daily vitamin A and beta-carotene supplement intake to within this range	
Extra zinc	35 mg to 60 mg	Increase your total daily zinc supplement intake to within this range. Use zinc lozenges when you have upper respiratory infections	
Extra copper	12 mg to 18 mg	Increase your total daily copper supplement intake to within this range	
Extra selenium	200 mcg to 400 mcg	Increase your total daily selenium intake to within this range	
Echinacea (4% phelolics or echinacosides)	450 mg to 900 mg	Use in cycles of 3 weeks on and 7 days off during cold and flu season. Use up to 3 months at a time for lingering respiratory tract ailments and lower urinary tract infections, along with drug therapy	
L-glutamine	1 g to 3 g	Take L-glutamine supplements to give a general boost to your immune system	
L-lysine	500 mg to 2,000 mg	Take a lysine supplement if you have or are prone to getting cold sores	
Additional Supplements to Consider for Boosting Immune System Function:			
Green tea extract (35% to 50% polyphenols)	100 mg to 300 mg	Increase daily intake of green tea supplements during periods of infection. Green tea is a mild immuno-stimulant	
Olive leaf extract (15% to 17% oleuropein)	Use as directed on product labels	This new dietary supplement product has been reported to exert antimicrobial activity. Use is as complementary antibiotic, along with your prescribed drugs, when infections persist	

When using herbs to stimulate your immune system, keep in mind that over-stimulation is not beneficial. Take immune-boosters such as echinacea in an on/off cycle: two to three weeks of supplements, followed by one or two weeks off, and use them during periods when you are likely to get sick or have already come down with something. Your core supplement program and healthy eating will promote healthy immunity the rest of the time.

Another supplement that has been shown to help reduce the incidence and duration of upper respiratory ailments is zinc, usually in the form of lozenges. Zinc actually inhibits viruses from establishing themselves in your throat. If you suffer from bouts of cold sores, add some lysine to your basic immune system–enhancing supplement program. Some newly popular immune system boosters include shiitake mushroom, maitake mushroom, and astragalus, all of which have a history of use in Asia.

Caution: If you have a serious disease, such as cancer, AIDS, or an autoimmune disease, taking certain supplements in support of your prescribed drug treatment may be beneficial—*but only if the individual who develops your nutrition and supplement program is experienced.* Taking supplements indiscriminately to help treat serious diseases can sometimes cause the disease to worsen. Make sure you seek out competent guidance from a naturopathic doctor, licensed acupuncturist, licensed herbalist, or other licensed health professional specializing in these often complex therapeutic nutrition programs.

Products
Bioenergy Echinacea
Bioenergy Olinacea
Echina Fresh
Goldshield Echinacea
Goldshield Echinacea with Zinc
Herbscience Echinacea
Herbscience Echinacea with Goldenseal
Medicine Shoppe Echinacea Extract
Medicine Shoppe Echinacea/Goldenseal
    Extract
Sundown Echinacea
Tree of Life C and Green Tea
Tree of Life Echinacea
Tree of Life Esta-C
Tree of Life Vitamin A
Tree of Life Zinc Lozenges
TruNature Echinacea
Windmill Beta-Carotene
Windmill L-Lysine
Windmill Vitamin A, C, E
Windmill Vitamin C
Windmill Vitamin E
Your Life L-Lysine
Your Life Vitamin A and Beta-Carotene
Your Life Vitamin C
Your Life Vitamin E

11

Joint and Bone Health Dietary Supplements

One of the most encouraging developments in the 1990s is the discovery that osteoporosis—a decrease in bone mass and bone density—can be prevented. In fact, bone strength and density can be restored through nutritional means. Similarly, connective tissues, such as cartilage and ligaments, respond favorably to nutritional supplements. Scientists have clearly determined that certain nutritional products can help successfully treat connective tissue disorders, including osteoarthritis. These supplements can also help restore the strength of connective tissues, maintaining or restoring strength and mobility in your joints. As a result of these phenomenal medical discoveries, many dietary supplement products targeted toward joint and bone health have appeared on store shelves. The table on page 100 summarizes the most popular joint and bone health nutrients.

It is well established that calcium builds bones and maintains bone density. The research is so conclusive that the FDA has approved a health claim for calcium and its role in preventing osteoporosis. While you will hear about different forms of calcium (see calcium entry in Part 3 for details), research has shown that calcium carbonate, when taken with food, is as fully absorbable as calcium citrate. Chewable calcium carbonate supplements also result in good absorption. The key is that for maximum absorbability, calcium carbonate needs to remain in the digestive system long enough to be fully dissolved in the gastrointestinal juices.

But there is more to the bone health story than just calcium. Vitamin D assists in the absorption and utilization of bone-forming calcium and phosphorus, and vitamin D itself is an essential precursor of a hormone that is required for normal bone growth in children, maintenance of bone in adults, and the prevention of osteoporosis. But even if you have an adequate intake of vitamin D, you may have low blood levels of this vitamin. In adults, low blood levels of vitamin D are a risk factor for osteoporosis and bone fractures. One way to increase blood levels of vitamin D is to take supplements. With this in mind, the Food and Nutrition Board of the Institute of Medicine recently recommended a new health standard for vitamin D intake that takes into consideration the needs of different age groups. The new recommendations are 200 IU a day for adults nineteen to fifty years old, 400 IU daily for adults fifty-one to seventy years old, and 600 IU a day for adults seventy-one years or older. (Keep in mind that adequate exposure to sunlight increases vitamin D levels in your body.)

Progressive health practitioners and health-minded consumers already know the importance of using supplements in their diet to promote optimal health, including stronger bones. In addition to vitamin D and calcium, there are other vitamins and minerals (magnesium, vitamin B_6, folic acid, vitamin B_{12}, vitamin K, boron, and silicon) that can help build and maintain bone health.

Concerning strong connective tissue and joints, two dietary supplement ingredients continue to dominate this category: glucosamine and chondroitin. As we age, our body's capacity to maintain and build connective tissues diminishes. If dietary measures are not taken to provide essential building blocks for these important tissues, degenerative diseases such as arthritis and osteoarthritis may develop. Clinical studies conducted throughout the world have shown that the body will respond positively to nutritional therapy and actually repair degenerated tissues over the course of several weeks to several months.

Glucosamine has been successfully used to stop and even reverse the progression of osteoarthritis in some people, and studies conducted on thousands of people show it is well tolerated. (Refer to the section on glucosamine in Part 3 for more information on using this product.) Scientists believe it works by enabling increased synthesis of collagen, a tough, stringy protein that is the major component of connective tissue. The building and rebuilding of collagen in the body is a constant process, related to normal wear and tear of the connective tissues. When the body is undergoing periods of stress or intensive exercise, the demand for the building blocks of collagen increases. Because there are no significant food sources of glucosamine, taking supplemental amounts of glucosamine will help support the production of collagen, which in turn will help your body maintain healthy connective tissues.

Research conducted on patients taking 400 mg to 1,500 mg per day of glucosamine have demonstrated the ability of dietary glucosamine to stimulate the production of connective tissue and its repair. Some of the benefits reported from these studies include improved joint structure and function, maintenance of cartilage, improvements in skin appearance and thickness, repair of worn and damaged connective tissues in joints, and increased manufacture of hyaluronic

Supplement Facts™

Buyer's Guide for Joint, Bone Health, and Botanical Pain Control Supplement Products

Try taking the following supplements to improve joint and bone health; follow this program for 4 to 6 months at a time.

Supplement Ingredient	Safe and Effective Daily Supplement Dosage Range	Comments	Your Personal Daily Supplement Intake Notes Section
Essential vitamins and minerals	Follow guidelines in Chapter 5	By following the guidelines in Chapter 5, you will attain adequate intake of minerals and vitamins required for bone growth and maintenance. Mega-doses of niacinamide are effective in arthritis, but must be given under medical supervision only. Patients taking this need regular blood tests to check for liver toxicity	
Joint and Connective Tissue Growth Factors: These are the primary supplements that will provide connective tissue matrix growth. In other words, increasing connective tissue growth greater than it is being broken down. While any connective tissue disorder will benefit from these nutrients, they are of particular use for individuals with osteoarthritis.			
Glucosamine sulfate or HCl	500 mg to 1,500 mg	Start with 1,500 mg for the first 3 months, then taper to 400 mg to 750 mg per day	
Chondroitin sulfate	600 mg to 1,200 mg	A cofactor to be used with glucosamine, not instead of it	
Methyl sulfonyl methane (MSM)	250 mg to 1,500 mg	Also include MSM into your connective tissue repair program if your budget permits	
Botanical Anti-inflammatories: If you are finding that your pain control medicine is not working effectively, or you are experiencing many annoying side effects, then it might be time to try one of nature's anti-inflammatories. In addition to helping relieve pain and inflammation, botanicals contain healing phytonutrients to help stop tissue breakdown and allow restoration to take place. The key consideration when selecting anti-inflammatory botanicals is to get a standardized, high-quality product.			
Curcumin (85% to 98% curcuminoids)	250 mg to 500 mg, 3 times per day	Try using one or more of these anti-inflammatory botanicals. If you find they cause upset stomach, start with small dosages for a few weeks, and work your way up to what is recommended on the product's directions	
Boswellia (40% to 65% boswellic acids)	100 mg to 400 mg		
Ginger (4% ginerols)	250 mg to 750 mg		
White Willow bark	500 mg to 2,000 mg	This herb contains salicylates; if you are taking aspirin, or one of the nonacetylated salicylates, like Diflunisal or Salsalate, make sure you keep track of your total salicylate intake and do not exceed a total daily dosage recommended by your doctor	

acid, the body's natural joint lubricant. Other clinical studies on the therapeutic use of glucosamine are equally impressive. When a total daily dosage of 1,500 mg was given to individuals with osteoarthritis, their condition improved in just a matter of weeks. Increased range of motion and a reduction in pain and inflammation were observed in patients taking glucosamine supplements. Glucosamine has also been shown to help with healing and repair of cartilage and ligament problems, including athletic injuries such as shoulder and knee problems involving the connective tissue.

If you already have an existing connective tissue or joint health problem, taking higher therapeutic nutritional dosages for several months, until results are seen—under a doctor's supervision, of course—is your first course of action. For those of you who are interested in maintaining and optimizing healthy connective tissues and joints and preventing problems from developing, taking a daily nutritional-level dose of glucosamine and/or chondroitin as part of your core supplement program can help prevent problems in the future.

People suffering from conditions such as osteoarthritis or injured joints often have to combat the inflammation that accompanies these problems. There are a number of dietary supplements that can help reduce inflammation and serve as an alternative to various drugs. Some of the products shown to reduce pain and inflammation include curcumin and boswellia. In addition, antioxidants, other vitamins and minerals, bioflavonoids, and perhaps enzymes such as bromelian may promote healing and reduce inflammation. If you use natural products to help with healing, it is very important to do so under your doctor's supervision, and also to follow the label directions carefully. Bromelian, for example, should not be taken in high amounts for long periods of time.

Products

Country Life MSM

Dr. Shari Lieberman's Soy Solution
  Bone Guard

Futurebiotics Methyl-Sulfonyl-Methane
  Biological Sulfur

Goldshield Glucosamine Hi-Strength
  with Chondroitin

Medicine Shoppe Glucosamine and
  Chondroitin Sulfate

Medicine Shoppe Glucosamine Sulfate

Nature's Plus RxJoint

Nutritionworks Glucosamine Drink

Schiff Joint Free Plus

Schiff Pain Free

Sundown Osteo Bi-Flex

Tree of Life Calcium and Magnesium

Tree of Life Chondroitin Sulfate

Tree of Life Glucosamine Sulfate with
  Devil's Claw

Your Life Glucosamine Sulfate
  Complex

Your Life Osteo-Joint

12

Liver Health
Dietary Supplements

The liver is one of the most important organs in the body because of the vital roles it plays in metabolizing nutrients, cleansing the blood of wastes and toxins, and many other functions essential to life. But today, all the artificial and toxic chemicals in our food, our environment, and our workplaces can stress the liver and cause disease. In addition to chemical insults, diseases such as hepatitis can damage the liver. Some of the drugs used to treat other diseases can have damaging effects on the liver; some commonly used ones are antidepressive and anticonvulsant medications, acetaminophen in excessive amounts, and drugs used for anesthesia during surgery.

One supplement on the shelves has a reputation in Europe as a potent liver protector and healer. It has been studied for decades, and more than 120 clinical studies have demonstrated its beneficial effects on the liver. This miraculous herbal product is called milk thistle. If the biggest pharmaceu-

tical companies spent billions of dollars on developing a product to promote liver health, they could not do any better than Mother Nature. Milk thistle has three major roles (see Part 3 for details): (1) Substances in milk thistle actually line up on the cells of the liver and protect them from damage. (2) Milk thistle stimulates growth of liver cells. (3) The antioxidants in milk thistle also contribute to protecting the liver from damage.

Clinical studies on people with liver damage, from disease or exposure to toxins, have demonstrated that milk thistle can help restore liver function. If you think your lifestyle, environmental exposure, alcohol consumption, or drugs you take may be affecting your liver, milk thistle is one supplement you should make sure you get every day. The effects of taking milk thistle are usually seen within only six to eight weeks. For those of you who are concerned about preventing and maintaining liver health, look for a comprehensive dietary

Supplement Facts™

Buyer's Guide for Liver Health Supplement Products

Maintain daily supplement intake of these supplements to promote or maintain liver health.

Supplement Ingredient	Safe and Effective Daily Supplement Dosage Range	Comments	Your Personal Daily Supplement Intake Notes Section
If you are at risk of liver damage from the chemicals you inhale at your workplace, if you drink alcohol, take drugs that are known or suspected of damaging your liver, or have hepatitis or other diseases of the liver, then try this supplement combination to complement your doctor's treatment, or as a protective measure against developing a liver problem in the first place.			
Milk thistle extract (70% to 80% silymarin)	420 mg to 800 mg	Milk thistle extract has been shown to reverse liver damage due to alcohol consumption and disease	
Curcumin (85% to 98% curcuminoids)	750 mg to 1,500 mg	Also shown to protect the liver and reduce inflammation	
Cysteine or N-acetylcysteine	300 mg to 600 mg	These nutrients will provide additional protective action in the liver	
L-methionine	500 mg to 1,000 mg		

supplement that contains milk thistle. Refer to the table above for other ingredients commonly found along with milk thistle in liver health formulas.

Products

Goldshield Natural Care Silymarin

Herbscience Milk Thistle Extract

Nature's Way Thisilgn

Solgar Herbal Liver Health

Solgar Milk Thistle Herb Extract

Sundown Milk Thistle

Tree of Life Milk Thistle

13

Mind Wellness, Memory, and Mental Clarity Dietary Supplements

Around 1994 a national advertising campaign for ginkgo products captured the attention of many. Ginkgo, which has its origin in Asia, has been used for many decades in Europe to help promote mental function and circulatory health. The success of these ginkgo products in the U.S. market paved the way for a variety of other dietary supplement ingredients purported to have additional beneficial effects on the mind.

Keeping the brain and nervous system in working order is essential to the health and proper functioning of the entire body. When these degenerate, thought, function, and movement are all negatively affected. What scientists have determined, as with other degenerative conditions, is that there is a nutrition connection. Inadequate intake of key nutrients is associated with speeding up the breakdown of brain and nervous system tissues, manifesting itself with symptoms of impaired mental function. As with the other nutritional-related degenerative dis-

orders, brain wellness can be maintained, and promotion of brain function can be restored in cases of mental dementias.

Remember that it is better to keep the mind and nervous system healthy in the first place. Starting to take products such as *Ginkgo biloba* extract as a young adult will help keep your mind healthy and vibrant. For those mature individuals who are experiencing a decline in mental function, ginkgo has been shown to restore mental function and alertness in the majority of people examined. Though it is not a cure for Alzheimer's disease, it can help slow the disease's progression and improve the patient's quality of life.

One way scientists believe ginkgo works is by protecting the nerves and brain from free radicals. This is possible because ginkgo contains a powerful antioxidant. Also, studies have documented that ginkgo extract is very effective in increasing microcirculation, treating venous insufficiency and edema of

Supplement Facts™

Buyer's Guide for Mental Wellness Supplement Products

Use some or all of the following supplements to help maintain and restore mental function. For serious conditions in adults such as dementias, memory loss, and Alzheimer's Disease, consider using all of the following brain wellness–enhancing supplement ingredients, under doctor supervision.

Supplement Ingredient	Safe and Effective Daily Supplement Dosage Range	Comments	Your Personal Daily Supplement Intake Notes Section
Ginkgo biloba extract (25% ginkgo flavo-glycosides, 6% lactones)	80 mg to 140 mg	Ginkgo and gotu kola help promote circulation to the brain and are neuroprotective	
Gotu kola (8% to 10% triterpenes or asiaticosides)	100 mg to 150 mg		
Phosphatidyl-serine	300 mg to 600 mg	Works to improve nervous system structure and function	
DHA	250 mg to 1,000 mg	DHA improves nerve structure. DHA is also suitable for improving intelligence in children, 250 mg to 750 mg	
Acetyl-L-carnitine (ALC)	1 g to 2 g	Like carnitine, ALC improves cellular energy and function. The ALC form has better bioactivity in brain tissues	
Vitamin E	800 IU to 1,600 IU	Increase vitamin E intake to improve nervous system tissue health from its neuroprotection activity	
Lipoic acid	120 mg to 240 mg		
Lecithin	6 g to 12 g		
For Sufferers of Migraine Headaches: Try using Feverfew extract, which has been shown to reduce the frequency of migraine headaches and their occurrence.			
Feverfew extract (0.2% parthenolide)	125 mg to 400 mg	It may take a few months for benefits to be experienced	

the lower limbs due to poor circulation, and improving physical endurance.

Other dietary supplement ingredients that you will see touted as having beneficial effects on brain wellness include phosphatidylserine, choline, the B vitamins, lipoic acid, DHA, and gotu kola, for example. So in addition to your core vitamin and mineral dietary supplement program, you may wish to try one or several of these mental-wellness-enhancing supplement ingredients. After only a few weeks of taking them you should see benefits such as better memory, increased rate of learning, improved concentration, and greater mental clarity and sharpness. The scientific evidence also suggests that use of these nootropics, or "smart nutrients," may protect against senile dementia and other nervous system and brain disorders that can occur later in life.

Products

Country Life Lecithin

Ginkoba

GNC Natural Brand Ginkgo

Goldshield Acumen

Goldshield Memoloba

Herbscience Ginkgo extract

Herbscience Gotu Kola with Guarana

Medicine Shoppe Feverfew Extract

Medicine Shoppe Ginkgo Extract

Nature's Way Feverfew

Quanterra Ginkgo

Solaray Phosphatidylserine 100 mg

Sundown Feverfew

Sundown Ginkgo Biloba

Sundown Gotu Kola

Tree of Life Feverfew

Tree of Life Kava Kava

Tree of Life Lecithin

Tree of Life Memoryplex with
    Phosphatidylserine

Tree of Life Neuromins DHA

Tree of Life St. John's Wort

Tree of Life Valerian

TruNature Ginkgo

Your Life Feverfew Concentrate

14

Men's Health Dietary Supplements

As men age, they experience changes in metabolism and hormone levels, and different types of problems can occur. Two that most men will experience involve the prostate gland and sexual function. Some natural products are sold as dietary supplements to help promote health of the prostate, and some advertise that they can restore sexual performance.

The major botanical extract you will encounter for promotion of health of the prostate gland is saw palmetto extract. A vast majority of men will experience difficulties with their prostate gland as they age, including enlargement of the prostate, which can cause pain when urinating and other related problems. In several well-controlled clinical studies saw palmetto was demonstrated to improve the health of the prostate gland and help restore proper urinary function. The most recent research has even shown that taking saw palmetto will help shrink an enlarged prostate. A word of

caution: Because prostate cancer becomes increasingly common as males age, any kind of disorder of the prostate gland should be evaluated by your doctor to make sure that your prostate problem is benign and doesn't escalate into a serious disease. If you are looking for relief of benign prostatic hyperplasia, it will comfort you to know that saw palmetto extract has been proven to be safe and effective for treatment of this condition. Improvement is usually seen within three to six weeks with regular use of a high-quality saw palmetto supplement. Some other ingredients to help with prostate health, including reduction of the risk of prostate cancer, are lycopene, pygeum, and nettle root.

With the advent of the drug Viagra, there have been many products positioned as natural Viagra alternatives. Let me clear up a few things concerning these male potency products. There are several nutritional strategies that can be used to help promote

Supplement Facts™

Buyer's Guide for Male Health Concerns

Use these supplements for prostate health and to promote healthy sexual function.

Supplement Ingredient	Safe and Effective Daily Supplement Dosage Range	Comments	Your Personal Daily Supplement Intake Notes Section
Ingredients for Prostate Health: The following supplement ingredients have been shown in clinical studies to improve prostate health and restore sexual performance due to prostate gland complications.			
Saw palmetto (80% to 95% phytosterols)	160 mg to 320 mg	Number one choice for prostate health; use to treat BPH. Saw palmetto works fine on its own, but pygeum and nettle root also have similar benefits and may provide extra benefits when taken together	
Pygeum (10% to 13% phytosterols)	100 mg to 200 mg	Also effective in maintaining prostate health; use to treat BPH	
Nettle root (0.8% to 2% phytosterols)	400 mg to 800 mg	Helps maintain prostate health; use to treat BPH	
Lycopene	10 mg to 60 mg	Higher intake is related to lower risks of prostate cancer	
Aphrodisiacs? Scientific research has determined that the following supplement ingredients can be effective in promoting male sexual function. However, be patient; it takes several weeks for improvements to be experienced.			
Ginkgo biloba (25% ginkgo flavoglycosides, 6% lactones)	40 mg to 120 mg	Use ginkgo and arginine for improving circulation	
Arginine	1,000 mg to 3,000 mg		
Ginseng (4% to 24% ginsenosides)	100 mg to 600 mg	Ginseng and tribulus improve hormonal balance and promote sexual function	
Tribulus (20% to 40% furanosterols)	250 mg to 600 mg		

healthy sexual function in males. However, at this time there are no clinically tested natural alternatives to Viagra. The drug Viagra has a very specific biochemical action in the body. When a male gets sexually aroused, the levels of a substance called cGMP begin to increase, allowing blood to accumulate in the penis and resulting in an erection. Some men experience erection problems because not enough cGMP is produced. Viagra works to prevent the breakdown of cGMP, and so enough can accumulate to allow a full erection to occur. At this time no natural products have been shown to do exactly the same thing that Viagra does.

Viagra aside, good circulatory system health, good energy levels, and proper body weight are all factors in healthy sexual performance, and nutritional strategies can help you achieve these goals. You may also wish to try supplements such as ginkgo, ginseng, tribulus, yohimbe, or products containing combinations of these.

Products

Goldshield Prostate Plus

Herbscience Saw Palmetto with Pygeum

Herbscience Yohimbe with Avena Sativa

Medicine Shoppe Saw Palmetto Extract

Quanterra Saw Palmetto

Spring Valley Men's One Daily

Sundown Nettle

Sundown Saw Palmetto

Tree of Life Saw Palmetto

TruNature Saw Palmetto

15

Relaxation, Antistress, and Sleep-Promoting Dietary Supplements

It is well known that in our fast-paced, hectic culture many people are over-stressed and have dysfunctional sleep patterns. Some of the most widely used drugs are those used for their calming effect, to reduce anxiety, and to promote restful sleep. Dietary supplement manufacturers have responded by formulating and marketing a variety of nutrition-based products to help promote relaxation, reduce stress, and encourage a good night's sleep.

One of my favorite products to help relieve stress and promote muscular relaxation while also improving mental focus and concentration is an herb called kava (or kava kava). Kava has been used for hundreds of years in the South Pacific as a beverage taken at night to help promote relaxation. In fact, as the story goes, some South Pacific cultures would give kava drinks to adversaries before they were brought together in court or at the negotiating table, to keep them from getting excited and to prevent arguments. I find kava is very useful during

times when I start to get edgy and feel my body becoming more reactive due to over-work and mental overload. Studies have shown that kava is an effective antianxiety herbal treatment; because it relieves anxiety, it also can help people who are having stress-related sleep problems. Another thing kava does is to relax muscles. Typically the muscle-relaxant benefits are felt after a short time—a day or two—and it takes about seven to ten days to experience the full antianxiety effects of kava, though studies have shown that anxiety-related symptoms tend to start to diminish within a few days. People using kava supplements report an improved sense of well-being and a feeling of having more control over their emotions.

There are a few sleep-enhancing dietary supplement products available on the market that have good science behind them and can be useful when used appropriately. One dietary supplement ingredient, melatonin, received some good press as a result of several clinical studies showing that it helps you get to sleep quicker, stay asleep, and reach a more restful deep sleep. This is no surprise if you understand how your body's own melatonin helps promote your natural sleep-wake cycles. Melatonin levels start to increase at night, in darkness. The increase in melatonin helps induce a restful state, which is most desirable for sleep. When your natural nighttime melatonin levels are reduced due to aging, staying up at night with the lights on, stressful conditions, exposure to a significant amount of electromagnetic radiation, or pathological or chemically induced conditions, it can result in sleep dysfunction. Melatonin may help in such cases.

Another botanical product that I employ sometimes myself is valerian. From its use in Europe, we know that valerian is a safe and effective natural way to induce and promote proper sleep. Physiologically, research has determined that valerian contains substances that help increase production of calming neurotransmitters in the brain and nervous system. When using natural sleep aids such as valerian, keep in mind that each individual will respond differently. Some people experience beneficial effects the very first night they take these products, while others may need several days to see a response.

One of the most popular products in the mood-altering supplements category is St. John's wort. In numerous clinical studies conducted in Europe, St. John's wort has been shown to be effective in treating mild to moderate depression, anxiety, and some sleep disorders. While St. John's wort is marketed for its antidepressive properties in Europe, such a claim is not currently permitted in the United States; rather, you will see it being marketed as a supplement for promoting positive mood or improving well-being. St. John's wort is best used under a doctor's supervision, and you should avoid using it in conjunction with other drugs, especially MAO inhibitors. When using St. John's wort, it usually takes a few weeks to start experiencing significant improvements in your mood. Refer to the table on the following page for a list of some of the other dietary supplement ingredients in this category, such as tyrosine, phenylalanine, and 5-HTP.

Products
Goldshield Natural Care St. John's Wort
Herbscience Kava Kava
Herbscience St. John's Wort
Herbscience Valerian
Herbscience Valerian with Passionflower
Kavatrol
Medicine Shoppe Kava Kava
Medicine Shoppe St. John's Wort
Medicine Shoppe Valerian Root
Movana
Natrol Melatonin
Natrol SAM-Sulfate
Natrol St. John's Wort
Nature Made SAMe
Now SAMe
Schiff Melatonin
Solgar SAM

Supplement Facts™

Buyer's Guide for Promoting Relaxation, Antistress, and Sleep

These are the clinically proven supplement ingredients shown to work to make you calmer, more relaxed, less depressed, and sleep better.

Supplement Ingredient	Safe and Effective Daily Supplement Dosage Range	Comments	Your Personal Daily Supplement Intake Notes Section
For antianxiety, kava kava has the best clinical track record. You will also find that some combination formulas contain some of the other ingredients contained in this list to work as cofactors. But the research confirms that kava kava reins supreme when it comes to combating anxiety.			
Kava extract (30% kavalactones)	200 mg to 400 mg	Use periodically for antianxiety effects	
For Sleep: If you are having trouble falling and staying asleep, give these supplements a try. They work gentler on your system than drugs and may take a few days for improvement to be experienced.			
Valerian (0.8% to 1% valernic acid)	200 mg to 400 mg	Use alone or in combination with melatonin and/or chamomile	
Melatonin	500 mcg	For short periods of time, a few weeks	
Chamomile (1.2% to 2% apigenin and 0.5% terpenoids)	250 mg to 500 mg	Chamomile can promote additional relaxation and sleep-inducing effects	
For Depression: If you think you experience mild to moderate depression, then St. John's wort is the most clinically verified botanical to help restore your positive mood. You can also try taking some of the central nervous system amino acids, known to help make neurotransmitters that may need a nutritional boost as well.			
St. John's wort (0.3% hypericin)	300 mg to 900 mg	Try St. John's wort first for a few weeks, then add in one or more of following amino acids or SAMe, which will help calm and relax. I don't recommend mixing St. John's wort with amino acids without medical supervision. People may develop hyperserotonergic symptoms (irritability, poor concentration, headache, etc.) from too much serotonin production, which is potentially fatal	
L-tyrosine	1,000 mg to 3,000 mg	Use especially if you think your depression is due to stress	
SAMe	400 mg to 1,600 mg	Use SAMe especially if you have depression as a side effect of arthritis	
D,L-Phenylalanine	1,000 mg to 3,000 mg		
5-HTP (hydroxy-tryptophan)	50 mg to 300 mg	Listed under tryptophan, 5-HTP helps restore serotonin levels. It can also help promote restful sleep	

Source Naturals Melatonin

Sundown Kava Kava

Sundown St. John's Wort

Sundown Valerian

TruNature St. John's Wort

YourLife Advanced Strength Kava Kava

YourLife St. John's Wort and Kava Kava

YourLife Valerian Concentrate

16

Urinary Tract Health Dietary Supplements

During the 1990s scientists finally confirmed the folk remedy of drinking cranberry juice to prevent or treat urinary tract infection. Now cranberry juice extract is sold as a dietary supplement to promote urinary tract and bladder health. It can help you avoid the high amounts of sugar found in many commercial cranberry juice drinks.

Clinical studies have shown that the phytochemicals in cranberry juice prevent bacteria from sticking to the inner wall of the urinary tract and thus reduce the incidence of urinary tract infection. It is important to understand that cranberry juice extract does not kill bacteria. If you do have a bacterial infection, make sure that you are undergoing proper medical supervision and treatment. For those who are under treatment, drinking cranberry juice and taking cranberry extract supplements can help facilitate recovery. Cranberry extract can also help reduce the frequency of urinary tract infections in some people.

Products
Goldshield Natural Care Cranberry
    Extract
Herbscience Cranberry Extract
Medicine Shoppe Cranberry Extract
Sundown Cranberry
Tree of Life Cranberry
YourLife Cranberry Concentrate

Supplement Facts™

Buyer's Guide for Urinary Tract Health Supplement Products

Research findings support the use of cranberry extract, uvi ursi, and immunostimulants in your quest for an infection-free urinary tract.

Supplement Ingredient	Safe and Effective Daily Supplement Dosage Range	Comments	Your Personal Daily Supplement Intake Notes Section
Cranberry extract (22% to 30% organic acids)	500 mg to 2,000 mg	Take cranberry extract supplements to combat urinary tract infections or help prevent them	
Uvi ursi extract (20% to 30% arbutin)	100 mg to 300 mg	Also include a uvi ursi supplement in your urinary tract health plan	
Immuno-stimulants	See Chapter 10	When you are experiencing infection, along with your doctor's prescribed medication, try taking the immunostimulates to boost your natural infection-fighting immune system	

17

Vision Health
Dietary Supplements

Bilberry has long had a folk reputation for improving vision. During World War II Royal Air Force pilots tried eating bilberries before flying their night missions, and in fact noticed an improvement in their night vision. Subsequently, scientific research has determined that bilberry contains certain phytonutrients that indeed help the eyes function better and also help protect the eyes from certain types of macular degeneration (deterioration of the center of the retina). Anyone concerned with maintaining eye function and preventing or treating eye disease may wish to add bilberry to the supplement regimen. Refer to the entry on bilberry in Part 3 for more details on exactly how it works to produce these phenomenal results.

Another key part of maintaining visual health is not to overstress your eyes. There are weeks when I have to read through literally thousands of pages of information, and so I know firsthand how the light reflected off white pages contributes to eye fatigue.

While bilberry will help ameliorate the symptoms of eye fatigue, you need to pay attention to how your eyes respond to different workloads. If you are suffering from eye fatigue, try to avoid long periods of intensive reading; spread out the work over a longer period, with frequent breaks. Look up now and then and focus for a minute or two at a longer distance.

Some other dietary supplement ingredients helpful for promoting eye health include lutein, beta-carotene, zeaxanthin, taurine, lipoic acid, and ginkgo, which has a high affinity for the retina and has been shown to prevent macular degeneration and other retinal diseases. These twenty-first-century antioxidants, along with the traditional antioxidants such as vitamin C and vitamin E, all effectively protect your eyes as well as other parts of the body; epidemiological evidence indicates that higher levels of these antioxidants may protect against macular degeneration.

Supplement Facts™

Buyer's Guide for Vision Health Supplement Products

Declining vision performance can be prevented or delayed with the regular intake of certain supplements. Give these a try if you are experiencing vision disorders such as eye fatigue, visual acuity problems, night vision, macular degeneration, and cataracts.

Supplement Ingredient	Safe and Effective Daily Supplement Dosage Range	Comments	Your Personal Daily Supplement Intake Notes Section
Bilberry (25% anthocyanidins)	80 mg to 280 mg	Use bilberry on a regular basis, and higher amounts if you are nutritionally treating an eye disorder	
		Add extra amounts of the key essential vision nutrients, and special nutrients to help promote/restore vision	
Lutein	25 mg to 100 mg	Especially useful for people experiencing macular degeneration	
Extra vitamin C	1,000 mg to 3,000 mg		
Extra beta-carotene	15,000 IU to 30,000 IU		
Extra vitamin E	600 IU to 1,000 IU		
L-taurine	500 mg to 1,500 mg		
Zeaxanthin (carotenoids)	15 mg to 40 mg		
Lipoic acid	15 mg to 60 mg		
Ginkgo biloba extract (25% ginkgo flavo-glycosides, 6% lactones)	80 mg	For added antioxidant protection of the retina	

Products

Futurebiotics Bilberry Extract

Goldshield Eye Formula

Medicine Shoppe Bilberry Extract

Solaray Lutein Eyes

Solgar Lutein Lycopene Carotene
    Complex

Twinlab OcuGard Plus with Lutein

Windmill L-Taurine

YourLife Bilberry Extract

YourLife Lutein

18

Weight Loss
Dietary Supplements

In fighting the proverbial battle of the bulge, the most important ammunition is the establishment of proper eating habits and appetite control. While there are many nutritional aids that can help you in this quest, my thirty years of experience in weight management, combined with much research on the dynamics of weight management and weight loss, make it clear that you must first and foremost approach eating as a skill. While it is true that exercise and certain supplements can help with appetite control and improving and maintaining a vibrant metabolism, they need to be used in conjunction with a proper eating plan. To assist you in this endeavor, and to help sort through the many misconceptions that are perpetuated in the numerous diet books on the market, I have included a special bonus section for you, the Natural-Thin program, in the Appendix.

Many people binge, or they skip meals during the day and tend to overeat at night.

Other people do okay during the week but live it up with an all-you-can-eat weekend buffet. You need to acknowledge the fact that regularly overeating at any meal will condition your body to more easily store the excess calories as fat. You need to exercise your willpower at every meal and during snack time. Stick to eating a smaller number of calories at each meal, which you will use up for energy and not store as body fat. Keep in mind, too, that as you age, your metabolic rate will be reduced and your body will burn fewer calories.

Try to include more fiber in your diet; this controls your appetite by slowing down the rate at which your stomach empties. Keep high-fat and high-calorie foods out of your house, so you won't eat them all up in a binge. Stock up on low-calorie, high-fiber foods such as vegetables; a pound of most vegetables contains only about 160 calories.

If you have a weight problem, you must first acknowledge that this can stem from many factors: eating the wrong foods, over-eating, inactivity, a reduced metabolism due to aging, or other lifestyle factors. On the bright side, it doesn't take that much effort to get on the right track toward a healthy weight. The beneficial side effects of finding and staying on this track include a slimmer, trimmer, more energetic, and more attractive body, and a healthy cardiovascular system.

There are many supplements that help improve your body's metabolic rate. The trace mineral chromium is a cofactor for the proper function of insulin, the hormone that signals cells to let in nutrients that are circulating in the bloodstream after a meal, and adequate amounts of chromium will ensure that more nutrients make it into your cells, where they can be used for energy and growth, instead of being circulated back to the liver and converted to fat.

Carnitine is one of the supplements sold as lipotropics. Carnitine has been shown to increase the rate of fat loss for many people as well. Carnitine optimizes the conversion of fatty acids to energy within the cell, stimulating your fat-burning metabolism. Recent clinical studies show that taking carnitine supplements resulted in study participants losing more fat than from diet and exercise alone. Other fat-fighting nutrients to look for include choline, inositol, and methionine.

Natural appetite suppressants are leading the category of weight loss supplements. A relative newcomer, 5-HTP (which can also help calm you down) can aid in appetite control. Next on the list is *Garcinia cambogia,* also called brindall berry. This botanical can help control appetite and may also help block the formation of fat from carbohydrates in the liver.

Supplement companies also offer botanical diuretics to help reduce excess water weight. Traditionally, diuretics are used in the treatment of menstrual distress, edema, and hypertension, but dieters have turned to diuretics to help reduce edema and the bloated feeling common to being overweight. You can purchase botanical diuretics such as uva ursi. I don't advocate the use of these types of supplements unless under a doctor's supervision. I know it is satisfying to see quick results on the scale; however, remember that the weight lost is just water, and it will return as fast as you lost it.

Fiber and fat-absorbing supplements also fall into the weight loss aid category. Eating more fibrous foods, such as non-starchy vegetables, and taking fiber supplements, including psyllium, guar gum, and citrus pectin, will help improve your digestion and appetite control and decrease the amount of fat absorbed in the intestines. Studies have shown that chitosan can help absorb and lock on to ingested fats, thereby keeping some of them from entering your body.

The last major type of weight loss aid, thermogenics, has been the subject of controversy in the media and at the FDA for

Supplement Facts™

Buyer's Guide for Weight Loss and Weight Management Supplement Products

Try one or more supplement weight loss aids, as you require. Remember that these nutritional weight loss aids can help improve your rate of fat loss and appetite control, but you need to additionally follow a calorie-restricted diet; see Natural-Thin Weight Loss Approach, Appendix.

Supplement Ingredient	Safe and Effective Daily Supplement Dosage Range	Comments	Your Personal Daily Supplement Intake Notes Section
L-carnitine	1 g to 3 g	Helps to burn more fat	
5-HTP	50 mg to 200 mg	Helps control appetite	
Garcinia (50% HCA)	500 mg to 750 mg, 3 times a day with meals	Helps control appetite and slows the conversion of carbohydrates to fats in the liver	
Extra chromium	400 mcg to 600 mcg	Can enhance fat metabolism in some people	
Fiber supplements	5 g to 25 g	Take with meals to slow digestion and reduce fat absorption	
L-tyrosine	500 mg to 1,500 mg	Helps with appetite control	
L-phenylalanine	500 mg to 1,500 mg	Helps with appetite control	
Chitosan	Use as directed with meals	Helps absorb fat in the intestines to prevent its absorption into the body. You usually need 500 mg to 1,500 mg taken with each meal. Loose bowel movements are a common side effect	
Caffeine containing thermogenic aids, such as green tea, guarana, and yerba mate.	Use as directed by manufacturer	Can help increase your metabolic rate (increases the calories you burn). But don't abuse or overdose	
7-KETO™	50 mg to 200 mg	A new compound, shown to aid in weight loss by stimulating thermogenesis without side effects.	

several years. Just as exercise will boost the rate at which you burn calories, so can the foods you eat (which are included in the Natural-Thin program) and botanical supplements. Supplements considered safe include guarana, yerba mate, and ginseng. Then there is the champion of thermogenic aids, ephedra, which is widely sold and used by millions; however, some people may experience potentially harmful side effects when using supplements containing ephedra (see Part 3 for details).

When losing weight, remember the golden rules:

- Do so under a doctor's supervision.
- Do not overeat.
- Do not skip meals.
- Spread out your calories over five or six meals/snacks.
- Follow a nutritionally balanced low-fat diet.
- Exercise regularly.
- Take your nutrition supplements.

- Maintain a healthy rate of weight loss, one to two pounds per week.
- Eliminate foods you are allergic to.
- Have fun! Eating less is not more work, it's less work (and it's cheaper).

Products

Dr. Shari Lieberman's For Women Only
   Advanced Weight Control System
Dr. Shari Lieberman's For Zero Fat
Goldshield Lipobind
Goldshield Results Meal Replacement
Goldshield 7-Keto Thermogenic
Goldshield SQ7 Slim Quick Programme
Lite Bites
Natrol Citramax Plus
Solgar L-Phenylalanine
Twinlab MegaCitrimax
Windmill L-Phenylalanine
YourLife Chitosan
YourLife L-Carnitine

19

Women's Health Dietary Supplements

Just as there are certain dietary supplement products that help promote men's health, there are products to help nutritionally improve women's health. These products consider a woman's unique metabolism and hormonal differences, monthly variations in hormone levels, and reproductive changes throughout the course of life. You will find a number of products that are marketed as reducing the discomfort associated with the menstrual cycle, products called PMS supplements, and products for easing the symptoms of menopause. There is a lot of good research backing the use of certain vitamins, minerals, and botanicals for each of these uses.

Women's health issues have become such an important national concern that the FDA has established the Office of Women's Health to test FDA-regulated products in women, support research and education to increase knowledge of women's health issues, and form partnerships with other govern-

ment agencies and advocacy groups to advance women's health concerns. Some of the most pressing issues of interest to the Office of Women's Health include cancer screening and treatment; sexually transmitted diseases; contraception, pregnancy, and childbirth; hormone replacement therapy for menopause; autoimmune diseases; cardiovascular disease; and osteoporosis and other diseases affecting older women. See their Web site at http://www.fda.gov/womens. Also see the Web site of the National Women's Health Information Center (http://www. 4women.org), a gateway for women seeking health information on over one hundred health topics from acne to weight loss. It also has current health news, dictionaries, phone numbers, and links to other Web sites. When visiting these and other self-help Web sites, keep in mind that they are not intended to replace supervision by a health professional. Also keep in mind that these sites are usually not on the cutting edge in terms of using supplements and nutrition to prevent or treat diseases and promote health and well-being.

The first step for women in improving their health is to follow a healthy diet, using the guidelines in Chapter 4 and the Appendix. Avoid substances known to cause health problems, such as alcohol, tobacco, and excessive caffeine intake. A daily multinutrient supplement is an important part of any health program as well; follow the guidelines in Chapter 5 for designing a daily supplement program that will help you live longer, stay healthy, and give birth to healthier children.

PMS AND MENOPAUSE

Among the plethora of women's health issues, reducing the side effects of PMS and menopause with dietary supplements ranks at the top of the list. A healthy diet with adequate intake of calcium and magnesium is the first step in combating discomfort from PMS and menopause. Also, there are two main botanical products that have been clinically shown to help reduce many of the adverse effects associated with menopause. Black cohosh has been shown to reduce hot flashes and other associated symptoms, such as sweating and nervousness, within three to four weeks of beginning its use. Reducing the amount of total fats in the diet and increasing the consumption of soy products has also been shown to alleviate these problems as well as reduce breast tenderness. Products that have been shown to

reduce feelings of depression or anxiety during menopause include St. John's wort and kava (see Chapter 15). If you find that you are still suffering from PMS after three months of eating right and taking appropriate supplements, then there are two other botanical supplements you can try. Chaste tree berry *(Vitex agnus-castus)* is said to have a normalizing effect on levels of sex hormones, particularly prolactin, which has been associated with some PMS symptoms, including swollen and tender breasts, and may help to reestablish normal menstruation. Another herb of Asian origin noted as a female health tonic is dong quai. Use of dong quai has been shown to normalize menstruation, improve blood flow, and reduce menstrual cramps. Dong quai is also an adaptogen associated with restoring energy levels, and may exert a mild laxative effect on some people.

There is accumulating evidence that soy products are especially helpful for women. Specific isoflavones found in soy, genistein and daidzein, exhibit phytoestrogenic activity. Phytoestrogens have been demonstrated to decrease the number and severity of hot flashes among menopausal women. In fact, in his review of this book, Dr. J. Zeuss pointed out that in his experience, menopausal symptoms, including hot flashes, etc., are completely eliminated just by drinking soy milk—two cups daily. Also, experimental data from animals and population studies suggest that the phytoestrogenic and antioxidant activity of isoflavones may lower a woman's risk of breast cancer and endometrial cancer. Analysis of several studies has shown that increased soy consumption is associated with reduction of total cholesterol levels, LDL cholesterol, and triglycerides; this may be due to the isoflavone content. Finally, phytoestrogens may also help reduce bone loss and the risk of osteoporosis, since genistein has been found to bind to estrogen receptors in bone, and we know that estrogen inhibits the activity of osteoclasts, cells that break down bone.

Green tea is another useful supplement with wide-ranging benefits that include reduction of cancer risk and improvement of cardiovascular health; brewed green tea and green tea supplements can be an important component of any woman's supplement program, especially during menopause.

PREGNANCY

Nutritional issues in pregnancy are a major concern for many women, and though they are beyond the scope of this book, there is no doubt that eating well, using appropriate supplements, and making sure your lifestyle is healthy are all important factors for a healthy pregnancy. Consult with your doctor to make sure you are getting enough of essential nutrients such as iron, zinc, copper, vitamin B_6, folic acid, vitamin C, and vitamin D. Additionally, pregnant women should supplement with omega-3's, too, or at least eat fish several times weekly. Make sure, too, that you are not taking too much

vitamin A in the form of acetate or palmitate; excessive intake of these forms of vitamin A are associated with certain types of birth defects.

You may wish to consult *Nutrition During Pregnancy,* published by the Institute of Medicine, National Academy of Sciences. This report contains a section on the use of supplements during pregnancy.

SKIN

One pioneering product that claims to help reduce the appearance of wrinkles, increase the thickness of the skin, and improve skin's overall appearance is Imedeen, a European product. Indeed, its active components are marine proteins that are basically similar to glucosamine and that stimulate the health of connective tissue, which is a major component of skin. Glucosamine also is a component in the body's production of hyaluronic acid, a natural internal moisturizer.

Other botanicals that can protect against breakdown of connective tissue, specifically elastin, are grape seed extract and Pycnogenol.

Products
Amerifit Estroven
Challenge Soy Solution
Dr. Shari Lieberman's For Women Only
    Advanced Changes for PMS and
    Menopause
Dr. Shari Lieberman's For Women
    Only Advanced Rejuvicare Skin
    Nutritional

Supplement Facts™

Buyer's Guide for Women's Health Supplement Products

In addition to following your healthy eating and supplement program, as presented in Chapters 4 and 5, here are some additional supplements women may wish to take for promoting female health.

Supplement Ingredient	Safe and Effective Daily Supplement Dosage Range	Comments	Your Personal Daily Supplement Intake Notes Section
For PMS: Try using either or both of these herbs to reduce PMS discomfort and menstrual irregularities. Include GLA if PMS pain persists.			
Chaste tree berry (0.5% agnuside, 0.6% acubin)	80 mg to 120 mg	If after 3 months of taking your core nutritional supplement program, eating right, and increasing physical activity you still have discomfort, then start taking chaste tree berry and/or angelica. You can expect to feel relief of annoying PMS symptoms within 3 months	
Angelica (1% ligustilide)	200 mg to 600 mg		
GLA	250 mg to 400 mg	Optional; if you are still experiencing PMS pain, give this a try. GLA can help reduce inflammatory substances in your body if you have low production levels. Usually supplied from evening primrose oil	
For Menopause: Most annoying menopausal symptoms are due to high leutinizing hormone levels and/or lower estrogen levels. Before turning to hormone replacement therapy, you may want to try taking black cohosh and soy isoflavones containing supplements.			
Black cohosh (2% to 2.5% triterpenes)	100 mg to 300 mg	Best for relieving hot flashes and other annoying discomfort associated with menopause. Note: black cohosh is also effective in the treatment of PMS and dysmenorrhea	
Soy isoflavones	40 mg to 60 mg	Also increases in soy protein from soy foods and soy protein drinks, 15 g to 25 g per day. Isoflavones and other phyto-chemicals exhibit phytoestrogenic activity and have been shown to compensate for low estrogen levels in some women	
For Better Skin: Aging, sagging, and wrinkled skin is due in part to the breakdown of connective tissues that support the skin and poor hydration. Providing your body with a connective tissue nutrient that can help maintain or rebuild the connective tissue matrix is the first step in promoting healthy, beautiful skin. Preventing skin damage from ultraviolet light and free radicals is also important. These supplements can help revitalize your skin.			
Glucosamine sulfate or HCl	500 mg to 1,500 mg	Glucosamine can thicken skin, reduce wrinkles, and improve hydration, all from within	
Pycnogenol	40 mg to 100 mg	A potent antioxidant that also contains phytonutrients, which protect collagen and elastin from being broken down	
Grape seed extract (50% to 85% pro-anthocyanidines)	60 mg to 120 mg	Similar functions to Pycnogenol. You can take both together, or just one	
Gotu kola (8% to 10% triterpenes or asiaticosides)	50 mg to 150 mg	Helps protect and support the growth of skin	
Varicose Veins: In Europe, one of the leading products for preventing and treating varicose veins is horse chestnut seed extract.			
Horse chestnut extract (13% to 24% aescin)	150 mg to 600 mg	Give this a try if you have varicose veins or believe you are susceptible to developing them. Also useful for treating hemorrhoids	

Supplement Ingredient	Safe and Effective Daily Supplement Dosage Range	Comments	Your Personal Daily Supplement Intake Notes Section
Ginkgo biloba (25% ginkgo flavoglycosides, 6% lactones)	80 mg to 140 mg	Ginkgo will also improve circulatory system health. Try taking both for a few months to help stimulate improvements in vein structure and function	

Dr. Shari Lieberman's For Women Only Soy Solutions Smoothie

Dr. Shari Lieberman's For Women Only Venipro

GNC Meno-Poise

GNC Natural Brand Soy Protein

GNC Phyto-Estrogen

GNC Women's EPO

GNC Women's Ultra Mega

Goldshield Equitem 40 Plus

Goldshield Evening Primrose Oil

Goldshield Super GLA

Herbscience Black Cohosh with Chaste Tree Berry

Herbscience Dong Quai with Soy Isoflavone

Hyperacine—A Special Formula for Treating Acne

Medicine Shoppe Black Cohosh Extract

Medicine Shoppe Evening Primrose Oil

Promensil—Isoflavones

Remifemin—Black Cohosh

Ricola Herbal Health Women's Formula

Shiff Breast Health

Shiff Menopause Nutritional System

Shiff PMS Nutritional System

Spring Valley Women's One Daily

Sundown Black Cohosh

Sundown Chasteberry

Sundown Dong Quai

Sundown Ginkgo Biloba

Tree of Life Evening Primrose Oil

Tree of Life Ultra Beauty Complex

Venastat—Horse Chestnut Extract

YourLife Black Cohosh

YourLife Dong Quai

YourLife Evening Primrose Oil

YourLife Healthy Legs Horse Chestnut Seed Extract

Your Life Soy Isoflavones

Part 3

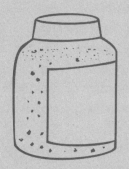

Alphabetical Guide to the Best Dietary Supplement Ingredients

Part 3 is your salvation for understanding the ingredients found in dietary supplements. It's your personal resource for determining which products contain ingredients that work, and what amounts to look for. This part contains a comprehensive alphabetical listing of both common and uncommon dietary supplement ingredients. Common ingredients are those found mostly in conservative national brands, such as Centrum or One-A-Day. Uncommon ingredients are usually seen in specialty brands found in health food stores and sold by direct sales companies.

Here is an example of how the information is presented for each nutritional supplement ingredient and its intended purpose. In order for an ingredient to make the list, it had to pass the criteria of having scientific substantiation that it works. But, please note that there are some ingredients included because they are found frequently in supplement products. In either case, the information found for each entry will enable you to decide if an ingredient is worth considering. Also, you can visit my Web site at supplementfacts.com for additional information.

Name(s). Each entry starts out with the most common name used on dietary supplement labels. Additional names are also included when applicable and may contain other common names and/or scientific names. All botanical entries contain the scientific plant name. This information allows you to be sure what you are buying, since common names may vary. It will also be useful when you discuss supplements with your doctor or pharmacist, whose reference books may not include common names used on supplement products.

Supplement Type. Identifies the supplement ingredient category to which it belongs: vitamins, minerals, amino acids, botanicals, metabolites, etc.

Overview. Under this heading you will find background information on the ingredient, and the ingredient's primary proven functions. I use the phrase "primary proven functions" specifically to indicate that independent clinical studies have been conducted to confirm the functions of the ingredients. There are a few exceptions for ingredients whose traditional use is well founded. I deliberately have not included a long list of "possible benefits," as many books do. I chose this approach in order to enable you to easily identify products that you will benefit most from. You do not need to waste your time and money experimenting.

Benefits. The information under this heading will describe the primary proven benefits of the ingredient supported by scientific consensus, in the "structure/function" language used on dietary supplement product labels. Note that there will be instances where therapeutic benefits are included, due to the reality that very often consumers take a supplement product to help prevent, manage, or treat a disease condition. Remember always to consult with your doctor when taking a supplement product as part of your treatment of a medical condition. Your doctor needs to know what you are ingesting, including drugs, food, and supplements, to monitor your progress and respond intelligently if problems arise. Even when you are taking supplements for the promotion of better overall health, it is wise to let your doctor know.

Ingredient Forms. When applicable, the most common forms of the ingredient are listed. For botanicals, I listed the plant part that the standardized extract is made from; included in parentheses is the phytonutrient the botanical extract is standardized to. In most cases, standardized botanicals are the best forms to use, because these extracts were used in clinical studies to confirm their beneficial effects and because without standardization, it is hard to ensure consistent dosage of the active botanical ingredients. Note that most herbalists and naturopaths will use a combination of products, including dried whole herbs that you make into a tea and nonstandardized herbs in capsule, liquid, and tablet form. But when it comes to mass-producing supplement products for over-the-counter sales, using standardized ingredients is preferred to ensure consistency. I sometimes list particular trade names, since the trend is for suppliers to create brand names for particular ingredients they sell to supplement manufacturers. For example, Activin is a special standardized extract of red grape seeds made by InterHealth Nutraceuticals; Ester-C is a nonacidic form of vitamin C from Inter-Cal; and L-carnipure is a purified form of L-carnitine made by Lonza. In most cases, the manufacturers of these branded supplement ingredients have conducted studies to demonstrate the product's safety and effectiveness.

Effective Supplement Dosages. Under this heading you will find dosages that are reported in the scientific literature to be safe and effective for their intended use. Some ingredients have been shown to be most beneficial when used every day, while others should be used for only short periods of time. Differences in these "nutritional" and "therapeutic" dosages are mentioned when applicable; therapeutic dosages are intended for short-term use only. Do not assume that if 50 mg of a product is supposed to have a beneficial effect, 100 mg is twice as effective; overdosing of any nutrient may cause side effects, sometimes serious ones. Always consult your doctor with questions about a particular supplement's proper dosage. Avoid megadoses of supplements, unless indicated for a particular reason and used under a doctor's supervision.

Cofactors. When applicable I include a list of supplement ingredient cofactors. Cofactors can have similar benefits, or may help the primary ingredient work better. In a few cases, cofactors may also be indicated to supply extra nutrition support due to the nutrient interference action of the primary ingredient. When I

list no cofactors, it means the ingredient alone is sufficient to provide the desired benefits. It does not mean that you will not encounter other ingredients along with it in some supplement formulations.

Concerns. This heading includes cautions associated with the use and abuse of the specific supplement ingredient, or the consequence of not getting enough of an essential nutrient. The term "concern" is used over toxicity or safety, because dietary supplement ingredients are food products that are inherently safe in the dosages found in products sold over the counter. Another reason is that ingredients that are known to be dangerous are not included in this book. This heading will also describe which age groups the ingredients are most suitable for.

Use Guidelines. Under this heading I include summary information to help you decide if you need to take supplements containing the particular ingredient on a regular basis or occasionally, and under what circumstances to take it.

L, D, AND DL-AMINO ACIDS

Molecules sometimes occur in a variety of configurations. To distinguish between the different forms, chemists have devised an elaborate system of nomenclature. As it applies to naming amino acids, when an amino acid has more than one configuration, a D or L may be used to identify which one is in your supplement product. As a general rule, most biologically beneficial amino acids are in the L form. However, there are some instances where the D forms have beneficial effects as well: D-methionine and D-phenylalanine. The difference between the D and L forms concerns how the elements making up the molecules are aligned. D and L forms of the same amino acids are essentially mirror images of each other; however, the official classification system is a bit more complicated and beyond the scope of this book. When you see a product containing DL-methionine or DL-phenylalanine, this indicates that there is approximately an equal mixture of D-phenylalanine and L-phenylalanine in the product. Other nutrients may also have D and L forms, but are most often found among amino acid names, for example, L-carnitine, which is technically not an amino acid. On a final note, some amino acids only exist in one form, and you will not see an L or D used in their name; this is the case with the amino acid glycine.

Acerola (also *Malpighis glabra*)

Supplement Type: Botanical

Overview: The fruit of acerola is high in vitamin C, beta-carotene, bioflavonoids, and other nutrients. It is sometimes used as a dietary supplement ingredient when manufacturers want to include a natural source of vitamin C. Acerola is also known as Barbados cherry and West Indian cherry. The fruit of this shrub is small and red like a cherry. Some people prefer acerola as a vitamin C supplement, because of the other naturally occurring vitamins, minerals, and phytonutrients it contains.

Benefits: Same benefits as vitamin C (refer to vitamin C for details), and those of bioflavonoids.

Ingredient Form: Acerola standardized to 5% or higher ascorbic acid (vitamin C) content, from dry fruit extract.

Effective Supplement Dosages: Safe and effective daily dosages of acerola range from 100 to 1,000 mg per day.

Cofactors: Acerola is commonly found in supplement formulas along with other antioxidants, rose hips, and vitamins and minerals.

Concerns: Acerola is not an essential nutrient, but contains the essential nutrient vitamin C. Refer to vitamin C entry for concerns when there is not enough or too much vitamin C in your diet. Acerola is considered nontoxic when used as directed.

Use Guidelines: Acerola can be consumed every day as part of your daily essential nutrient supplement program. It provides the added benefits of naturally occurring bioflavonoids along with the benefits of vitamin C.

Acetyl-L-Carnitine (ALC): *see* Carnitine

Acidophilus: *see* Probiotics

Adaptogens

The term *adaptogen* was coined by Russian researchers to describe a substance that helps increase the body's resistance to adverse influences, both physical and environmental. An adaptogen is a type of general prevent-all and cure-all. To be a true adaptogen, a substance must be safe for daily use, increase the body's resistance to a wide variety of factors, and have a normalizing action on the body's systems. Some commonly used adaptogens include Arctic Root, ashwaganda, ginseng, reishi mushroom, and siberian ginseng. Adaptogens are useful to healthy individuals as an aid for coping with daily stresses and as a tonic to help maintain normal body functions. They are also used by people suffering from illness in support of therapeutic treatment.

Adrenal extracts: *see* Glandulars

Alanine (also L-alanine)
Supplement Type: Amino acid
Overview: Alanine is classified as a nonessential amino acid because it can be made by the body in adequate amounts to meet metabolic needs. Alanine is involved in an important biochemical process that occurs during exercise, the glucose-alanine cycle. During energy production from glucose, pyruvate is formed, some of which is converted to alanine, which is transported from the exercising muscles to the liver, where it is converted to glucose. Sports physiologists believe that this cycle helps maintain plasma glucose levels during exercise. Likewise, clinical nutritionists recognize alanine's importance in the regulation of glucose metabolism. As more clinical research is performed using alanine-containing dietary supplements, conclusive benefits and dosages will become better established.

Benefits: Use of dietary supplements containing alanine can be useful in sparing muscle glycogen in athletes, and as nutritional support for individuals who experience hypoglycemia due to low body alanine status.

Ingredient Form: Alanine occurs in protein-containing dietary supplements as a part of the protein molecules. It also is added to supplement products in its free form as L-alanine.

Effective Supplement Dosages: Alanine is not commonly added to dietary supplements, but occurs naturally as part of proteins. Some sports nutrition energy formulas contain 500 mg or more of alanine per serving.

Cofactors: Pyruvate, B vitamins, and other amino acids.

Concerns: Alanine is considered a nonessential amino acid, but dietary intake may be beneficial. Alanine is found in meats and other protein-containing foods, and is considered safe for ingestion. L-alanine supplements should be used by children and pregnant or lactating women only under a doctor's supervision.

Use Guidelines: Consider using L-alanine supplements periodically during athletic season.

Aloe (also *Aloe vera, Aloe Barbadensis*)
Supplement Type: Botanical
Overview: Aloe contains several kinds of phytochemicals that have two primary functions.

The mucilaginous gel obtained from the center of the leaf contains polysaccharides, chiefly glucomannan. A bitter yellow latex is obtained from just beneath the skin of the leaves. This bitter yellow latex contains anthraquinones and other similar chemicals, collectively referred to as aloin. Topical use of aloe gel is well known for promoting healing of the skin. Internally, aloe gel is used to promote a healthy stomach lining and normal digestion. The soothing, healing, moisturizing, emollient properties of aloe gel are attributed to the polysaccharides. The bitter anthraquinone-containing aloin fraction of the aloe leaf has been used for centuries as a cathartic. A cathartic, or purgative, functions as a laxative by stimulating the peristaltic action of the intestines and bowel evacuation. Peristalsis is the rhythmic contractions of the intestines, which move digested food along the long journey from the stomach to the rectum. People who have mild gastrointestinal problems report improvements in stomach and intestinal health and function after a few weeks of taking high-quality aloe gel drinks, capsules, or tablets. For individuals with chronic constipation problems, use of aloe products under a doctor's supervision may help restore normal function. Health practitioners speculate that the polysaccharides have a positive effect on the lining of the gastrointestinal system.

Benefits: Aloe gel promotes a healthy digestive system. Whole-leaf aloe, containing aloin, promotes regularity of the digestive system.

Ingredient Form: There are no official regulatory or scientific standards in the United States to categorize dietary supplement aloe products using aloe gel for soothing of the gastrointestinal system; there are concentrated aloe health drinks available, as well as aloe-containing tablets and pills. Look for products that use *Aloe vera* gel 40:1 concentrates and *Aloe vera* gel powder 200:1 extract. For laxative products containing aloin, look for products that use standardized extracts of whole-leaf aloe (containing the gel and aloin), or just aloin.

Effective Supplement Dosages: Each person will respond differently to aloe products depending on the quality and potency of the product ingested. It is best to follow the directions provided by the manufacturer. *Aloe vera* gel products are considered safe. However, exercise caution when using whole-leaf aloe (which contains aloin) and concentrated aloin-containing products, which exert a laxative effect. When using botanical products as laxatives, remember that this is an unregulated drug use and that the products are not governed by FDA regulations concerning potency, dosage, proper use, duration of use, and warnings. It is best to seek medical supervision if you are looking for a natural alternative to over-the-counter or prescription laxatives.

Cofactors: *Aloe vera* gel health drinks contain other "health tonic" herbs and nutrients. Concentrated aloin-containing products may contain other botanical laxatives such as rhubarb, plantago seed, cascara sagrada, buckthorn, and senna.

Concerns: Aloe is not an essential nutrient and there are no nutritional deficiencies associated with not ingesting aloe supplements. When using aloe gel products, make sure to use high-quality products that do not contain aloin (anthraquinones). Use laxative aloe preparations with caution, and for short periods of time, only until your gastrointestinal regularity is restored. Aloin-containing aloe products can cause severe gastrointestinal cramping and should not be used by pregnant or lactating women, children, and individuals with known gastrointestinal disorders or diseases. As with all botanical products, allergic reactions can occur with use of any aloe products. Consult your doctor if constipation or other gastrointestinal problems persist for more than a few days.

Use Guidelines: Many people find that the daily consumption of a liquid or tablet aloe gel supplement helps promote and maintain gastrointestinal health. Use aloin-containing products only periodically.

Androstenedione (also andro, 4-androstene-3, 17-dione)

Supplement Type: Metabolite

Overview: Androstenedione functions as an androgen hormone in the body. It also acts as a prohormone and is made into testosterone in the body. Androstenedione is an example of one of the "loophole ingredients" now allowed in dietary supplements as a result of passage of the DSHEA in 1994. Prior to passage of the act, it was not allowed in dietary supplements and was considered a new drug. As an androgen and a precursor of testosterone, androstenedione causes masculinizing characteristics in males (and females, but it should not be used by females). The exact benefits are not fully known, but androstenedione is used in sports nutrition formulas taken by strength athletes, and is used by mature males in an attempt to naturally boost their testosterone levels and improve vitality and virility. Proper use of androstenedione-containing supplements requires a doctor's supervision.

Benefits: At this time there is a lack of scientific data on the benefits of using androstenedione supplements.

Ingredient Form: Used in dietary supplements as androstenedione.

Effective Supplement Dosages: Dietary supplement dosages of androstenedione range from 5 to over 50 mg per day.

Cofactors: Other male virility and vitality herbs and prohormones, such as tribulus, DHEA, yohimbe, and ginseng.

Concerns: Androstenedione is not an essential nutrient. Its use as a hormone/prohormone in dietary supplements is speculative. There is a lack of data to determine the exact guidelines for safe and effective androstenedione use. It should not be used unless under a doctor's supervision. It should not be taken by females or children. The documented side effects for androgens are numerous and include liver cancer, infertility, testicular atrophy, confusion, dizziness, skin problems, acne, mental depression, aggression, mood swings, unusual bleeding, increase in urination, gynecomastia (development of dormant breast tissue in males), insomnia, and unusual decrease or increase in sexual desire.

Use Guidelines: Consult your doctor for proper use of androstenedione-containing supplements.

Angelica (also Chinese angelica, *Angelica sinensis,* dong-quai, dong-qui, dang-qui, dong-kwai)

Supplement Type: Botanical

Overview: Angelica is traditionally used to regulate female hormone balance, increase energy, and treat gynecological conditions such as PMS and symptoms of menopause. It has also been shown clinically to have an effect on stimulating the uterus. The primary phytochemicals contained in angelica include ligustilide and ferulic acid. Other functions of angelica include improved peripheral blood circulation, reduction of muscle spasms, and relaxation of blood vessels. Angelica is one of the preferred health-promoting herbal supplements for women.

Benefits: Promotes female health, restores regular menstruation.

Ingredient Form: Standardized angelica root extract (1% ligustilide).

Effective Supplement Dosages: Dosages for regular use in dietary supplements range from 200 to 800 mg per day of standardized angelica root extract. Higher dosages of unstandardized root powder are also used, 3 to 5 g per day. Use angelica in cycles of three to four months, with a two- to four-week interval of nonuse.

Cofactors: Black cohosh.

Concerns: Angelica is not an essential nutrient but can help promote, maintain, and restore female health. Angelica is considered safe when used as directed. Not for use if you have gastrointestinal problems, hemorrhagic disease, or during pregnancy, during infection with the flu, and in cases of hypermenorrhea. Angelica should be used by adult females only and under a doctor's supervision when taken in conjunction with other drugs or being treated for illness. Not for use by children.

Use Guidelines: Use of angelica supplements can be beneficial for restoring female balance, in particular among females thirty years or older. Use on a periodic basis, when needed.

Arctic Root (also *Rhodiola rosea*)

Supplement Type: Botanical

Overview: Arctic Root is considered an adaptogen (see page 132), which works by stimulating and maintaining the body's metabolic functions to help it remain healthy under unfavorable conditions. It has also been shown to restore the body's serotonin balance. Arctic Root is a recent addition to the botanical products available in the U.S. market. It is preferred by many people over ginseng and other adaptogens because it is generally milder and does not cause nervousness. It is interesting to note that Arctic Root (as part of a complex herbal formula) was tested by Russian scientists in the 1990s to measure its performance-enhancing effects on a group of cosmonauts. Short-term use was found to be effective in improving mental and physical working capacity in conditions of simulated space flight, consisting of long periods of monotonous work designed to induce the development of fatigue. There were no side effects reported during the several-week study. Therefore it is likely that Arctic Root can have beneficial effects for everyone in the workplace, especially under conditions of monotonous work.

Benefits: Some of Arctic Root's beneficial effects include increased resistance to stress and illness, improved work performance, improved mental function, stimulation of immune function, and increased physical (athletic) performance. Also, Arctic Root acts as an antidepressant, along with other antidepressant herbs.

Ingredient Form: Standardized *Rhodiola rosea* (standardized for Rosavin and salidrosides).

Effective Supplement Dosages: Use in dietary supplements ranges from 100 to 200 mg a day of standardized *Rhodiola rosea*. Rosavin is the brand name of a certain type of standardized rhodiola, which is modeled after the extracts used in clinical studies. Lower amounts of rhodiola are also used in multiherbal formulas, 35 to 100 mg per day.

Best used in cycles of three to four months, with two to three weeks off between cycles.

Cofactors: For depression: St. John's wort. For immunity: astragalus, reishi mushroom, shiitake mushroom, and echinacea. For physical performance and as an adaptogen: ginseng (American and Korean), Siberian ginseng, carnitine, and coenzyme Q_{10}.

Concerns: Arctic Root is not an essential nutrient. It has a history of safe and effective use in Europe and Russia and is considered safe and effective when used as directed. Consult your doctor if you are considering taking Arctic Root for depression or other diseases, which should be treated under a doctor's supervision. Not for children or for pregnant or lactating women without a doctor's supervision.

Use Guidelines: Use supplements containing Arctic Root as part of your daily botanical health-promoting program. Use is recommended for individuals who are under periods of physical or emotional stress.

Arginine (also L-arginine) *— found in peanuts & peanutbutter + at lower levels of other nuts except almonds.*

Supplement Type: Amino acid

Overview: Arginine is classified as a nonessential amino acid because the body can make enough for its own needs. Arginine is involved in several metabolic functions in the body, such as elevating growth hormone levels; creatine manufacture; wound healing; circulatory system health; fertility, and in the detoxification of the metabolic waste product ammonia. Arginine is becoming a popular longevity nutrient due to its ability to increase growth hormone levels and promote a healthy circulatory system.

Benefits: Arginine dietary supplements can promote overall well-being, increase growth hormone levels, stimulate wound healing, increase fertility, stimulate immune system function, and promote circulatory system health.

Ingredient Form: L-arginine HCl.

Effective Supplement Dosages: Arginine is found in a wide range of dosages in dietary supplements. For short-term use for elevating growth hormone levels and wound healing, 1 to 3 g per day of L-arginine is required. Lower daily dosages, 500 to 1,000 mg per day, have beneficial effects for long-term use.

Cofactors: Used with lysine, ornithine, phenylalanine, or glycine in growth-hormone-stimulating supplement formulas.

Concerns: While arginine is considered a nonessential amino acid, it has very important roles in the body, and beneficial health effects are observed when it is taken as a supplement. When taken in the recommended dosages, there are no major side effects associated with arginine supplement intake. There is some concern that increasing arginine intake may aggravate cold sore episodes in people who normally experience outbreaks. That's one reason why lysine is often included with arginine, to offset any potential cold-sore-stimulating effects. For adult use only; not for use by pregnant or lactating women or for those with liver or kidney disease, unless under a doctor's supervision.

Use Guidelines: Taking arginine supplements on a regular basis is recommended for athletes, individuals forty years and older, and people with concerns about cardiovascular health.

Asparagine: *see Aspartic acid*

Aspartic acid (also L-aspartic acid)

Supplement Type: Amino acid

Overview: Aspartic acid is a nonessential amino acid that has been shown to help reduce blood ammonia levels after exercise. Aspartic acid is metabolized from glutamic acid in the body. It is involved in the urea cycle and the energy-producing Krebs cycle. Aspartic acid also functions as an excitatory (stimulating) neurotransmitter in the brain. Aspartic acid is one of the amino acids that shows potential use for athletes. Asparagine is another nonessential amino acid that is manufactured from aspartic acid. Its use as a dietary supplement is under investigation.

Benefits: Supplemental aspartic acid can be beneficial for improving energy levels and promoting mental alertness. However, more clinical studies are needed to determine its exact beneficial role as a dietary supplement for regular use.

Ingredient Form: L-aspartic acid

Effective Supplement Dosages: Currently aspartic acid is used in high dosages, 2 to 4 gs a day, for short periods, under a doctor's supervision for medical reasons.

Cofactors: Asparagine and glutamine.

Concerns: Aspartic acid is a nonessential amino acid, produced by the body. Short-term use may be beneficial for improving athletic performance. Should only be used by healthy adults, for short periods (a few weeks) at a time. Not for use by children or by pregnant or lactating women, unless under a doctor's supervision.

Use Guidelines: Aspartic acid supplement use is optional and intended for periodic use by individuals looking to increase athletic performance or energy levels.

Astragalus (also *Astragalus membranaceus*)
Supplement Type: Botanical
Overview: Astragalus is a traditional Chinese medicine with a long history of use, taken primarily to improve and maintain immune function. It is used in restorative and preventative botanical preparations. It has been used with promising results as a supportive botanical therapy to treat cancer and AIDS, and it is especially useful to help restore immune system function after chemotherapy. If you have an immune-related disease or recurring infections, talk to your doctor about giving astragalus a try along with your prescribed drug therapy.

Benefits: Stimulates and restores the immune system function.

Ingredient Form: Standardized astragalus root extract (0.5% to 1% 4-hydroxy-3-methoxyisoflavone).

Effective Supplement Dosages: Astragalus is used as a dietary supplement to stimulate and support immune system function using 200 to 800 mg of standardized extract per day, for intervals of several weeks. Lower dosages, under 100 mg per day, are sometimes found in daily combination health-promoting products. Up to 4 gs per day of unstandardized astragalus root powder is also a common dosage used for short periods of time.

Cofactors: Sometimes used with other immune-stimulating or adaptogenic herbs, such as echinacea, garlic, reishi mushroom, cat's claw.

Concerns: Astragalus is not an essential nutrient, but has been demonstrated to produce beneficial health effects when used as directed. It is considered one of the safest botanicals, with no reported toxicity, making it safe for adult use when used correctly. Always use astragalus under a doctor's supervision when taking it as supportive nutritional therapy to help treat a disease condition. Not for use by children or by pregnant or lactating women unless under a doctor's supervision.

Use Guidelines: Use astragalus-containing supplements periodically when you want to stimulate immune system function, such as during flu and cold season, during times of emotional and physical stress, and at times of the year when you typically fall victim to illness. Also for athletes during the preseason and season.

Barley grass powder: *see* Greens powders

Beta-carotene (also β-carotene, carotaben)
Supplement Type: Botanical

Overview: Beta-carotene is an antioxidant, displays vitamin A activity as a vitamin A precursor, and enhances immune system response. Its vitamin A activity makes it an essential nutrient, with additional semiessential health functions. In plants, beta-carotene functions as a pigment; for example, it gives carrots their characteristic orange color. Because your body can make as much vitamin A as it needs from beta-carotene, with any excess beta-carotene being excreted, any potential side effects of taking vitamin A are avoided unless your vitamin A intake from other sources is already high. This is especially important for children and women, who tend to be more susceptible to potential vitamin A toxicity effects. When you take a close look at your supplements, you will notice that many supplements include beta-carotene as their source of vitamin A, either alone or in combination with vitamin A acetate or vitamin A palmitate. Foods high in beta-carotene include apricots, asparagus, beet greens, broccoli, Brussels sprouts, cantaloupe, carrots, chicory leaf, and endive.

Benefits: Beta-carotene's antioxidant activity protects the body from free-radical damage, which is important for maintaining proper biological structure and function and lowering the risk of developing degenerative diseases (see Chapter 5 on the benefits of antioxidants). Beta-carotene is considered a safe way to take vitamin A, because once in the body, beta-carotene is converted to vitamin A as needed.

Ingredient Form: Synthetic beta-carotene is the most common form of beta-carotene used in dietary supplements and has an impressive safety record. Some dietary supplement products contain natural beta-carotene, which can be derived from palm oil or sea algae. The natural beta-carotene products usually will also contain other carotenoids that occur naturally with beta-carotene, such as alpha-carotene, lycopene, zeaxanthin, cryptoxanthin, and lutein. Betatene and FloraGlo are examples of brand name ingredients.

Effective Supplement Dosages: Daily dietary supplement intake of beta-carotene, measured as vitamin A activity, between 5,000 and 20,000 IU is well tolerated. Higher beta-carotene intakes may be indicated for athletic people or for therapeutic reasons; 25,000 to 50,000 IU of vitamin A activity from beta-carotene can be safely taken for short periods of time under a doctor's supervision. It is not unusual for doctors to use even higher dosages of beta-carotene to treat nutritional disorders or diseases.

Cofactors: Vitamin C and vitamin E can enhance the antioxidant function of beta-carotene.

Concerns: Regular intake of beta-carotene in amounts equivalent to 25,000 IU of vitamin A activity or more may cause yellowing of the skin. This is a harmless condition, which disappears when beta-carotene intake is reduced. Reduce the amount of supplemental vitamin A you take if you are also taking high amounts of beta-carotene. Beta-carotene is considered safe for both sexes and all age groups.

Use Guidelines: Obtain a daily supply of beta-carotene from eating fruits and vegetables, and from your daily multinutrient supplement. Increase beta-carotene intake as required by increased activity or for special medical reasons.

Bee pollen

Supplement Type: Botanical

Overview: Pollen is the flowering plant's counterpart of animal sperm. Bee pollen is collected from beehives; sometimes pollen is collected directly from flowers. It is thought to be high in nutrients and energy-promoting phytonutrients. While bee pollen is touted throughout the world for its energy-promoting effects, there is currently a lack of scientific verification to support this claim. However, many people report improvements in energy and stamina when taking bee pollen products.

Benefits: Traditionally used to stimulate energy.

Ingredient Form: Due to the lack of standardization, there are currently no agreed-upon industry guidelines being followed at this time. There is an inherent problem with standardization of bee pollen products, due to the fact that it is virtually impossible to know what plants the pollen was collected from.

Effective Supplement Dosages: Because the quality of bee pollen supplements varies widely, it is best to follow dosage guidelines on specific products.

Cofactors: Other bee products, such as honey, bee propolis, and royal jelly.

Concerns: Bee pollen is not an essential nutrient. It may cause allergic reactions in some individuals. Bee pollen should not be used by children, pregnant or lactating women, or individuals with known allergies to plant pollens, unless under a doctor's supervision.

Use Guidelines: Optional daily use in a multinutrient supplement product or energy-promoting supplement product.

Bee propolis

Supplement Type: Concentrate

Overview: Bee propolis is a natural sticky plant substance collected by bees from plants, specifically particular conifers. Propolis contains many phytochemicals, including substances that have been shown to display antimicrobial and anti-inflammatory activity. Bee propolis has a long history of use dating back over two thousand years. In addition to possible internal benefits, bee propolis is used in topical products for a variety of soothing and healing purposes, as in treating bruises, burns, and skin blemishes.

Benefits: Bee propolis has been traditionally used internally to promote gastrointestinal wellness, in particular to reduce inflammation and heal certain types of ulcers.

Ingredient Form: There are currently no industry standards for bee propolis quality.

Effective Supplement Dosages: Follow directions on the particular product you are taking.

Cofactors: Honey, bee pollen, royal jelly.

Concerns: Bee propolis is not an essential nutrient. Benefits are speculative; however, emerging scientific evidence supports its use for treating gastrointestinal disorders. For adult use only; not for pregnant or lactating women unless under a doctor's supervision. If you choose to use bee propolis products as nutritional support of medical therapy for gastrointestinal disorders, do so only under the supervision of a doctor. Allergic side effects may occur in individuals sensitive to bee products.

Use Guidelines: Use bee propolis periodically to support gastrointestinal system health.

BHMB (also **HMB,** Beta-hydroxy-beta-methylbutyrate)

Supplement Type: Metabolite

Overview: Scientific studies have demonstrated that BHMB improves nitrogen balance, reduces muscle damage, and can improve strength and muscle mass in some individuals who are undertaking a weight-training program. BHMB is especially useful for strength and power athletes. But make sure you are also maintaining adequate intake of essential vitamins and minerals, as well as ensuring adequate intake of protein and other nutrients.

Benefits: Regular use of BHMB as a dietary supplement in conjunction with weight training may promote increases in muscle mass and strength. It reduces muscle soreness in exercisers and athletes.

Ingredient Form: BHMB is available in dietary supplements as calcium beta-hydroxy-beta-methylbutyrate.

Effective Supplement Dosages: Clinical studies have verified that a dosage ranging from 1,500 to 4,000 mg per day of BHMB can produce the desired results in improving muscle size and strength.

Cofactors: BHMB is sometimes formulated along with other nutrients beneficial to athletic performance, such as creatine and protein.

Concerns: BHMB is not an essential nutrient but is beneficial for supporting the metabolism, particularly in athletes. There have been no reported side effects in short-term clinical studies. For use by healthy adults only; not for pregnant or lactating women unless under a doctor's supervision. Use for short intervals, up to three months, until long-term studies confirm long-term safety. BHMB is expensive—a month's supply costs about $105.

Use Guidelines: For athletes and individuals exercising to increase muscle size and strength, use in three-month cycles, with three to four weeks off between cycles.

Beta-glucan (also Beta-1,3-D-glucan)

Supplement Type: Botanical, fiber

Overview: Beta-glucan is a soluble dietary fiber that has been shown to have a cholesterol-lowering effect. The FDA has approved a health claim for certain foods high in beta-glucan, such as oatmeal and oat bran, stating that ingestion of beta-glucan-containing foods may reduce the risk of heart disease. Increasing intake of dietary fiber also improves appetite control. Officially, the FDA health claim is allowed only for *whole foods* naturally containing beta-glucan from oats or psyllium seed husks, and dietary supplements containing psyllium seed husks. Since the approval of this health claim, dietary supplement companies have begun to market isolated beta-glucan supplements from other sources, such as barley. If you are using a beta-glucan supplement, take it with meals, and also include foods high in naturally occurring beta-glucan for best results. This is a good example of a nutraceutical.

Benefits: Promotes healthy cholesterol levels and coronary health. Can reduce the risk of heart disease. Increases appetite control.

Ingredient Form: Foods and dietary supplements containing naturally occurring beta-glucan fiber. Beta-glucan contained in dietary supplements may be from concentrated plant sources, such as oats or psyllium seed husks.

Effective Supplement Dosages: The FDA has established that at least 3 g of beta-glucan soluble fiber per day is required for coronary-health-promoting effects.

Cofactors: Other plant fibers, such as guar gum and pectin.

Concerns: Dietary fiber is an important part of the diet. The soluble fiber beta-glucan will promote coronary health and reduce the risk of coronary heart disease as part of a diet low in saturated fat and cholesterol. No side effects are expected with regular use. However, note that some people may experience temporary gastrointestinal upset during the first few days upon increasing their intake of dietary fiber. To reduce the possibility of fiber-induced gastrointestinal upset, you can start with small daily dosages during the first week and slowly increase to the recommended daily dosage over a period of a few weeks. This will give your digestive system a chance to adjust to the increased fiber intake.

Use Guidelines: Include a fiber supplement in your diet each day.

Beta-sitosterol

Supplement Type: Botanical

Overview: When taken with meals, beta-sitosterol can help reduce the amount of cholesterol absorbed into the body from food. Also, studies of botanicals high in beta-sitosterol, such as saw palmetto berries, indicate that beta-sitosterol contributes to prostate health. Use of beta-sitosterol can be beneficial in your quest for lower cholesterol levels. Always first try to reduce the saturated fat and cholesterol in your diet. If you are having problems maintaining a diet low in saturated fat and cholesterol, use of beta-sitosterol supplements can be a wise strategy.

Benefits: Beta-sitosterol supports heart health, promotes healthy cholesterol levels, and promotes a healthy prostate.

Ingredient Form: Contained in dietary supplements as beta-sitosterol.

Effective Supplement Dosages: Take 100 to 200 mg of beta-sitosterol with meals, three times per day, as a dietary supplement.

Cofactors: Chitosan and plant fibers for lowering cholesterol.

Concerns: Beta-sitosterol is not an essential nutrient. It can be beneficial for people who are looking to maintain healthy cholesterol levels. It is considered safe when used as directed; there have been no reports of toxicity. For adults only. Use under a doctor's supervision if you have coronary heart disease or are being treated for high cholesterol levels.

Use Guidelines: Use beta-sitosterol supplements if you are concerned about maintaining a healthy circulatory system.

Bilberry (also *Vaccinium myrtillus, Myrtilli fructus*)

Supplement Type: Botanical

Overview: Bilberry contains high amounts of bioflavonoids called anthocyanosides. Anthocyanosides possess collagen-stabilizing action and promote collagen synthesis; display antioxidant activity; suppress the release of anti-inflammatory chemicals such as prostaglandins, leukotrienes, and histamine; reduce excessive blood platelet aggregation; and promote visual function. Bilberry supplements improve and maintain eye health and vision. Bilberry extract, along with vitamin E, can slow the progression of cataract formation in some individuals. It has been shown to reduce progression of macular degeneration as well. It can be used to help prevent eye fatigue, due to the role of anthocyanosides in replenishing rhodopsin, a pigment found in the eye. Bilberry is also used to maintain circulatory system health. Use bilberry supplements every day if you have concerns about maintaining eye health and good vision, and for maintenance of vascular health.

Benefits: Bilberry improves and maintains good vision. It also maintains circulatory system structure and health.

Ingredient Form: For best results, use bilberry dietary supplements that contain bilberry fruit extract standardized to at least 25% anthocyanidins. VmA25+ is an example of a brand used in supplements.

Effective Supplement Dosages: Safe and effective daily dosages of standardized bilberry extract (25% anthocyanidins) range from 60 to 240 mg per day. If you are using bilberry to improve eye function, use the higher dosages for a few months until improvements occur. Lower daily dosages are beneficial for support of eye health and function as well.

Cofactors: Bilberry is sometimes included in comprehensive antioxidant formulas and circulatory system formulas.

Concerns: Bilberry is not an essential nutrient, but contains phytonutrients shown to be beneficial to health and body function. Bilberry is considered nontoxic and safe when used at recommended dosages. Safe for both sexes and all ages.

Use Guidelines: Look for multinutrient and antioxidant formulas that contain standardized bilberry for daily consumption. Use a separate bilberry supplement to increase intake for improving vision and circulatory system health.

Bifidus: *see* Probiotics

Bioflavonoids (also Flavonoids)

Supplement Type: Botanical

Overview: Bioflavonoids are a group of naturally occurring plant compounds that act primarily as plant pigments and antioxidants. In humans bioflavonoids exhibit a host of biological activities, most notably powerful antioxidant activity. The term *bioflavonoid* was first used by pioneering researchers who used this term to distinguish flavonoids displaying biological activity. Bioflavonoids are present in all botanical supplement products and foods. In fact, many medicinal herbs owe their curative actions to the bioflavonoids they contain. There are over several thousand flavonoids, and perhaps a few hundred or so have been discovered to exert biological activity in humans. Bioflavonoids help the body maintain health and function in many ways besides the important antioxidant effects. Bioflavonoids have been shown to be antimutagenic and anticarcinogenic, to block enzyme activity, and to promote structure and function in the circulatory system, for example. Make sure your daily supplement contains most or all of the important bioflavonoids listed below. You may also want to take extra amounts of particular bioflavonoids depending on your specific goals (see individual bioflavonoid listings). The different classes of bioflavonoids include catechins, anthocyanidins, leucoanthocyanidins, flavonones, flavones, flavanonols, flavonols, isoflavones, flavans, dihydrochalcones, aurones, and chalcones. Specific kinds of bioflavonoids belong to one of these classes. For example, quercetin belongs to the flavonol class; genistein belongs to the isoflavone class; catechin belongs to the catechins class; and cyanidin belongs to the anthocyanidins.

Benefits: High dietary bioflavonoid intake has been associated with reduction in risk of many diseases, in particular degenerative illnesses. Different bioflavonoids tend to have different health effects on the body. Some of the health effects include improving eyesight, promoting cardiovascular health, protecting connective tissues, increasing capillary strength, improving the structure and appearance of skin, boosting immune system function, having a vitamin C and vitamin E potentiating effect (boosting their function), and offering protection from degenerative diseases such as atherosclerosis, cancer, arthritis, and gastrointestinal disorders. Therapeutic benefits of bioflavonoid use include: treating a variety of diseases and disorders, such as inflammation, hemorrhoids, coronary diseases, allergies, respiratory diseases, viral infections, and peptic ulcers.

Ingredient Form: As there are many types of bioflavonoids, some of the main ones will be listed here, with more detailed entries found under individual alphabetical listings. Some of the common bioflavonoid ingredients you will find in supplements include quercetin, quercetin dihydrate, quercetin chalcone, Pycnogenol (the brand name of a special bioflavonoid extract from the French maritime pine tree [*Pinus pinaster*], grape seed extract (Activin is the brand name of one grape seed extract), green tea extract, citrus bioflavonoids (hesperidin, rutin, and narignin), soy bioflavonoids (isoflavones), and bilberry extract.

Effective Supplement Dosages: Bioflavonoid dosages will vary considerably depending on the type of bioflavonoid, its purity, and the intended use. Nutritional dosages are typically under 300 mg per day. For short-term therapeutic uses, bioflavonoid intake can be as high as 500 mg or more three times per day. Here are some typical daily intake ranges found in dietary supplement products intended for nutritional use: Pycnogenol, 20 to 100 mg; grape seed extract, 20 to 80 mg; green tea extract, 50 to 200 mg; citrus bioflavonoids, 100 to 500 mg; quercetin, 20 to 60 mg; soy isoflavones, 20 to 60 mg.

Cofactors: Other bioflavonoids, vitamin C.

Concerns: While there is no official reference daily intake (RDI) established for any bioflavonoid, many researchers consider them semiessential, in that they maintain health, prevent disease, and promote longevity. Studies from around the world support the fact that diets high in bioflavonoids are associated with lower incidences of most diseases. Along with other phytonutrients, the health benefits of bioflavonoids is one reason why the National Institutes of Health and the U.S. Surgeon General's office advocate the consumption of several servings of fruits and vegetables per day. Bioflavonoids are nontoxic and have an excellent safety record as dietary supplements. However, there are rare instances where sensitive individuals may develop an allergic reaction. They are safe for all ages and both sexes.

Use Guidelines: Include a good dose of bioflavonoids in your daily supplement program to optimize health and longevity.

Bioperine (also *Piper nigrum*)

Supplement Type: Botanical

Overview: Bioperine is the brand name for an extract made from the fruit of the black pepper plant. It is used in dietary supplements for its role in stimulating the intestinal absorption of nutrients. The increased absorption effects of Bioperine may be of special interest to people who take coenzyme Q_{10} and vitamin C dietary supplements. Studies have reported greater uptake of these nutrients in supplements that also contained Bioperine. However, keep in mind that the studies examined the improved nutrient absorption when taken on an empty stomach.

Benefits: Bioperine can result in greater uptake of vitamins and minerals.

Ingredient Form: Bioperine is a special extract manufactured and tested by Sabinsa and sold to dietary supplement makers.

Effective Supplement Dosages: Bioperine is contained in dietary supplements at 5 mg per dose. However, note that in the studies in which Bioperine was shown to improve absorption of some vitamins and minerals, it was taken on an empty stomach. It is unknown whether Bioperine will promote greater nutrient uptake when supplements are taken with meals.

Cofactors: None.

Concerns: Bioperine is not an essential nutrient. It is considered safe when ingested in small amounts.

Use Guidelines: If you are looking for ways to improve nutrient absorption from your supplements, try taking supplements that contain Bioperine.

Biotin (also Coenzyme R, hexahydro-2-oxo-1H-thieno[3,4-d]imidazole-4-pentanoic acid)

Supplement Type: Vitamin

Overview: A water-soluble essential vitamin that is a member of the B vitamin group, biotin is involved in new cell growth, glucose formation, fatty acid synthesis, energy production, and urea formation. Biotin also assists in the metabolism of the other B vitamins. Maintenance of adequate biotin intake is essential to good health. During stressful times, increase your intake of biotin and other B vitamins.

Benefits: Supplemental intake of biotin will ensure adequate dietary biotin status and prevent biotin deficiency. Biotin deficiency can lead to loss of appetite, anemia, baldness, high blood sugar, nausea, vomiting, depression, muscular pain, increased serum cholesterol concentration, loss of muscle tone, soreness of the tongue, and a dry scaly dermatitis.

Ingredient Form: Supplements contain pure biotin.

Effective Supplement Dosages: A dose of 100 to 400 mcg per day is well tolerated. Higher intake may be indicated for therapeutic purposes, as determined by your health care practitioner. The adult RDI for biotin is 300 mcg.

Cofactors: Best taken as part of a complete vitamin-mineral formulation.

Concerns: Biotin is safe and effective for all ages and both sexes when taken in the recommended nutritional dosages.

Use Guidelines: Biotin-containing supplements are recommended for daily consumption.

Black cohosh (also *Cimicifuga racemosa*)

Supplement Type: Botanical

Overview: Black cohosh has two main functions particularly useful for women. Its active phytochemicals reduce levels of luteinizing hormone, and they exhibit weak estrogenic activity. Studies have confirmed that intake of standardized black cohosh reduces menopausal symptoms such as hot flashes, nervousness, anxiety, and depression. During menopause, estrogen levels begin to decrease steadily, and levels of luteinizing hormone increase. The increase in luteinizing hormone is believed to be responsible for these symptoms. Black cohosh has been shown to also be effective for relieving premenstrual discomfort and dysmenorrhea. Improvements are seen after several weeks to three months of daily use. Black cohosh has a long history of use in Europe, and is taken safely by millions of women each year. In fact, a European company recently introduced its standardized black cohosh product, Remifemin, into the U.S. market. Remifemin has been used in Europe for over thirty years and has undergone clinical studies to verify its safety and effectiveness. In premenopausal women, its luteinizing hormone suppressing effects may interfere with conception. A rise in luteinizing hormone (along with follicle stimulating hormone) is required for follicle ripening and release of the egg into the oviduct. If you are taking black cohosh for management of PMS or dysmenorrhea, you should discontinue using it a few months before you plan on becoming pregnant, or avoid its use until after your childbearing years.

Benefits: Black cohosh supplements promote and maintain balance and health in women, reduces menopausal side effects.

Ingredient Form: Black cohosh root/rhizome extract standardized to 2% to 2.5% triterpenes or 27-deoxyaceteine.

Effective Supplement Dosages: Clinical studies have demonstrated that 6 mg of total triterpenes (as 27-deoxyaceteine) per day is a safe and effective dose for short-term use in relieving menopausal symptoms, which can be obtained from 240 mg to 300 mg of standardized product. Lower dosages can also be found in formulas intended for daily use by women.

Cofactors: Other female health botanicals such as chaste tree berry and soy isoflavones.

Concerns: Do not use black cohosh supplements during pregnancy or lactation. Black cohosh may complicate estrogen therapy due to its weak estrogenic effect. No studies have been conducted on the effects of long-term use

of black cohosh, so limit use to up to six months unless otherwise advised by your health care practitioner. Excessive dosages can result in vomiting, dizziness, occasional gastric discomfort, headaches, visual disturbances, and nausea. Black cohosh should be used only by adult females who do not have heart, liver, or blood clotting problems; it is not for children or men.

Use Guidelines: Women who are approaching menopausal age should include black cohosh in their supplement program; women who are going through menopause should definitely give black cohosh a try.

Boron
Supplement Type: Mineral

Overview: Boron is an essential trace mineral that occurs in the body in small amounts. It plays an important role in bone formation and maintenance. Boron is a recently discovered essential mineral and has therefore not been extensively studied. One major study conducted by the United States Department of Agriculture in 1987 was performed on postmenopausal women using 3,000 mcg of boron per day. It was found to help prevent loss of bone mass.

Benefits: Supports bone health and normal metabolism.

Ingredient Forms: Boron trichelate, boron citrate, boron glycinate.

Effective Supplement Dosages: Daily dosages found in supplements generally range from 500 to 3,000 mcg per day. Higher dosages may be indicated in individuals being treated for bone loss and osteoporosis.

Cofactors: Boron should be taken as part of a complete vitamin-mineral formula, or as part of a bone health formula that includes calcium, magnesium, vitamin D, and other bone-forming nutrients.

Concerns: No adverse health effects have been reported from people taking the recommended daily dosage of boron. Excessive intakes, such as 5,000 mg per day, can cause nausea, diarrhea, dermatitis, lethargy, nervous system irritability, renal failure, dermatitis, and shock. Boron is safe and effective for all ages and both sexes at the suggested dosage.

Use Guidelines: Boron should be consumed as part of your daily multinutrient supplement program.

Boswellia (also *Boswellia serrata*)

Supplement Type: Botanical

Overview: Boswellia is an herb used in the traditional Ayurvedic medicine of India. Boswellic acids, one of the active phytonutrients found in boswellia, exhibit antiarthritic and anti-inflammatory properties. Used in clinical studies, boswellia extract has been shown to be effective in the treatment and management of osteoarthritis, rheumatoid arthritis, gout, low back pain, myositis, fibrositis, and chronic inflammatory conditions. Like other herbs, boswellia contains other phytonutrients, including bioflavonoids, that add to the beneficial health effects. If you have or are prone to

developing inflammatory disease, give boswellia a try. It is best used under a doctor's supervision, especially if you are being treated for a disease. Boswellia has a long history of use in India, and its use in the United States is growing in popularity. Expect to start feeling results in one to four weeks.

Benefits: Boswellia promotes connective tissue health and reduces inflammation.

Ingredient Form: Standardized *Boswellia serrata* extract (40% to 65% boswellic acids), in tablets and capsules.

Effective Supplement Dosages: For use as part of your dietary supplement program to promote joint health and reduce inflammation, use 100 to 400 mg of standardized boswellia per day. In clinical studies for treatment of arthritis and other conditions, 200 mg, taken three times per day for four weeks, produced improvements in the majority of subjects tested.

Cofactors: Curcumin, glucosamine, and chondroitin sulfate to benefit joint health and healing.

Concerns: Boswellia is not an essential nutrient, but can have beneficial health effects for some people. For the treatment and management of inflammatory diseases, it should be used under a doctor's supervision. In clinical studies boswellia has been shown to be safe and effective when used properly. For adult use only; not for pregnant or lactating women.

Use Guidelines: Use boswellia dietary supplements periodically for therapeutic purposes to reduce pain and inflammation.

Bovine cartilage: *see* Chondroitin sulfate

Branched-chain amino acids: *see* Isoleucine, Leucine, Valine

Brewer's yeast: *see* Yeast

Bromelain (also *Ananas comosus*)

Supplement Type: Botanical

Overview: Bromelain is a proteolytic enzyme derived from pineapple. Proteolytic enzymes digest or break apart proteins. In fact, bromelain and other proteolytic enzymes are used in food tenderizers to soften meat. In the body, bromelain can decrease the time needed to recover from injury by enhancing the breakdown of fibrin. While fibrin plays a vital role in the body as a clotting agent, after an injury occurs, too much fibrin in the damaged tissues can block blood flow, resulting in poor oxygen supply, buildup of metabolic waste products, and increased swelling and inflammation. Bromelain can function to minimize fibrin buildup in injured tissues. Studies also show that bromelain exhibits other actions to reduce fibrin formation, improve blood flow by inhibiting platelet aggregation and anti-inflammatory action. Bromelain can be useful in reducing injury healing time. Use of bromelain for treating injury should be conducted under a doctor's supervision. For people with problems digesting protein, bromelain taken with meals can help promote normal digestion. Only use bromelain as directed; with high dosages, take only for short periods, up to a few weeks at a time.

Benefits: Bromelain can aid in the digestion of proteins when taken with meals. Bromelain and other proteolytic enzymes are used by many alternative medicine doctors for treating chronic low-grade inflammatory conditions, like chronic back pain. They are best used for chronic, lingering inflammation, and not in the acute injury situation, since they inhibit the natural healing function of inflammation. Bromelain has been shown in clinical studies to shorten recovery time from injury, accelerate tissue repair, and reduce swelling, inflammation, and pain.

Ingredient Form: Bromelain with a guaranteed potency of 2,400 gelatin-digesting units, or other equivalent enzyme activity.

Effective Supplement Dosages: As a digestive aid for regular use, bromelain is included in dietary supplements in amounts ranging from 5 to 30 mg, along with other digestive enzymes. For nutritional support as part of a total treatment for injuries, the dosage found to be effective in clinical studies is 500 mg of standardized bromelain, three times per day; take thirty minutes before meals. Use under a doctor's supervision to ensure proper treatment of injuries.

Cofactors: For injury recovery, papain and curcumin; in digestive enzyme formulas, proteases, cellulases, and lipases.

Concerns: Bromelain is not an essential nutrient, so there is no possibility of bromelain deficiency. Use of bromelain is not recommended for individuals with known gastrointestinal disorders. Bromelain can cause reversible side effects such as gas, nausea, diarrhea, and allergic skin reaction. For adult use, not for pregnant or lactating women.

Use Guidelines: Use low-dosage bromelain-containing supplements on a daily basis, taken with meals, to aid digestion. Use high-dosage bromelain-containing supplements for short periods of time for nutritional treatment of certain injuries.

Butcher's broom (also *Ruscus aculeatus*)
Supplement Type: Botanical

Overview: Butcher's broom contains phytonutrients called saponins, which are reported to display anti-inflammatory action and are vasoconstrictive. Butcher's broom has a long history of use, particularly by European women to treat capillary fragility and reduce edema resulting from prolonged standing. While these traditional benefits are acknowledged, more clinical studies are needed to make a conclusive evaluation of the beneficial effects.

Benefits: Used to promote circulatory system health. Used to reduce edema in the legs, and as a natural medicine to treat varicose veins and hemorrhoids.

Ingredient Form: Standardized butcher's broom extract (8% to 12% ruscogenins).

Effective Supplement Dosages: Taken in dosages of 40 to 160 mg per day of standardized butcher's broom extract.

Cofactors: Other botanicals beneficial to the circulatory system, such as bilberry, ginkgo, gotu kola, and horse chestnut seed.

Concerns: Butcher's broom is not an essential nutrient. It can be beneficial to promoting the health of the circulatory system and in the natural treatment of venous disorders. Butcher's broom is considered a safe botanical but should be taken only as directed. For adult use only; not for use by children or by pregnant or lactating women. Use under a doctor's supervision for medical conditions.

Use Guidelines: Take butcher's broom supplements on a periodic basis to strengthen your circulatory system, or as a natural treatment for venous disorders.

Caffeine (also 1,3,7-trimethylxanthine)
Supplement Type: Botanical constituent

Overview: Caffeine is a central nervous system stimulant, increases glycogenolysis and lipolysis, is a mild diuretic, and stimulates the heart. It is found naturally in some botanicals, such as coffee, tea, and guarana. It is also made synthetically and added to foods or sold as a drug. Caffeine is a common ingredient in herbal energy formulas and thermogenic weight loss formulas. Its overuse can result in mild to severe side effects. Recently caffeine consumption has been linked to depletion of calcium from the body; however, many studies do not find bone loss in people who maintain adequate calcium intake. Moderate caffeine intake is relatively safe, but heavy caffeine intake, equivalent to five cups or more of coffee per day, should be avoided. Women who have concerns about osteoporosis should avoid caffeine and take appropriate actions to ensure adequate intake of calcium and other bone-building nutrients.

Benefits: Caffeine is primarily used as a stimulant to improve mental alertness, shorten reaction time, improve performance of attention-requiring tasks, temporarily sustain performance during continuous physical exertion, restore mental alertness, and keep people awake.

Ingredient Form: Some dietary supplements contain naturally occurring caffeine from botanical ingredients such as guarana and yerba mate, standardized to 4% to 80% methylxanthines, or also reported as caffeine.

Effective Supplement Dosages: Dosages in over-the-counter drug products range from 100 to 200 mg caffeine. Lower dosages of 25 to 100 mg are typically found in herbal caffeine-containing products and foods. Because there is quite a variation in caffeine-containing supplements, refer to specific products for proper dosage instructions.

Cofactors: None.

Concerns: Caffeine is not an essential nutrient. It is used widely in beverages such as coffee, tea, and soda. Caffeine can cause adverse effects, such as gastrointestinal irritation, nervousness, insomnia, restlessness, tinnitus, muscle tremor, headache, mild delirium, nausea, excitement, tachycardia, or cardiac arrhythmia. Not for use by children or by pregnant or lactating women. Caffeine should not be ingested every day in excessive amounts; in fact, its use should be limited or avoided. Because caffeine ingestion may cause an increase in calcium excretion, make sure you maintain adequate calcium intake, and avoid regular caffeine consumption if you are at risk for bone disorders such as osteoporosis.

Use Guidelines: For people who can tolerate caffeine, use caffeine-containing supplements periodically to increase mental and physical performance.

Calcium (also Calcium carbonate, calcium citrate, calcium malate, calcium citrate-malate, calcium lactate, calcium gluconate, calcium glycinate, and calcium phosphate. Other forms of calcium include bone meal, dolomite, hydroxyapatite, and oyster shell.)

Supplement Type: Mineral

Overview: Calcium is an essential mineral and a major component of bones and teeth. It activates a number of enzymes, regulates muscle contraction and relaxation, aids in vitamin B_{12} absorption, is required for acetylcholine synthesis, is needed for blood clotting, and is essential for regulation of heartbeat. Weight-bearing exercise is important to maintain bone mass. If you are taking corticosteroids, which inhibit calcium absorption and have been associated with onset of osteoporosis and bone fractures, higher daily dosages of calcium may be needed.

Benefits: Calcium builds strong bones and teeth, prevents bone loss and osteoporosis, and promotes blood pressure regulation and normal physiology.

Ingredient Forms: The digestion and absorption of calcium are related to its solubility. Inorganic forms such as calcium phosphate and calcium carbonate tend to be less soluble, especially in mature adults. The organic forms, such as calcium citrate, calcium citrate-malate, and calcium gluconate, are more absorbable when taken on an empty stomach, and are also more expensive. Refined calcium carbonate is a good choice and is sometimes found combined with the more expensive forms. Use of the expensive forms is preferred for children and for special therapeutic reasons, such as during menopause or while bone fractures are healing. You can also select one of the many brands of calcium supplements that have undergone clinical research. Calcium carbonate is one of the most clinically researched forms of calcium and has been shown to be safe and effective for all ages.

Dosages: Calcium's estimated total dietary safe range of intake is 1,200 to 4,000 mg per day, depending on your size and activity level. The typical adult dietary supplement calcium intake ranges between 500 and 1,500 mg per day. Children's dosages range from 350 mg to 1,000 mg per day. Calcium supplements are available in tablets, capsules, chewable wafers, and liquids. Calcium supplements may contain one or more forms of the mineral, and can contain other minerals and vitamins. As individual needs vary, always check with your health care practitioner and follow the directions on the products you purchase.

Cofactors: Vitamin D, vitamin K, boron, and magnesium can enhance calcium absorption.

Concerns: Poor calcium intake can lead to bone deformation, growth retardation, bone fractures, muscle spasms, leg cramps, high blood pressure, and osteoporosis. Excessive calcium intake for long periods of time can cause constipation and calcium deposits in the kidneys and can inhibit absorption of iron, zinc, and other minerals. The adult RDI for calcium is 1,000 mg. Naturally occurring lead has been found to occur in some forms of calcium, in particular dolomite, bone meal, oyster shell, calcium phosphate, and unrefined calcium carbonate. Forms of calcium supplements reported to have less problem with lead contamination include refined calcium carbonate, calcium citrate, calcium citrate-malate, calcium glycinate, and other chelated calcium forms. The best way to be sure is to check with the manufacturer. Lead contamination is a major concern with children, as it can adversely affect mental function.

Use Guidelines: Use calcium-containing supplements daily.

Calcium sulfate: *see* Excipients

Carnitine (also L-carnitine, 3-carboxy-2-hydroxy-N,N,N-trimethyl-l-propanaminium hydroxide, inner salt)

Supplement Type: Metabolite

Overview: Carnitine is an organic compound made in your body. It is sometimes mistakenly referred to as an amino acid, but chemically it is classified as a quaternary amine. The biologically active form of carnitine, L-carnitine, functions to transport fatty acids into the cells' mitochondria, where energy is produced. Carnitine is essential for the proper functioning of all living cells in the human body. The more research that is done on people taking L-carnitine dietary supplements, the more health benefits are reported. Carnitine's role in energy production is essential to maintaining vibrant health. It is useful for all athletes, especially those participating in endurance sports. Start taking carnitine if you are concerned about maintaining your cardiovascular or brain wellness, or if you have a family history of heart or brain illness. Recently medical studies have reported improvements in individuals with Alzheimer's and other senile dementias who took 2,000 to 4,000 mg per day of acetyl-L-carnitine, a modified form of L-carnitine. By adding the acetyl molecule to L-carnitine, the new molecule, acetyl-L-carnitine, has enhanced activity in the brain. Research indicates that acetyl-L-carnitine is better absorbed by brain and nervous system tissues, and should be the dietary supplement of choice for people with brain wellness concerns. Ask your doctor about using this supplement as part of treatment of senile dementias.

Benefits: Even though your body can make carnitine, over forty clinical studies have reported various health benefits from taking carnitine supplements. These include improved weight loss results, increased exercise and athletic performance, enhanced heart and circulatory system wellness, brain wellness, effective nutritional therapy for chronic fatigue syndrome, and improved sperm count and motility. It is essential for optimal health in infants and children.

Ingredient Form: L-carnitine HCl, L-carnitine tartrate, and L-carnitine magnesium citrate. Avoid products containing D-carnitine, which can have adverse health effects. L-Carnipure is the brand name of a certified pure form of L-carnitine.

Dosages: For nutritional purposes, 250 to 500 mg every day is useful; 500 to 1,500 mg is more beneficial taken every day. Higher dosages, ranging from 2,000 to 4,000 mg per day, taken in divided dosages, have been used for up to several months for therapeutic purposes under a doctor's supervision, and have been well tolerated.

Cofactors: L-carnitine can be taken alone or along with other ingredients in special-use formulas. For example, it is found with coenzyme Q_{10} and magnesium in heart wellness formulas, and with choline, inositol, methionine, and betaine in fat-metabolizing formulas.

Concerns: Carnitine is not an essential nutrient, but is beneficial when ingested as a supplement. Carnitine dietary supplements have a good safety record with no major adverse side effects reported using nutritional dosage ranges. Take high dosages of L-carnitine for therapeutic purposes only under the supervision of a doctor. Use by children and pregnant or lactating women should be under a doctor's supervision.

Use Guidelines: Make carnitine part of your daily supplement program. Use higher daily dosages when needed.

Carotenoids

The principal carotenoid that research has focused on during the 20th century is beta-carotene (see entry for details). Its health-promoting effects are well known, due to beta-carotene's action as an antioxidant, which primarily deactivates destructive free radicals that can harm the body's cells. During the 1990s, scientists began to widen the focus of their research and quickly discovered that there are other biologically important carotenoids that occur in food and the human body. These "new carotenoids" offer similar health benefits as their relative, beta-carotene. By preventing free radical damage, people who have higher body levels of carotenoids and other antioxidants are less likely to develop a degenerative disease, in particular cancer and cardiovascular diseases. These new carotenoids include alpha-carotene, lycopene, lutein, zeaxanthin, and beta-cryptoxanthin. However, researchers have focused their studies on lutein and lycopene in particular. Lutein functions as an antioxidant, but has shown to have selective benefits in improving vision, circulatory system health, and immune system function. Lycopene offers similar benefits, but has been touted for its suspected benefits in preventing cancers, especially prostate and lung cancers.

Future research will continue to provide insights on the benefits carotenoids have to offer. In addition to taking a supplement containing some or all of these carotenoids (beta-carotene, alpha-carotene, lutein, and lycopene being the most commonly encountered), you should consume foods that are good sources of these antidisease nutrients. Some good food sources of carotenoids include amaranthus leaves, broccoli, Brussels sprouts, carrots, Chinese cabbage, green beans, kale, spinach, sweet potatoes, tomatoes and tomato products, and winter squash.

Cascara sagrada (also *Rhamnus purshiana*)
Supplement Type: Botanical
Overview: Cascara sagrada contains anthraquinones, which function in the digestive system as stimulant laxatives. Cascara sagrada has a long history of use as a traditional natural laxative. Some people find that use of cascara sagrada offers advantages over over-the-counter drug laxatives and other more stimulatory herbal laxatives, such as senna. It is known for gentle, restorative action when taken in low dosages. It is best used under a doctor's supervision, in case side effects or complications develop.

Benefits: Cascara sagrada promotes intestinal regularity. It is considered a mild herbal laxative that helps restore intestinal function and tone.

Ingredient Form: Standardized cascara sagrada dried bark (7% to 30% total hydroxyanthracene derivatives [HAD]).

Effective Supplement Dosages: Cascara sagrada tablets or capsules, 40 to 160 mg for the treatment of constipation. Use as directed on the product labels to ensure proper dosage of the HAD active ingredients, which can vary from product to product. You can also take cascara sagrada in liquid extract form, but it is extremely bitter.

Cofactors: Other herbal laxatives may be included in cascara sagrada formulas, such as senna, plantago seed, aloin, rhubarb, and buckthorn.

Concerns: There is no essential nutritional need for cascara sagrada. Use with caution as a herbal laxative. Extended use should be avoided. It should not be used by pregnant or lactating women, children, or individuals with gastrointestinal diseases, unless under a doctor's supervision. Do not use with other laxative drugs, especially other stimulant laxatives. If constipation persists for two or more days, consult your doctor.

Use Guidelines: Use cascara sagrada periodically to promote gastrointestinal regularity.

Cat's claw (also *Unicaria tomentosa*)
Supplement Type: Botanical
Overview: Cat's claw is reported to stimulate the immune system. More research needs to be done to determine the exact benefits of cat's claw. Popular use in dietary supplements is based on South American Indian traditional use.

Benefits: Supports immune system function. Used in South America to help maintain health.

Ingredient Form: Standardized cat's claw bark (15% polyphenols, 3% alkaloids).

Effective Supplement Dosages: Daily dosage of 400 to 800 mg per day as capsules or tablets for short-term use, to promote immune system function and good health. Do not use to treat diseases.

Cofactors: Other immune-stimulating herbs, such as echinacea, garlic, astragalus, and reishi mushroom.

Concerns: Cat's claw is not an essential nutrient. Its usefulness in supporting immune system health is based on traditional use by Peruvian Indians. Limited clinical research corroborates an immune-stimulating effect and usefulness in treating digestive system ailments. More research is needed to determine the exact benefits of stimulating the immune system with cat's claw. It is not to be used by pregnant or lactating women, children, or people with serious diseases. No major side effects have been reported.

Use Guidelines: Use supplements containing cat's claw periodically to boost your immune system, along with other immune-stimulating supplements.

Cellulose: *see* Excipients

Chamomile (also *Matricaria chamomile*)
Supplement Type: Botanical

Overview: Chamomile contains phytochemicals with antispasmodic, anti-inflammatory, calming, and sedative actions on the body. Chamomile has a long history of use for these applications. Chamomile can be very useful for individuals with gastrointestinal spasms and inflammatory diseases of the gastrointestinal tract. If you are experiencing gastrointestinal problems, seek immediate medical attention for the proper treatment or management of your condition. Chamomile is also used in sleep, calming, and relaxation herbal formulations for its reported sedative effects.

Benefits: Chamomile supplements have traditionally been used to promote digestive system health. Chamomile is also used to reduce gastrointestinal spasms and inflammation of the gastrointestinal tract caused by some diseases.

Ingredient Form: Chamomile tea, made from chamomile flowers, is the most widely used form of chamomile to provide relief for the digestive system. Standardized liquid extracts are also common. Recently tablets and capsules have been developed using standardized chamomile flower extract (1.2% to 2% apigenin and 0.5% terpenoids).

Effective Supplement Dosages: For chamomile tea, three to five cups per day between meals is a common daily dosage range. Common dosages for tablet and capsule supplement forms are 250 to 1,000 mg per day of the standardized chamomile flower extract. Do not overdose on chamomile products, and follow the directions provided on the product labels carefully.

Cofactors: Chamomile formulas sometimes contain other herbs beneficial to the digestive tract, such as ginger, licorice root, and aloe gel.

Concerns: There is no essential nutrition requirement for chamomile, and no nutritional deficiencies result from insufficient intake. Chamomile products can be used periodically as needed to provide the desired gastrointestinal benefits. In rare cases allergies have been reported; people with known allergies to ragweed and other members of the Asteraceae family of plants should be cautious about ingesting chamomile products. Use by children and pregnant or lactating women should be under a doctor's supervision.

Use Guidelines: Use chamomile supplements periodically as needed.

Chaste tree berry (also *Vitex agnus-castus*)
Supplement Type: Botanical
Overview: Of the many phytochemicals in chaste tree berry, some inhibit prolactin release by binding to dopamine receptor sites. This prolactin-inhibiting effect is what makes chaste tree berry useful to many adult females. Chaste tree berry extract is a safe and effective choice for premenopausal women with menstrual problems and PMS discomfort. It has been used in Europe for over thirty years by millions of women.

Benefits: It is used to support female health and hormonal balance, especially in premenopausal women. Elevated prolactin levels are sometimes associated with PMS symptoms, such as swollen and tender breasts. Chaste tree berry's prolactin-lowering effect is thought to play a vital role in restoring a normal menstrual cycle and relieving PMS discomfort.

Ingredient Form: Standardized chaste tree berry extract (0.5% agnuside, 0.6% acubin) in tablets and capsules.

Effective Supplement Dosages: The daily dosage for periodic use by women who are not pregnant or lactating is 20 to 120 mg of standardized extract, in tablet or capsule forms. Chaste tree berry is also available as an aqueous-alcoholic extract.

Cofactors: A variety of botanicals or nutrients, depending on the product's intended use.

Concerns: Chaste tree berry is not an essential nutrient, but its use can be beneficial. Side effects that may occur include itchy rash due to allergic reaction, headaches, and gastrointestinal upset. Not to be used by children or by pregnant or lactating women unless under a doctor's supervision. This ingredient is recommended for periodic use only by adult females. If you have persistent breast or abdominal pain, consult a doctor for supervised medical treatment. Do not use with dopamine-receptor antagonist drugs.

Use Guidelines: For periodic use by adult females as needed to promote balance and reduce discomfort associated with PMS and menstrual problems.

Chitosan (also N-acetyl-D-glucosamine)

Supplement Type: Metabolite

Overview: Chitosan is a fibrous substance of animal origin. It is derived from a compound called chitin, found in the exoskeletons of shellfish such as crabs, lobsters, and shrimp. Chitosan absorbs fats in the digestive system, thereby lowering the amount of fat and cholesterol that goes into the bloodstream. Chitosan has a history of use in cosmetic and pharmaceutical products, but its use in dietary supplements is relatively new.

Benefits: Chitosan binds to fats and reduces the absorption of cholesterol and fats from the digestive system into the body. It helps maintain healthy cholesterol levels and can function as a weight loss aid.

Ingredient Form: In dietary supplements as N-acetyl-D-glucosamine (chitosan).

Effective Supplement Dosages: For use as a diet aid or cholesterol-lowering agent, take 500 to 1,500 mg three times a day with main meals.

Cofactors: A multivitamin-mineral supplement should be taken between meals to ensure adequate nutrient bioavailability, as chitosan may reduce the absorption of certain essential nutrients. Take other dietary supplements between meals as well to minimize the possibility that chitosan may interfere with their absorption.

Concerns: Chitosan is not an essential nutrient. Its popularity is mostly as a novel weight loss aid, due to its fat-binding effects. Chitosan is considered nontoxic but should not be overused, as nutrient deficiencies may develop. Persons who are allergic to shellfish should consult a doctor before using it. For use by adults only; not for use by children or by pregnant or lactating women unless under a doctor's supervision.

Use Guidelines: Use chitosan-containing supplements periodically.

Chloride

Supplement Type: Mineral

Overview: Chloride is important to the body as an anion (a negatively charged molecule) in extracellular fluid (any fluid that is found in the areas of the body outside the cells, such as blood, lymph, and interstitial fluid, or fluid between cells and tissues). Chloride plays a role in both fluid and blood acid-base balance. It is also a component of the stomach's digestive juice secretions, required in the formation of hydrochloric acid. Chloride is also one of the electrolyte minerals, which, along with sodium and potassium, regulates the flow of water between cells and the bloodstream. Due to the fact that most people ingest too much sodium and not enough potassium, you should consider using a potassium chloride salt substitute so that you ensure adequate intake of both potassium and chloride.

Benefits: Chloride promotes normal body function. It maintains the body's water balance. Promotes normal digestion in the stomach.

Ingredient Form: Chloride is rarely added to dietary supplements because of its prevalence in foods. It is provided in the diet primarily as part of the sodium chloride (salt) molecule, but it is also found in salt substitutes as potassium chloride. Chloride is also contained in supplements as part of the hydrochloric acid molecule (HCl), commonly combined with other nutrients such as thiamine, pyridoxine, and arginine.

Effective Supplement Dosages: The adult Reference Daily Intake (RDI) for chloride is 3,400 mg. Chloride is sometimes added to athletic fluid replacement drinks to compensate for the chloride lost through increased sweating. Chloride is also found in supplements for the elderly, whose dietary intake can be deficient in this important mineral. When chloride is added to dietary supplement products it is usually in small amounts, under 100 mg. Also, remember that when you add salt to food (and you should do so sparingly, if at all), you are supplementing your diet with both chloride and sodium.

Cofactors: The other electrolytes, potassium and sodium. Note, however, that the typical American diet is too high in sodium and too low in potassium. Refer to the individual sections on these other ingredients for tips on lowering sodium intake and increasing potassium intake.

Concerns: Chloride is an essential nutrient. A deficiency is rarely reported but may occur under conditions of severe dehydration, renal disease, or malnutrition; the symptoms include dizziness, fainting, and weakness. Excessive intake of chloride may result in side effects such as hypertension and problems with fluid balance. Chloride is safe for use by all ages and both sexes, as directed.

Use Guidelines: Chloride-containing supplements may be useful for active people or individuals who are at risk for nutrient deficiencies due to poor dietary habits.

Chlorophyll: *see* Greens powders

Choline (also 2-hydroxy-N,N,N-trimethylethanaminium)

Supplement Type: Vitamin

Overview: Choline functions as a precursor for betaine, acetylcholine, and phospholipids such as phosphatidylcholine. It is a lipotropic agent, involved in fatty acid metabolism and the prevention of fat deposits in the liver. Choline is a component of lecithin and a part of all cell membranes. In the nervous system, choline is important in the synthesis of the neurotransmitter acetylcholine, which is involved in memory, muscle control, and other functions. Choline supplements have a long history of safe use. Make sure your daily vitamin supplement includes choline as an ingredient. Increase your intake of choline if you are concerned about maintaining brain wellness or are athletic, or for other therapeutic reasons determined by your health care practitioner.

Benefits: Choline intake is associated with improved brain and nervous system wellness and with maintenance of healthy cellular structure and function. It is essential for efficient fatty acid metabolism and health of the liver. It is also important in infant formula to ensure proper brain and nervous system development and overall growth and development.

Ingredient Forms: Choline is found in dietary supplements as choline bitartrate, choline dihydrogen citrate, choline citrate, and phosphatidylcholine. It is also contained in lecithin, as phosphatidylcholine.

Effective Supplement Dosages: In 1998 choline was officially classified as an essential vitamin and recommended daily intakes were designated for the first time. The adequate intake for adult males is 550 mg per day, and for adult females is 425 mg per day, 450 mg per day during pregnancy, and 550 mg per day during lactation. The tolerable upper intake level for adults is 3.5 g per day. Nutritional use dietary supplement intake typically ranges from 25 to 500 mg per day. Athletes, people on weight loss programs, and individuals trying to improve or maintain brain function will typically take 500 to 1,200 mg per day without reported side effects.

Cofactors: Choline is found in vitamin-mineral formulas; in lipotropic formulas along with methionine, inositol, carnitine, and betaine; and in memory formulas with various mind-enhancing nutrients and herbs, such as phosphatidylserine and ginkgo.

Concerns: Choline is an essential nutrient, required for the promotion and maintenance of health. High intakes of choline supplements for prolonged periods of time, over 2,000 mg per day, may cause diarrhea, depression, dizziness, body odor, sweating, salivation, reduced growth rate, hypotension, and hepatotoxicity. Choline supplements are safe for all ages and both sexes when used as directed.

Use Guidelines: Take choline-containing supplements each day.

Chondroitin sulfate (also Chondroitin 4-sulfate, chondroitin 6-sulfate, chondroitin sulfuric acid, chonsurid, glycosaminoglycan, mucopolysaccharide)

Supplement Type: Metabolite

Overview: Chondroitin sulfate is a biological polymer, which is an important component of connective tissues. It gives cartilage and ligaments their flexibility and attracts water to these tissues, thereby maintaining proper hydration. Chondroitin sulfate is also an important component of the circulatory system. Chondroitin sulfate is a long molecule made up of repeating molecules of N-acetylgalactosamine and glucuronic acid. The research on using chondroitin sulfate supplements to improve joint and bone health is promising. However, researchers point out that because chondroitin sulfate is poorly absorbed by the body, it should be taken with glucosamine to ensure best results in treating osteoarthritis and other connective tissue conditions.

Benefits: As we age, our connective tissues can become increasingly worn, causing joint mobility problems and degenerative diseases. Chondroitin sulfate supplementation has been shown to improve the condition of connective tissues, improve tissue repair and wound healing, treat osteoarthritis by restoring joint function and reducing pain, and also cause improvements in circulatory system wellness by increasing structure of the inner lining of blood vessels.

Ingredient Forms: Chondroitin sulfate is derived from cartilage from different animal sources. Purity and quality vary considerably. Select products that contain purified chondroitin sulfate or hydrolyzed chondroitin sulfate.

Effective Supplement Dosages: For nutritional support of joint and cardiovascular system health, use 400 to 600 mg per day. Concerning therapeutic use of chondroitin sulfate, several clinical studies have reported that taking 600 to 1,200 mg per day for several months caused improvements in joint function in cases of osteoarthritis and rheumatoid arthritis.

Cofactors: For best results, chondroitin sulfate should be used with glucosamine. Additional nutrient cofactors include vitamin C, manganese, zinc, copper, bioflavonoids, and vitamin E.

Concerns: Chondroitin sulfate is not an essential nutrient, but it can be beneficial to health. Use under a doctor's supervision for treatment of diseases such as osteoarthritis and coronary heart disease. Minor side effects observed with long-term use include allergic reactions and gastrointestinal upset. Take with meals to reduce gastrointestinal upset. Safe for all ages and both sexes, but children and pregnant or lactating women should use it under a doctor's supervision.

Use Guidelines: Chondroitin sulfate supplements can be taken every day at nutritional dosage levels. Use therapeutic dosages for short periods of time, several months at a time.

Chorella: *see* Greens powders

Chromium

Supplement Type: Mineral

Overview: Chromium is an essential mineral. Its major biological role is as a potentiator of insulin; that is, it helps insulin do its job. It is important in carbohydrate metabolism. Chromium also functions in the maintenance and metabolism of nucleic acids. Because most diets are lacking in chromium, make sure chromium is included in your daily supplement program.

Benefits: Studies report that taking chromium supplements can help in weight management by increasing fat loss and by maintaining or increasing muscle tissue; stabilize blood sugar levels; improve insulin functioning; and help in the nutritional management of diabetes.

Ingredient Forms: Chromium dinicotinate glycinate, chromium picolinate, chromium polynicotinate, chromium chloride, chromium arginate, chromium gluconate, Chromax, and Chromemate.

Effective Supplement Dosages: The adult RDI for chromium is 120 mcg. Daily dosages of between 200 and 600 mcg per day are well tolerated. Most complete supplements include 50 to 200 mcg of chromium. It is used in higher dosages for weight loss, body building, and other special circumstances.

Cofactors: Chromium should be part of a complete vitamin-mineral supplement.

Concerns: Chromium is an essential nutrient. It is safe and effective when used as recommended. Chromium deficiency can result in elevated blood cholesterol, insulin resistance, fatty deposits in arteries, and overall poor health. Chromium toxicity is rarely reported. It is safe for all ages and both sexes in recommended dosages.

Use Guidelines: Use chromium-containing supplements daily for optimal health.

Citrimax: *see* Garcinia

Citrin: *see* Garcinia

Citrus seed extract: *see* Bioflavonoids

Coenzyme Q_{10} (also coQ_{10}, ubiquinone, ubiquinol, mitoquinone)

Supplement Type: Metabolite

Overview: Coenzyme Q_{10} is involved in energy production in all cells, and functions as an antioxidant. It plays a particular role in the proper function and maintenance of a healthy heart and circulatory system. Take a separate supplement to add extra amounts to your diet as required. If you have a cardiovascular condition, ask your doctor about using coenzyme Q_{10} as part of your nutritional therapy.

Benefits: Supplemental intakes of coenzyme Q_{10} have been associated with the following benefits: improved heart function, reduced free radical damage of LDL cholesterol, greater reduction of body fat in dieting obese females than with diet alone, immune system enhancement, improved athletic performance in endurance sports, and lowering of blood pressure.

Ingredient Form: Coenzyme Q_{10} is sold as capsules, tablets, softgels, and powders. A new lipid-based form of coQ_{10} has recently been developed and is available in some products. It is called CoQsol, and the marketers report that an independent clinical trial concluded that CoQsol has an intestinal absorption rate three times faster than the same amount of coenzyme Q_{10} taken in capsule form. Q-Gel is another special form of coenzyme Q_{10} that has been shown to have improved bioavailability.

Effective Supplement Dosages: As an antioxidant, 10 to 60 mg is effective. For boosting heart health, weight loss, and athletic performance, higher dosages are required, from 60 to 300 mg per day.

Cofactors: It is found along with vitamins and minerals in daily supplements.

Concerns: Coenzyme Q_{10} is not an essential nutrient, but promotes good health. It has a good record of safety and effectiveness for all ages and both sexes.

Use Guidelines: Coenzyme Q_{10} should be part of your daily supplement program.

Colloidal Minerals

During the 1990s dietary supplement companies began to market mineral supplements containing "colloidal minerals." These mineral supplement products were mostly in liquid forms, but as the popularity of colloidal minerals grew, they began to be available in tablets and capsules as well. Colloidal minerals are actually complexes of seventy or more minerals obtained from certain kinds of earth formations, such as shale and clay. The mineral particles are so small that when added to water, they become suspended in it. Currently there are no medical studies reporting on the beneficial health effects of their ingestion. While these products can supply a vast array of minerals and trace minerals important to health, they also may contain toxic minerals such as aluminum, lead, lithium, mercury, and titanium, albeit in very small amounts. Many people report feeling better and having more energy when using colloidal mineral products, and no adverse health effects have been reported. However, keep in mind that some forms of mineral toxicity can take years to develop.

Colostrum

Supplement Type: Concentrate

Overview: Colostrum is the special milk that is secreted for a short period of time by mammals after they give birth. It contains growth factors, immune system compounds, and other nutrients that help give offspring a jump start on the road to a healthy life. Commercially, colostrum is collected from cows. Its use as a dietary supplement is increasing, based on reported benefits to gastrointestinal health and potential immune-stimulating effects. Recent research has been conducted on colostrum's benefits for helping promote and maintain the population of healthy microflora in the intestines. Studies with adults and children have shown that colostrum intake helps normalize the gastrointestinal system and combats severe diarrhea. Dr. Bernard Jensen, a pioneer in the field of nutrition, is one of the great proponents of colostrum, which he calls "white gold."

Benefits: Colostrum helps support gastrointestinal health.

Ingredient Form: Defatted, concentrated colostrum, standardized to 26% to 33% Ig (immunoglobulin) content.

Effective Supplement Dosages: As a dietary supplement, colostrum is taken in amounts between 100 and 500 mg a day. Higher dosages, 1,000 to 3,000 mg per day, are sometimes used initially for up to two to three months for colostrum's gastrointestinal restorative health benefits.

Cofactors: None.

Concerns: Colostrum is not an essential nutrient. Its use as a dietary supplement can be beneficial to gastrointestinal health. Colostrum is considered nontoxic, but no long-term studies exist to verify its long-term impact on the body. For adult use only. Use by children and pregnant or lactating women should be under a doctor's supervision.

Use Guidelines: Use colostrum-containing supplements periodically as required.

Conjugated linoleic acid (also CLA)

Supplement Type: Fatty acid

Overview: CLA occurs naturally in our diets in small amounts. It is made from the essential fatty acid linolenic acid. Interest was attracted to CLA during the 1990s when research showed anticarcinogenic effects in animal models. Subsequent research revealed CLA's involvement in promoting a reduction in body fat when used with proper diet and exercise. CLA is gaining in popularity among individuals wanting to lose weight or maintain lean bodies. Recent scientific studies on humans report conflicting results on the effectiveness of CLA in reducing body fat. CLA may be useful for athletes who need to burn fat while maintaining muscle mass.

Benefits: CLA stimulates metabolism of fatty acids, making it a useful nutritional weight loss aid.

Ingredient Form: Conjugated linoleic acid; one brand is Tonalin.

Effective Supplement Dosages: Studies indicate that in order to get the benefits of CLA, high daily dosages must be taken, ranging from 2 to 6 g per day.

Cofactors: Other nutritional weight loss aids, such as carnitine, garcinia, and fiber.

Concerns: CLA is not an essential nutrient. It is a metabolite, made by the body. Increasing dietary intake through supplementation may improve the body's fat-burning ability. While there are no major reported side effects from using CLA in short-term studies, long-term studies are needed to confirm safety and health benefits. Gastrointestinal upset is a temporary side effect reported in the research. Recommended for use by healthy adults only. Always consult your doctor before starting any weight loss program.

Use Guidelines: Use CLA periodically as part of your weight management program.

Copper

Supplement Type: Mineral

Overview: Copper is an essential mineral needed (along with iron) for the formation of hemoglobin, which carries oxygen in the body. It is present in many enzymes and is important in the formation of collagen, melanin synthesis, immune function, and energy production. It helps keep blood vessels, nerves, and bones healthy. There are no special uses for copper besides its essential nutrient roles.

Benefits: Supplement intake ensures adequate copper for maintenance of health.

Ingredient Forms: Copper lysinate, copper gluconate, copper aspartate, copper oxide, and copper arginate.

Effective Supplement Dosages: The adult RDI for copper is 2 mg. For daily supplement use in adults, dosages range from 0.5 to 3 mg per day.

Cofactors: It is found along with other minerals and vitamins in most complete dietary supplement formulations. Make sure that adequate iron and zinc intake is maintained as well.

Concerns: Copper is an essential nutrient, but do not take megadoses of it. Inadequate copper intake can cause bone abnormalities, anemia, reproductive system failure, abnormal skin pigmentation, decreased arterial elasticity, malformation of connective tissues, and low superoxide dismutase (SOD) activity. Safe and effective for all ages and both sexes when used as directed.

Use Guidelines: Use copper-containing multinutrient supplements daily.

Cranberry (also *Vaccinium macrocarpon*)

Supplement Type: Botanical

Overview: Cranberry has a history of use for combating urinary tract infections. Medical research has recently confirmed that phytonutrients in cranberry reduce the ability of infectious bacteria to cling to the inner surfaces of the urinary tract and cause infection. Regular consumption of cranberry juice has been associated with reducing urinary tract infections, bladder infections, and chronic kidney inflammation. Keep in mind that you need to maintain a high intake of cranberry supplements and/or juice to experience the health benefits. Health food stores also carry cranberry juice concentrate, which can be used to make your own low-calorie beverage or in cooking. Cranberry supplements offer a nice alternative to the calories in sugary cranberry juice drinks.

Benefits: Promotes and maintains bladder and urinary tract health.

Ingredient Form: Dietary supplements containing standardized cranberry fruit extract (22% to 30% organic acids). Drinking cranberry juice beverages is also effective.

Effective Supplement Dosages: The daily dosage is 500 to 3,000 mg of standardized cranberry fruit extract, or 12 to 24 ounces of high-quality cranberry juice beverages.

Cofactors: None.

Concerns: Cranberry is not an essential nutrient, but has beneficial effects on the urinary tract. It is safe, with no concerns about toxicity. However, consumption of large amounts of cranberry supplements or cranberry juice may cause gastrointestinal upset. If this occurs, reduce the daily dosage, and slowly increase it again over one week until the desired daily dosage is tolerated. Always treat infections under the supervision of your doctor. Remember that urinary tract infections can migrate to the bladder and kidneys and cause significant health problems. Use cranberry supplements and juice as supportive therapy in conjunction with medically supervised drug treatment. Safe for all ages and sexes when used as directed.

Use Guidelines: Take a cranberry-containing supplement on a regular basis if you are concerned about maintaining urinary tract health.

Creatine (also Creatine monohydrate)
Supplement Type: Metabolite
Overview: Creatine is manufactured in the body, and is used to make the high-energy molecule creatine phosphate. During periods of strenuous exercise, creatine phosphate is used to immediately replenish the muscles' supply of ATP, which helps sustain powerful muscle contractions. Creatine is therefore an important nutrient for maximizing short-term anaerobic strength and athletic performance. Of all the athletic supplements, creatine has received the most attention from researchers in recent years for its ability to improve muscle strength and power, increase muscle mass, improve performance in short-duration high-intensity exercise, and reduce muscle fatigue with short-term use. It is important for people who use creatine supplements to realize that it is not an essential nutrient and does not provide essential nutrition to the body, so eat well and take multinutrient, protein, and carbohydrate supplements for best results. Weight-lifting women frequently report that creatine helps them improve their workouts but makes them feel bloated and retain water. The "cell volumizing" effect referred to in magazine articles is in part due to the extra creatine and creatine phosphate content in muscle, which causes greater water retention. This is also one explanation why creatine causes muscle cramps in some individuals.

Benefits: Improves strength and power performance. Reduces fatigue experienced during strenuous strength exercise. Promotes increases in muscle mass when used along with a muscle-building training program.

Ingredient Form: Creatine monohydrate is currently the most clinically researched form of creatine.

Effective Supplement Dosages: Using creatine supplements involves a two-step procedure. Step one is the creatine loading phase, which involves ingesting 5 to 10 g of creatine three to four times per day, for a total daily intake of 20 to 40 g, for three to four days. Step two is the creatine maintenance phase, with daily ingestion of 5 to 15 g of creatine, depending on body size and hours of activity. Larger or more active athletes may need higher maintenance dosages.

Cofactors: Simple carbohydrates have been shown to improve creatine absorption, as have effervescent creatine beverages. Note that caffeine has a negative effect on creatine absorption and should be avoided.

Concerns: Creatine is not an essential nutrient. Its use as a dietary supplement has been shown to increase strength and power. Over twenty clinical studies using creatine for short periods of time, up to three months, have found it to be safe and effective. Minor side effects include gastrointestinal upset and muscle cramping. Creatine should be used only by well-nourished, healthy adults in good physical condition. Creatine nutrition therapy has been used to help improve creatine status in individuals with creatine metabolism disorder. One area of concern is that prolonged excessive creatine intake causes increased build-up and elimination of its breakdown product, creatinine. The health effects of this are unknown, and long-term studies are needed to determine the health effects of regular intake of high amounts of creatine supplements. For now, short-term use by strength and power athletes will produce beneficial performance effects. Not for use by children or by pregnant or lactating women.

Use Guidelines: Take creatine supplements periodically as required.

Croscarmellose sodium (Ac-Di-Sol): *see* Excipients

Curcumin (also Turmeric, *Curcuma longa*)
Supplement Type: Botanical
Overview: Curcumin has a long history of use in Ayurvedic medicine and as a spice. Recently scientists have determined that phytonutrients in curcumin have various beneficial health effects, such as potent antioxidant function, anti-inflammatory action, anti-platelet-aggregation activity, and natural antiseptic activity. While there are several traditional health roles attributed to ingestion of curcumin, recent research has discovered its role in maintaining liver health and function. Curcumin has also been tested in clinical studies and found to be an effective anti-inflammatory agent, useful for injury recovery and as supportive therapy for rheumatoid arthritis. In Europe, curcumin is used to treat peptic disorders. Curcumin is a great botanical supplement to try if you have liver, cholesterol, or digestive system

THE COMPLETE NUTRITIONAL SUPPLEMENTS BUYER'S GUIDE

concerns. For people who are suffering from inflammatory diseases, make sure to let your doctor know you are using curcumin, to ensure adequate medical supervision. Keep in mind that curcumin's anti-inflammatory action will take several days to become apparent. There is some indication that regular intake of curcumin, as a supplement or spice, can help reduce the risk of certain degenerative conditions and protect against cancers.

Benefits: Curcumin promotes liver health and circulatory system health. Curcumin protects against inflammatory disorders such as arthritis. Curcumin stimulates secretion of bile and reduces cholesterol levels.

Ingredient Form: Standardized curcumin (turmeric) root extract (85% to 98% curcuminoids). A special form of curcumin, called Curcumin C3 Complex, is manufactured by Sabinsa and used by dietary supplement manufacturers as an ingredient in the products they make.

Effective Supplement Dosages: As a dietary supplement for daily use, take 50 to 200 mg two to three times a day, of standardized curcumin root extract. For short-term nutritional therapeutic use, higher dosages in the range of 250 to 500 mg, three times per day, have been shown to be safe and effective. Some botanical antioxidant formulations contain smaller amounts, 15 to 60 mg, in consideration of the combined antioxidant actions of the other botanical ingredients.

Cofactors: Other antioxidants; milk thistle for liver health; and boswellia, bromelain, ginger, devil's claw, and yucca.

Concerns: Curcumin is not an essential nutrient, but it has beneficial effects. Turmeric has a long history of use as a spice and is considered nontoxic. However, long-term safety studies of high dosages have not been undertaken, so limit use of high dosages to a few months. Curcumin use is contraindicated in cases of obstructed bile ducts and gallstones, in which case a doctor's supervision is required, as with any medical condition. Curcumin dietary supplements should be used by adults only; they are not for use by pregnant or lactating women unless under a doctor's supervision.

Use Guidelines: Curcumin-containing supplements can be taken every day at nutritional dosages, or used at higher therapeutic dosages for short periods of time.

Cysteine (also L-cysteine)
Supplement Type: Amino acid
Overview: Cysteine is a nonessential amino acid made from methionine in the body. It is used in the manufacture of proteins and helps form glutathione, an important antioxidant and detoxifying compound. Cysteine is one of the less common dietary supplement ingredients, but more supplements are now using a modified form of cysteine, N-acetyl cysteine, for its reported glutathione-enhancing effects, leading to better antioxidant status throughout the body. Recent attention has been directed toward N-acetyl cysteine for its use in the management of angina and respiratory system problems. Consult your doctor

about using N-acetyl cysteine for these conditions. Cystine is another, less commonly encountered nonessential amino acid, important in hair and skin formation. Cystine is rarely used in dietary supplements.

Benefits: Maintenance of good health and well-being.

Ingredient Forms: Cysteine is sometimes used in dietary supplements as L-cysteine.

Effective Supplement Dosages: Cysteine is in most protein foods. As a dietary supplement, some antioxidant and detoxifying formulations will contain cysteine: 250 to 500 mg per day. Higher dosages of cysteine may be used for medical reasons under a doctor's supervision.

Cofactors: Selenium, which is also important for glutathione function; vitamin B_6, vitamin C, vitamin E, and calcium.

Concerns: Cysteine has attracted attention recently for its role in glutathione function and status. While cysteine is considered nontoxic, it is recommended that cysteine supplements not be taken in megadoses. For adult use only. Caution: Individuals with the metabolic disorder cystinuria should not take cysteine supplements due to an increased risk of cysteine-related gallstone formation.

Use Guidelines: Take cysteine-containing supplements on a regular basis as needed.

Dahlulin: *see* Fructans

DHEA (also Dehydroepiandrosterone)
Supplement Type: Metabolite

Overview: DHEA is a hormone made by the adrenal gland, and has become a popular ingredient in dietary supplements marketed as longevity products. As we get older, levels of DHEA decline in the body; this decline is thought to contribute to the aging process. Some studies conducted on adults over age forty have shown that DHEA contributes to improvements in body composition, energy levels, immune system activity, mood, and a youthful mental outlook. DHEA supplements have been used by millions of people since 1994. DHEA can therefore play a vital role in maintaining youth when used properly.

Benefits: Promotes normal DHEA levels in the body. DHEA has been clinically shown to improve body composition, function, and mental well-being.

Ingredient Form: Dietary supplements contain DHEA as dehydroepiandrosterone.

Effective Supplement Dosages: Keep in mind that DHEA is a hormone and is not for everyone. Its use should be monitored by your doctor. For people over forty years old, daily dosages of 25 to 50 mg have been shown to be effective. Dosages as high as 100 mg have been studied for several months; they provide benefits with only minor side effects.

Cofactors: Antioxidants, adaptogenic herbs, and other longevity nutrients.

Concerns: DHEA is not an essential nutrient. Its use as a dietary supplement should be under a doctor's supervision. Do not use DHEA if you have a preexisting medical condition, are under forty years old, are on hormone therapy, or are sensitive to hormone therapy. Women need to exercise extreme caution when using DHEA, as research studies report that DHEA has a weak androgenic effect and may induce growth of body and facial hair. Not for use by children, young adults, or pregnant or lactating women. Do not use DHEA if you are a male who may have prostate cancer or a female who may have breast cancer, a reproductive system cancer, or a reproductive system disorder. Other adverse effects of DHEA include acne, liver enlargement, irritability, and prostate hypertrophy. The IOC, USOC, NCAA, and NFL have banned its use.

Use Guidelines: Use of DHEA supplements by adult males under a doctor's supervision is optional.

7-KETO TM DHEA

In response to providing a dietary supplement ingredient that has the benefits of DHEA without the potential side effects, researcher Dr. Henry Lardy set out to develop a better raw material to be used in supplement products. The result of his research is contained in a new dietary supplement ingredient known as 7-KETO TM DHEA. What's so special about 7-KETO? Dr. Lardy points out that it does not convert to testosterone or estrogen, like DHEA does. Most of the unwanted side effects of taking DHEA supplements are due to overproduction of these metabolic products. Tests on

humans have been conducted using 7-KETO, which report that it is safe and effective. So far studies using 7-KETO show a beneficial effect on improving immune system function and promoting weight loss. A recent study reported that 7-KETO supplements promoted significant weight loss through a thermogenic effect, which stimulated increased fat utilization. In only eight weeks, people taking 7-KETO lost an average of over six pounds while following a balanced 1,800 calorie-per-day diet. The researchers report that the safe and effective daily dosage of 7-KETO is 50 mg to 200 mg. While additional studies are needed to clearly establish 7-KETO's safety for longer-term use, the current research findings indicate that 7-KETO can be used safely and effectively as part of short-term weight loss programs.

Desiccated liver: *see* Glandulars

Devil's claw (also *Harpogophytum procumbens*)

Supplement Type: Botanical

Overview: Devil's claw, so named because of its large claw-shaped fruit, contains phytonutrients with varied biological effects. The harpogosides have been shown to have anti-inflammatory activity and are considered the most biologically active components of devil's claw. In Europe devil's claw is also used as an appetite stimulant, digestive stimulant, and analgesic, and for dyspepsia, gallbladder dysfunction, and rheumatism.

Benefits: Devil's claw is an anti-inflammatory botanical, useful in the nutritional treatment of inflammatory diseases or inflammation from injuries.

Ingredient Form: Standardized devil's claw extract (5% harpogosides).

Effective Supplement Dosages: As a dietary supplement to nutritionally support anti-inflammatory therapy, take 100 to 150 mg per day of standardized devil's claw extract.

Cofactors: Ginger.

Concerns: Devil's claw is not an essential nutrient. There have been only limited human studies testing the effects of devil's claw. Long-term safety has not been established, but based on a long history of use, devil's claw is considered safe and effective for short-term use, up to several months at a time. For use by adults only; not for use by children or by pregnant or lactating women. Best used under a doctor's supervision for supportive treatment of inflammatory diseases. Not for use by individuals with stomach or duodenal ulcers.

Use Guidelines: Use devil's claw supplements periodically when needed.

Echinacea (also *Echinacea purpurea, Echinacea angustifolia*)

Supplement Type: Botanical

Overview: Echinacea extracts have been shown to stimulate immune system function by causing an increase in white blood cells and spleen cells, as well as improved phagocytosis (removal of foreign material from the blood). Echinacea is used worldwide, and is even recommended by the World Health Organization. It is best used for short periods of time. Only the higher dosages listed below have been found to be effective. The immune-system-enhancing effects of lower daily dosages has not been established.

Benefits: Echinacea stimulates and supports immune function. Clinical studies have verified that taking echinacea extract will reduce the incidence of and duration of flu symptoms. It supports immune function during times of physical or emotional stress. As an herbal drug, it is effective as supportive therapy for colds and flu and for chronic infections of the lower urinary tract and respiratory tract, along with appropriate drug therapy.

Ingredient Form: Standardized *Echinacea purpurea* (4% phenolics or 4% echinacosides) in tablets or capsules. Liquid tinctures and other preparations are also effective, and have been clinically verified. Echinacea extracts are variously made from the flower, the roots, or from the entire plant.

Effective Supplement Dosages: As a dietary supplement during cold season or periods of emotional or physical stress, use 450 to 900 mg of standardized tablets or capsules per day, or an equivalent liquid dosage, for three weeks, then discontinue use for seven to ten days. Use only periodically, when the immune system may be compromised by stress or exposure to infection.

Cofactors: Sometimes other immune system herbs will be found in echinacea preparations, such as goldenseal, garlic, astragalus, cat's claw, and reishi mushroom.

Concerns: Echinacea is not an essential nutrient. For use by adults only. Do not use for serious diseases or autoimmune diseases. Some people may experience flulike symptoms when taking echinacea. Always consult your doctor when illness sets in.

Use Guidelines: Use echinacea supplements periodically to help prevent or treat colds and flu, or during periods of emotional or physical stress, to help boost your immune system response.

Eleuthero (also Siberian ginseng, *Eleutherococcus senticosus*)

Supplement Type: Botanical

Overview: Eleuthero contains a variety of phytoactive substances grouped under the name eleutherosides. Eleuthero has long been used in traditional Chinese medicine as an energizer. In the twentieth century, research by Russian scientists determined its immunostimulating effects (it increases the number of T lymphocytes), its improvement of weak nervous system function, its contribution to increased energy, and other generalized health-promoting effects. Eleuthero is considered an adaptogen, which is a substance that causes a general improvement in the body's ability to withstand adverse influences and stress. Use eleuthero if you are feeling run-down and fatigued. Some supplements may use the traditional Chinese names for various parts of eleuthero, such as ciwujia (root) and ciwujiapi (bark). Eleuthero is a member of the ginseng plant family (Araliaceae), but it is not equivalent to the other ginsengs of the *Panax* genus.

Benefits: Eleuthero improves the general state of health, normalizes the body, improves nonspecific immune function, increases the ability to do work, stimulates mental alertness, and improves resistance to certain diseases. It is used as a daily health tonic; to improve physical and mental performance in stressful jobs, jobs demanding high performance, or in athletic performance; or for invigoration during times of fatigue or reduced capacity for work or concentration.

Ingredient Form: In dietary supplements, standardized *Eleutherococcus senticosus* root, stem, or leaves (0.8% or higher eleutherosides). A 33% ethanol extract was used in the Russian research studies.

Effective Supplement Dosages: Eleuthero has been used in studies for intervals of up to sixty days, followed by a two- to four-week period of nonuse. As with other herbs, when it is taken for therapeutic purposes, supervised short-term use is advised. In dietary supplements 100 to 1,000 mg per day of standardized eleuthero extract in tablet or capsule form is commonly used.

Cofactors: Other ginsengs.

Concerns: Eleuthero is not an essential nutrient. It is best used for two to three months at a time during periods of increased physical or emotional stress. It is not recommended for people with high blood pressure, pregnant and lactating women, or for children. It may cause feelings of nervousness or excitation. It may cause dizziness, due to a slight hypoglycemic effect after ingestion, in some people.

Use Guidelines: Use eleuthero supplements on a regular basis to improve energy levels and overall health.

Enzymes

Two types of enzyme ingredients are commonly encountered in dietary supplements: enzymes to aid in digestion, and enzymes to aid in healing and in cases of inflammation. Digestive enzymes include amylase, cellulase, lactase, lipase, and protease. Because potencies vary for digestive enzymes, consult the directions provided on the product label for proper use. Always take digestive enzymes with meals. If you have a gastrointestinal disorder, do not use digestive enzymes unless under a doctor's supervision.

Healing enzymes found in dietary supplements include bromelain, papain, and trypsin. Refer to the entry on bromelain for details of these types of enzymes.

Ephedra (also Ma huang, *Ephedra sinica*, and other *Ephedra* species)

Supplement Type: Botanical

Overview: Ephedra contains the drugs ephedrine, pseudoephedrine, and other alkaloids. It is traditionally used in China for the treatment of bronchial asthma, related ailments, and diseases of the respiratory tract with bronchospasms. Ephedra has gained popularity in the United States during the 1990s as a weight loss aid. Research studies using the drug ephedrine showed that ephedrine increased weight loss and appetite control. This spurred dietary supplement manufacturers to promote ephedra, which contains ephedrine, for similar uses. Despite all the potential side effects, the bad press, and the Food and Drug Administration's attempts to ban or severely limit the use of ephedra- and ephedrine-containing products, ephedra is still one of the most popular weight loss aid ingredients on the market. Perhaps it is because in people who do not experience the negative side effects, ephedra can promote a more energetic feeling, improve appetite control, and give you a "buzz." But if you are using ephedra products as a weight loss aid, keep in mind that there are no formal manufacturing controls to ensure that you are getting a safe and effective dosage. Products can contain higher dosages of ephedrine than are listed on the label, which is potentially dangerous. If you choose to use ephedra for any reason, do so under the supervision of your doctor.

Benefits: As a dietary supplement, it is used experimentally as a weight loss aid; as an herbal medicine, it is used for supportive treatment of bronchial asthma, and to relieve bronchospasms.

Ingredient Form: Standardized *Ephedra sinica* (8% to 12% alkaloids or naturally occurring ephedrines). The total amount of ephedrine per dosage should be listed on the label.

Effective Supplement Dosages: As a weight loss aid, ephedra-containing dietary supplements with 12 mg per tablet of ephedrine are taken with meals, two to three times per day. Some products recommend higher dosages, but with higher dosages side effects and adverse health effects increase. For bronchial treatment, a daily dosage of 15 to 30 mg per day of ephedrine is used under medical supervision. Only use ephedra products for short periods of time.

Cofactors: In herbal weight loss aids, caffeine-containing herbs such as guarana are frequently included with ephedra, due to caffeine's reported ability to enhance ephedra's weight loss effects. Other ingredients are commonly found in ephedra products for a host of alleged companion effects.

Concerns: Use of ephedra products can be dangerous to your health if misused. The drug ephedrine (one of the alkaloids in ephedra) is potentially addictive, and is one of the most highly controlled over-the-counter drug products. Do not use without a doctor's supervision. If side effects develop, discontinue use and consult your doctor immediately. Side effects include nausea, loss of appetite, tremors, sleeplessness, tachycardia, urinary retention, insomnia, irritability, anxiety, high blood pressure, vomiting, and cardiac arrhythmia. Chronic use or overdose can result in severe cardiac toxicity or psychosis. Long-term use can have permanent adverse health effects. Do not use ephedra if you are pregnant, lactat-ing, or have any diseases. Do not use ephedra with other drugs, especially monoamine oxidase inhibitors (MAOIs). Definitely not for use by children. Note that in his review of this book, Dr. J. Zuess pointed out, "I never prescribe ephedra. There are other medications that can do everything ephedra can, with much less toxicity. Many herbalists agree with me."

Use Guidelines: Ephedra-containing products should be used only on a periodic basis, under a doctor's supervision.

New Concerns About Ephedra-Containing Products

In May 1999 the Texas Board of Health published a warning statement that must appear on dietary supplement products containing the herb ephedra.

Persons using ephedra-containing products should consult a physician or other licensed qualified health care professional before taking the product if they have heart disease, thyroid disease, diabetes, high blood pressure, recurrent headaches, glaucoma, difficulty urinating, prostate enlargement, seizures or depression or other psychiatric condition, or a family history of any of these conditions. Ephedra-containing products are not for use by those who are pregnant, nursing, or under age 18. Exceeding the manufacturer-recommended dosage may cause serious health effects, including heart attack and stroke, and persons who consume caffeine while taking ephedra-containing products may experience serious adverse health effects.

It is interesting to note that the Texas Board of Health chose not to place restrictions on the amount of ephedrine (the active ingredient in ephedra) per single dosage and total daily dosage (though such restrictions were proposed, with a limit of 25 mg per single dosage and up to 100 mg of ephedrine per day). This leaves consumers' health vulnerable to what manufacturers think are safe dosages. If you are going to use ephedra-containing products, you should consult your physician.

Essential Fatty Acids

Essential fatty acids (EFAs) include linoleic, linolenic, and arachidonic acids. Linoleic acid is considered a primary EFA. It is necessary for normal growth and health. The body cannot manufacture it, so it must be obtained from the diet. Arachidonic acid, on the other hand, is made by the body from linoleic acid. However, dietary intake of this EFA may become essential if dietary linoleic acid intake is low. Arachidonic acid is therefore considered conditionally essential. Alpha-linolenic acid is the other important essential fatty acid. Among its important functions is that the body uses it to make two important health-promoting fatty acids, eicosapentaenoic acid (EPA) and docosahexaenoic acid (DHA). The body prefers to use EFAs for structural roles instead of fuel or fat deposits. Structural fatty acids are

important in forming and maintaining all cell membranes, for example. Therefore a diet that is low in nonessential fatty acids, such as saturated fatty acids, and contains moderate amounts of EFAs is healthier for you, assuming you are not overeating. Overeating forces the body to convert excess nutrients, like carbohydrates, to fatty acids and be stored in fat cells. Some of the functions of EFAs include:

- Growth enhancement
- Wound healing
- Maintenance of brain and nervous system cells and function
- Cell formation
- Serving as precursors of eicosanoids, which are involved in regulating a variety of metabolic processes
- Forming part of phospholipids, which are the building blocks of cellular and subcellular membranes

EFAs are vital to overall health, but too much of them can make you fat or lead to what I call the EFA health paradox. The EFA health paradox comes from ingesting too much linoleic acid and arachidonic acid. In the body these two fatty acids make a certain type of prostaglandin that can encourage inflammation, blood platelet aggregation, arteriosclerosis, and cancer cell growth. On the other hand, alpha-linolenic acid ingestion leads to beneficial products such as EPA and DHA, which have well-known cardiovascular effects. Alpha-linoleic acid results in production of beneficial prostaglandins, which reverses arteriosclerosis, decreases inflammation, promotes fat-burning metabolism, and inhibits cancer cell growth. Our modern processed food diets are too high in linoleic acid and too low in alpha-linolenic acid. Refer to the Natural-Thin diet for guidelines on correcting common fatty acid imbalances.

Ester C: *see* Vitamin C

Evening primrose oil: *see* Plant oils

Excipients

In addition to the nutrient ingredients contained in dietary supplements, a number of non-nutrient ingredients are usually present. Called excipients, these inert ingredients have various roles in the manufacture of dietary supplements and provide them with characteristics important to digestion and absorption into the body. The following lists some of the major types of excipients you will see listed on product labels. Note that some of the excipient ingredients can have more than one function.

Binders. Binders are added to tablets to help hold the ingredients together after the tablet is compressed. Examples of some common binders include dextrose, cornstarch, sugar, hydrogenated vegetable oil, carboxymethyl-cellulose, gums, gelatin, and methylcellulose.

Coatings. Coatings are used on tablets to make them smoother, to act as a barrier to moisture and oxygen, and to give them color. Some coatings are slowly poured on the tablets as they are tumbled about in a drum-like machine. The other major tablet-coating process is spray coating, which is done in a machine that looks like a big clothes dryer, with spray nozzles inside. Examples of common coatings include: pharmaceutical glaze, BetaCoat, and shellac. Shellac is a resin that serves as an enteric coating—it resists being dissolved in the stomach's acidic gastric juices but will dissolve in the more alkaline intestinal digestive juices.

Colors. Colors are sometimes added to supplements to give them a consistent look and improve their appearance. They can also be used in spray coatings. The ingredients used in supplements that add color can be natural but are usually synthetic. Synthetic colors used in dietary supplements, foods, drugs, and cosmetics must be approved by the FDA, and their designated uses are indicated by letters and numbers. For example, if you see "FD&C Red No. 3" on the label, the product contains a red coloring agent approved for use in foods, drugs, and cosmetics.

Diluents. Because the main ingredients of tablets and capsules may be present in very small amounts, diluents are often needed in tablet and capsule formulations to increase the tablet to a reasonable size. Most tablets contain some diluents. Some of the commonly used diluents include dibasic calcium phosphate dihydrate, hydrogenated vegetable oil, tribasic calcium phosphate, and microcrystalline cellulose.

Disintegrants. Disintegrants are added to tablet and capsule formulations to help them break up after ingestion. Some examples of disintegrants include croscarmellose sodium, microcrystalline cellulose, and colloidal silicon dioxide.

Flavors. Flavors are added to chewable tablets and to powder and liquid dietary supplements. Sometimes a flavoring agent, such as vanilla or peppermint, is added to tablet or capsule supplements to mask the smell of vitamins or herbs and make it more pleasant to the nose upon opening the bottle. Flavors used in dietary supplements can be natural or synthetic. The exact kind of flavor used in a product is usually not disclosed; it is just listed on the label as "natural flavor" or "artificial flavor."

Glidants. Glidants are excipients that improve the flow properties of the powder blends so that they move through the machines smoothly. Some glidants include colloidal silicon dioxide, magnesium trisilicate, and tribasic calcium phosphate.

Lubricants. Lubricants are added to tablet and capsule formulations for a number of reasons—to keep the dry powder formulation from sticking to the tablet/capsule manufacturing equipment; to improve the rate of flow through the machines; and to decrease sticking of the finished tablets to the dies in which they are compressed. Some examples of lubricants include magnesium stearate, stearic acid, and hydrogenated vegetable oils.

Feverfew (also *Tanacetum parthenium*)

Supplement Type: Botanical

Overview: The primary phytoactive component of feverfew, called parthenolide, is a serotonin antagonist—that is, it inhibits serotonin release. Increased serotonin levels are associated with headaches, so use of feverfew supplements can reduce the incidence of migraine headaches. It can take several weeks to notice a decrease in migraine occurrences and duration, which is well worth the wait for sufferers of migraine headaches.

Benefits: The most noted benefit of feverfew is to prevent or reduce the occurrence of migraine headaches. In clinical studies a daily dosage of feverfew has been shown to reduce the frequency and intensity of migraine headaches.

Ingredient Form: Standardized feverfew leaves (0.2% or higher parthenolide).

Effective Supplement Dosages: An effective dosage of parthenolide per day is obtained from 125 to 400 mg of standardized feverfew leaf per day.

Cofactors: Ginkgo, white willow.

Concerns: Feverfew is not an essential nutrient. It has been proven to be effective as a prophylactic treatment for migraine headaches. Occasional gastrointestinal upset can occur. For adults only; not for use by those with a clotting disorder, or pregnant or lactating women, unless under a doctor's supervision. In one study where the subjects ate feverfew leaves each day, some individuals developed mouth ulcerations. However, this does not occur with tablets or capsules. If side effects occur, discontinue use.

Use Guidelines: Feverfew should be used by people who suffer from migraine headaches.

Flaxseed oil: *see* Plant oils

Fiber (also Insoluble fibers: cellulose, hemicellulose, lignin. Soluble fibers: gums, mucilages, pectins.)

Supplement Type: Botanical

Overview: Insoluble dietary fiber promotes normal elimination by providing bulk for stool formation and thus hastening the passage of the stool through the colon. Insoluble fiber also helps to satisfy appetite by creating a full feeling. Soluble fiber can help to reduce cholesterol levels in the blood; see entry on beta-glucan for details. Adequate fiber in the diet will prevent many diet-related health disorders, such as diabetes, coronary heart disease, obesity, high blood pressure, and certain cancers. While fiber supplements can help, you need to eat right, which means ingesting several servings of high-fiber, low-calorie vegetables per day, and one to three servings of fruit. Grains also contain fiber, but don't overconsume them, because they are higher in calories.

Benefits: Promotes gastrointestinal health and normal bowel function.

Ingredient Form: Dietary supplements contain a variety of plant and fruit fibers. However, psyllium husk fiber is recognized by the FDA for its cholesterol-lowering ability. Bios Life 2 is a clinically tested fiber drink that has been shown to reduce cholesterol levels; it is available from Rexall Showcase International.

Effective Supplement Dosages: The daily reference value for total fiber intake is 25 g per day from fruits and vegetables. Experts estimate that the average American diet provides about 17 g per day or less. Other experts calculate that dietary fiber intake should be over 40 g per day. If you think your fiber intake needs a boost, try taking dietary supplements containing 4 to 12 g of fiber a day and see how your system responds.

Cofactors: A healthy diet.

Concerns: Dietary fiber is considered essential to optimal health. When using fiber supplements, make sure not to take too much too fast. Bloating, cramping, gas, and other gastrointestinal distress can occur. Give your body a chance to adjust to the increase in dietary fiber consumption by slowly increasing fiber intake over a three-week period. Adequate fiber intake is essential for adults and children. Also be aware that some dietary fibers, such as guar gum and glucomannan, can swell and cause esophageal obstruction. To prevent this, use fiber supplements in the form of beverages, especially for children.

Use Guidelines: Use fiber supplements on a daily basis.

Flavonols: *see* Bioflavonoids

Flower Pollen: *see* Bee pollen

Folate (also Folic acid, folacin)

Supplement Type: Vitamin

Overview: Folate is a water-soluble vitamin. It functions in the formation of genetic compounds (DNA and RNA) and participates in metabolic processes. When consumed by pregnant women, folate has been linked with prevention of certain birth defects and reduces the incidence of premature birth. Folate, along with vitamins B_6 and B_{12}, helps lower homocysteine levels; high levels of homocysteine can damage blood vessel walls and increase the risk of coronary heart disease.

Benefits: Maintenance of health, reduction in neural tube birth defects, improved cardiovascular health.

Ingredient Form: Folic acid.

Effective Supplement Dosages: The adult RDI for folate is 400 mcg. Maintain supplement intake of folate between 400 and 1,200 mcg per day. Take higher dosages of folate before and during pregnancy, as directed by your doctor. Athletes and people who lead stressful lifestyles should also consider maintaining higher folate supplement intake; 800 to 1,200 mcg per day.

Cofactors: Vitamins B_6 and B_{12}.

Concerns: Folate is an essential nutrient. Supplemental intake of folic acid is mandatory for all children and adults who want to optimize their health.

Use Guidelines: Take folate-containing supplements every day.

FOS (also Fructans, fructooligosaccharides, inulin)

Supplement Type: Botanical; however, note that some brands are made through microbial production

Overview: A dietary complex carbohydrate, consisting of mostly chains of fructose.

Virtually indigestible by the body, but a preferred food of the beneficial bacteria living in the intestines. In Japan FOS is added to hundreds of food products for its beneficial health effects. Scientists have determined that eating refined sugar increases the intestinal population of the less desirable bacteria and reduces the number of beneficial bacteria. FOS supplements can therefore be used to restore intestinal balance, function, and health.

Benefits: Clinical studies have shown that 1 g of FOS per day will increase the amount of the beneficial intestinal bacteria; such as bifidobacteria and lactobacilli. These are the bacteria that produce vitamins in the intestines, assist in digestion, deter the formation of pathogenic bacteria, relieve constipation, promote and maintain healthy intestinal function, lower blood cholesterol and triglyceride levels, and help maintain blood sugar levels. Dietary FOS is sometimes referred to as a prebiotic.

Ingredient Form: FOS as inulin, which is from natural plant sources, is often found in supplements. Some companies will just list fructooligosaccharides on the label. Some products contain a special patented form of FOS called Dahlulin, which is naturally derived from plants.

Effective Supplement Dosages: FOS content in dietary supplements will typically range from 250 to 4,000 mg. A daily dosage between 500 and 2,000 mg will produce good results. It takes about three to four weeks for the FOS to promote an increase in the beneficial intestinal bacterial, so be patient.

Cofactors: FOS is added to other digestive health formulas, usually products that contain the probiotic bacteria lactobacilli and bifidobacteria.

Concerns: FOS are not essential nutrients, but they are beneficial ones. Some people may experience temporary intestinal gas the first few days of taking FOS dietary supplements. This passes as your intestinal bacteria adjust.

Use Guidelines: Take FOS-containing supplements on a regular basis.

GABA (also Gamma-aminobutyric acid)

Supplement Type: Amino acid

Overview: GABA is a nonessential amino acid that functions primarily as an inhibitory neurotransmitter. Inhibitory neurotransmitters are substances produced in the nervous system that have calming effects. GABA has been demonstrated in clinical studies to be safe and effective. Some people use GABA supplements for a few months, in order to become a calmer person; others use GABA for a few days before meetings, public speaking, and other situations that they know make them nervous, to relax.

Benefits: GABA promotes relaxation and combats feelings of stress.

Ingredient Form: GABA.

Effective Supplement Dosages: GABA is taken in daily dosages ranging from 500 mg to 2 g. Higher dosages may sometimes be used under a doctor's supervision for behavioral disorder treatment.

Cofactors: Vitamin B_6, manganese, taurine, and lysine.

Concerns: GABA is a nonessential amino acid. It is considered safe and effective when taken in the recommended dosages. For adults only; not for pregnant or lactating women unless taken under a doctor's supervision. Some people may experience temporary side effects when taking GABA for the first time on an empty stomach; these include feelings of anxiety, increased rate of breathing, headache, and nausea. These side effects can last for a few hours.

Use Guidelines: If you are stressed out or feel edgy or nervous, try using GABA for a few months to help calm your nerves.

Gamma-linolenic acid: see GLA

GLA (also Gamma-linolenic acid)

Supplement Type: Fatty acid

Overview: GLA is a fatty acid that is made in the body from linoleic acid. GLA is an important precursor of the series-1 prostaglandins, a group of hormones that regulate many cellular activities. For example, the series-1 prostaglandins keep blood platelets from sticking together, control cholesterol formation, reduce inflammation, make insulin work better, improve nerve functioning, regulate calcium metabolism, and promote immune system functioning. Remember that a proper balance of fatty acids is required for optimal health, which means keeping total lipid intake under about 25 percent of total daily calories and not overeating. Also reduce cholesterol intake, and maintain proper body weight for best results. Recent research has determined that diets high in fats can even cause migraine headaches in some people.

Benefits: GLA promotes health and well-being, cardiovascular health, and immune system function. GLA reduces inflammation and relieves symptom associated with PMS.

Ingredient Form: Gamma-linoleic acid.

Effective Supplement Dosages: Typical daily dosages of GLA range from 100 to 500 mg per day. For nutritional treatment of specific conditions such as PMS, inflammatory diseases, and coronary heart disease, take higher dosages, 500 to 1,500 mg per day.

Cofactors: EPA, DHA, and alpha-linolenic acid.

Concerns: While GLA is not an essential fatty acid, it is important to good health. Dietary supplement intake of GLA is safe and effective. There are no known toxic or adverse effects reported for GLA; it is safe for all ages and both sexes. GLA has been reported to aggravate temporal lobe epilepsy. It is otherwise quite safe.

Use Guidelines: Make GLA-containing supplements a part of your daily nutrition program. Use higher amounts as required for nutritional management of specific health conditions.

Gamma-oryzanol

Supplement Type: Botanical

Overview: Gamma-oryzanol is a substance extracted from rice bran oil. The gamma-oryzanol molecule consists of phytosterols and ferulic acid. Gamma-oryzanol or its metabolites display a variety of biological activities in the body, such as antioxidant function, encouragement of endorphin release, lipotropic action, stress reduction, increased rate of growth, and improved recovery from exercise. Clinical studies have reported beneficial effects with gamma-oryzanol supplementation, such as reduction in serum cholesterol levels, reduction in menopausal symptoms including hot flashes and nervousness, improved gastrointestinal function, and improved physical performance. Gamma-oryzanol has been studied in several countries, with good results. It is especially useful for people concerned about circulatory system health, menopausal women, people with gastrointestinal problems, and physically active people and athletes.

Benefits: Gamma-oryzanol promotes wellness and improved health during menopause, improves physical performance, and promotes circulatory system health and function.

Ingredient Form: Purified gamma-oryzanol.

Effective Supplement Dosages: The dosages used in clinical studies and found to be safe and effective range from 300 to 900 mg per day. Small amounts (10 to 100 mg) are commonly found in multiple-ingredient dietary supplements, and these can be effective in promoting health when taken on a consistent basis. However, if you are taking gamma-oryzanol for a specific reason, use the higher dosages until improvements are seen, usually within one to three months.

Cofactors: Other daily supplements, such as vitamins and minerals.

Concerns: Gamma-oryzanol is not an essential nutrient, but is beneficial to health. Clinical studies report that gamma-oryzanol is well tolerated, safe, and effective for all ages and both sexes.

Use Guidelines: If you are athletic or looking to improve energy levels, include gamma-oryzanol in your daily nutrition program.

Garcinia (also *Garcinia cambogia*)

Supplement Type: Botanical

Overview: Garcinia contains a substance called HCA, (-)-hydroxycitric acid or (-)-hydroxycitrate. During the 1970s, in their search for a novel weight loss aid, the pharmaceutical company Hoffmann-La Roche discovered that HCA displays a few intriguing antiobesity functions in the body. For example, HCA reduces the rate of formation of fat from carbohydrates by interfering with an enzyme called ATP-citrate lyase; HCA has been found to decrease appetite, and may stimulate thermogenesis. Garcinia is now one of the most widely used nutritional weight loss aids. If you are having trouble losing weight, give garcinia a try; it may be effective for you, and it does not have the side effects found with weight loss drugs or some of the other herbal weight loss aids.

Benefits: Garcinia is useful as a nutritional weight loss aid and in the maintenance of desirable body weight.

Ingredient Form: Standardized *Garcinia cambogia* (50% or higher HCA). Some ingredient brand names include Citrimax and Citrin.

Effective Supplement Dosages: Standardized garcinia should be taken before meals, 500 to 1,000 mg, three times per day.

Cofactors: Garcinia is found in combination nutritional weight loss aids.

Concerns: Garcinia is not an essential nutrient. Its use as a nutritional weight loss aid is thought to be borderline effective; a few studies demonstrate a significant increase in weight loss, and some studies do not show a significant difference. More research is needed to provide additional dosage and use insights. Garcinia is considered safe and nontoxic. It is not for use by children or by pregnant or lactating women unless under a doctor's supervision.

Use Guidelines: Use garcinia supplements periodically as part of your weight management program.

Garlic (also *Allium sativum*)

Supplement Type: Botanical

Overview: The phytoactive ingredients in garlic, in particular allicin, display antioxidant activity, slow the development of atherosclerosis, have a mild blood pressure–lowering effect, reduce blood cholesterol, lower triglycerides, inhibit platelet aggregation, lower blood viscosity, stimulate immune system function, and exert mild anti-inflammatory effects. In some individuals, garlic may cause a temporary rise in triglycerides, due to the fact that it liberates fatty acids from adipose tissue (body fat); this usually passes in a few weeks to two months. Garlic supplements are particularly useful when used by older people to help maintain fluidity of blood flow, promote heart and circulatory system health, and stimulate well-being. Garlic is also recognized for its immune system–stimulating properties, and it is traditionally used as an antimicrobial agent; however, more clinical studies are needed to verify the exact dosages for these antimicrobial benefits.

Benefits: The main benefits of garlic as a dietary supplement are to maintain circulatory system health, promote healthy cholesterol and triglyceride blood levels, and build healthy immune system function. It protects blood vessels from the effects of free radicals, increases the good HDL cholesterol, lowers the bad LDL cholesterol, lowers mild elevated blood pressure, increases fibrinolysis (which results in a reduction in blood clots and plaques), and keeps the blood fluid.

Ingredient Form: Garlic supplements are typically standardized to 0.6% to 1% allicin. They may also be standardized to 1.3% alliin. Some products list "total allicin potential" on the label because the current scientific thinking on how garlic works is that

alliin is converted to allicin in the body, and it is allicin that has the primary biological activity. Pure-Gar is a brand of standardized garlic used in some products.

Effective Supplement Dosages: For use as a dietary supplement to lower cholesterol levels, mild blood pressure, and triglycerides, and improve immune function, a daily dosage of between 400 and 1,200 mg per day of standardized garlic is considered safe and effective, with dosages of 600 to 900 mg being commonly used. This is equivalent to about one-half to one clove of fresh (raw) garlic a day. (Cooking garlic reduces its effectiveness.) For promotion of a healthy circulatory system, 200 to 400 mg per day is sometimes used. However, if you have high cholesterol, triglycerides, or mild high blood pressure, use the higher dosages for two to four months until improvements are seen, as determined by your doctor.

Cofactors: Garlic is sometimes used with other circulatory system nutrients, such as ginkgo, hawthorn, and grape seed extracts.

Concerns: Garlic is not an essential nutrient. Its beneficial use has been established in many clinical studies to improve cardiovascular health, promote healthy blood lipid levels, and improve immune system function. Side effects are rare, and include garlic odor, occasional gastrointestinal upset, and allergic reactions. Consult a doctor for use of garlic supplements for children or for pregnant or lactating women.

Use Guidelines: Include garlic supplements as part of your daily supplement program if you are concerned about promoting circulatory system health.

Germanium

Supplement Type: Mineral

Overview: Germanium is an obscure trace mineral with no established essential functions in humans. Japanese researchers found that germanium supplements increase energy levels, improve circulation, stimulate immune function, and improve the body's adaptogenic response. Germanium is found in very small amounts in several common botanicals, such as ginseng, garlic, aloe, shiitake mushroom, onions, comfrey, and boxthorn seed.

Benefits: Current research does not support the use of germanium as a dietary supplement for daily intake. Clear benefits have not been determined.

Ingredient Form: Germanium sesquioxide, GE-132.

Effective Supplement Dosages: Supplemental amounts of 100 to 300 mg have been used; however, note there are reports of rash and kidney failure with germanium.

Cofactors: None.

Concerns: Should only be used under the supervision of your health care practitioner, to ensure safety.

Use Guidelines: Germanium supplements should not be used on a regular basis.

Ginger (also *Zingiber officinale*)

Supplement Type: Botanical

Overview: Ginger promotes saliva and gastric juice secretions, reduces stomach and intestinal gas, stimulates intestinal function, and has mild normalizing effects on the nervous system. Ginger can be useful to restore GI function if you are experiencing discomfort after eating. Its use to prevent motion sickness has been shown to be effective in some studies, and ineffective in others. Recent studies demonstrate that some of the bioactive substances in ginger extract can inhibit production of inflammatory compounds, such as PGE2 and leukotriene. This makes ginger a promising candidate for relieving inflammation and pain in people with arthritis and musculoskeletal disorders.

Benefits: The best-documented benefits of ginger supplements are in stimulating digestion, reducing GI gas, treating upset stomach, and preventing or reducing nausea due to motion sickness in some people. Ginger contains antioxidants and is thought to have health-promoting effects on the circulatory system.

Ingredient Form. In supplements, ginger root extract (standardized to 4% gingerols). You will also find whole unstandardized ginger powder used as well.

Effective Supplement Dosages: For use with meals to reduce nausea and stomach upset or for motion sickness, 250 to 750 mg per day of standardized ginger root extract. Ginger may occur in some dietary supplements at lower dosages, 20 to 100 mg, intended to support digestive system health. Ginger is sometimes added along with other herbs to help reduce their common GI upset side effects. Also, 1 to 4 g of unstandardized ginger root powder per day may be used as directed.

Cofactors: Ginger can be found mixed with a variety of other botanicals.

Concerns: Ginger is not an essential nutrient. Its use for GI disturbances, appetite stimulation, and motion sickness is usually restricted to a few days at a time, in the large dosages presented above. Ginger is considered safe, but you should consult your physician before using it for children, for pregnant or lactating women, or for GI disturbances.

Use Guidelines: Use ginger periodically as needed. Some multinutrient formulas may contain small amounts of ginger, 5 to 50 mg, for daily use.

Ginkgo (also Maidenhair tree, *Ginkgo biloba*, GBE, *Ginkgo biloba* extract)

Supplement Type: Botanical

Overview: Standardized extracts of ginkgo leaf have been shown to improve blood flow to the brain, increase microcirculation, exert antioxidant action, inhibit blood platelet aggregation, reduce capillary fragility, and improve neurotransmitter function. Ginkgo's circulation-improving and antioxidant actions can be beneficial to all individuals interested in maintaining health and promoting longev-

ity. Studies on patients undergoing walking rehabilitation experienced significant improvements after three weeks of taking ginkgo; improvements included increased walking distance, reduced time to perform walking exercise, and reduced leg pain. This may indicate that ginkgo supplement use is of benefit to exercisers and athletes.

Benefits: Scientific studies have reported a variety of benefits from using ginkgo: improved memory, improvements in senile dementia, treatment of headaches, reduction of vertigo and tinnitus, reduction of intermittent claudication.

Ingredient Form: Most of the clinical studies used a standardized *Ginkgo biloba* extract, consisting of 24% ginkgo flavoglycosides and 6% lactones. Only use ginkgo products that list the 6% lactone ingredients, as these are the ginkgolides, which play a major role in improving circulatory system function. Supplements and teas containing unstandardized ginkgo powder can be a source of ginkgo's phytonutrients; however, there are no clear guidelines for their most effective use due to a lack of studies using unstandardized ginkgo products. Ginexin and Gbe 24/6 are brand names of ginkgo extracts used in some supplement products.

Effective Supplement Dosages: Studies use mostly 120 mg of standardized ginkgo a day, usually divided among two or three dosages. Therapeutic dosages of 80 to 140 mg have been used for months at a time with no major side effects. Ginkgo supplements are available as tablets, capsules, and liquid extracts. Some ginkgo supplements may contain other ingredients. As individual needs vary, always check with your health care practitioner and follow the directions on the products you purchase for the safe use of ginkgo supplements.

Cofactors: Some formulas may also contain other ingredients to improve brain function or circulation, such as gotu kola, lecithin, choline, phosphatidylserine, and carnitine.

Concerns: Ginkgo is not an essential nutrient, but has beneficial health effects. Rare and minor side effects observed during clinical studies include gastrointestinal upset, headache, or skin rash. Due to ginkgo's blood-thinning action, caution should be exercised if you are taking anticoagulant drugs. Use by children or by pregnant or lactating women should be under a doctor's supervision.

Use Guidelines: If you are interested in improving the health of your mind and circulatory system, use ginkgo-containing supplements on a regular basis.

Ginseng (also Korean ginseng, Chinese ginseng, *Panax ginseng* [Korean ginseng, also called Chinese ginseng], *Panax quinquefolium* [American ginseng])

Supplement Type: Botanical

Overview: Ginseng has adaptogenic properties that increase the body's resistance to physical and emotional stress. It restores metabolic balance. Red Korean ginseng is *Panax ginseng* that has been steamed during processing, activating some of the phytonutrients (specifically antioxidants) in the ginseng roots and giving them a reddish tint, compared to the pure white of unsteamed ginseng root. In epidemiological studies in South Korea, a reduction in the risk of degenerative disease was reported with daily consumption of red Korean ginseng, which is thought to be due in part to the increase in dietary antioxidants. Korean ginseng is thought to be more stimulating than American ginseng because it contains a higher proportion of Rg1-type ginsenosides, which have weak central-nervous-system-stimulating effects, while American ginseng has a higher proportion of Rb1-type ginsenosides, which are calming. However, most clinical studies used Korean ginseng, and report the antistress, energy-boosting, and other benefits listed above. American ginseng has developed an identity as the "female ginseng"; this stems from its traditional use by American Indians as a tea to increase female fertility, but both men and women can take and benefit from both types. Finally, ginseng has been traditionally regarded as a weak aphrodisiac, and regular use is thought to promote longevity. Ginseng is reported to be of increasing benefit as you get older.

Benefits: This botanical improves physical and mental energy, reduces feelings of fatigue and burnout, increases work capacity, improves concentration, stimulates the immune system, increases alertness, improves reaction time, and increases coordination.

Ingredient Form: Standardized ginseng dietary supplements that contain *Panax ginseng* root (4% to 24% ginsenosides) or *Panax quinquefolium* root (5% to 14% ginsenosides). Note that the stem and leaves also contain ginsenosides and may be used in some formulations or in ginseng tea products.

Effective Supplement Dosages: Both Korean and American ginsengs are used in various amounts in dietary supplement formulas. Daily-use formulas with ginseng contain between 50 and 200 mg of the standardized root. Larger dosages, up to 1,000 mg per day of standardized ginseng, are used for shorter periods of time, up to a few months. For unstandardized ginseng root powder, 1 to 2 g per day in capsules is a common dosage. For ginseng products that contain higher standardized ginsenoside content than listed above, use lower daily dosages.

Cofactors: Ginseng is used in various combinations with other herbs and in vitamin-mineral dietary supplement formulas.

Concerns: Ginsenosides are not essential nutrients, but are beneficial. Ginseng is considered safe and nontoxic when used as directed; however, some people may experience nervousness, restlessness, or hypertension if excessive dosages are taken for long periods of time. Keep in mind that *Panax ginseng* has a history of safe use in Asia dating back two thousand years, and *Panax quinquefolium* was regarded as one of the most useful herbs by North American Indians. Also, keep in mind that when you are taking an adaptogenic herb, it may take a few weeks to produce the desired effects. During this period you may feel overstimulated or in some cases understimulated; this is a temporary condition, a result of the ginsenosides' various balance-restoring effects. Ginseng dietary supplement use should be restricted to adults; it is not recommended for children or for pregnant or lactating women unless under a doctor's supervision.

Use Guidelines: Use supplements containing low dosages of ginseng on a regular basis, while restricting use of higher dosages to intervals of a few months.

Glandulars

You will sometimes encounter processed animal glands as part of a dietary supplement formula. Liver is one of the most commonly encountered. Some other common glandular ingredients include adrenal glands, pancreas, spleen, thymus, and thyroid. In my experience, most high-quality glandular products are intended for use by a trained naturopathic doctor, chiropractor, or herbalist. At this time, I recommend that you select and use glandular products only as directed by your health care practitioner.

Glucosamine (also 2-amino-2-deoxyglucose, chitosamine)

Supplement Type: Metabolite

Overview: Glucosamine is manufactured by the body from glucose, nitrogen, and two molecules of hydrogen. It is used for the production of a group of compounds called glycosaminoglycans, which are needed to make cartilage and build strong connective tissues throughout the body. Glucosamine sulfate is not a sulfa drug, and people allergic to sulfa drugs should not be concerned; however, check with your physician to verify this if you have a known allergy to sulfa drugs or sulfites.

Benefits: Supplemental intake of glucosamine has been shown to stimulate production of connective tissues, improve joint repair and function, treat arthritis (osteoarthritis), promote healing of injuries and wounds and after surgery, strengthen the circulatory system, improve joint lubrication, and improve the thickness of skin, nails, and hair.

Ingredient Form: Most of the clinical studies used the glucosamine sulfate form, but most products contain the glucosamine HCl form; the benefits of the HCl form have been observed and confirmed by a recent clinical study.

Effective Supplement Dosages: The dosage regimen studied is 500 mg of glucosamine sulfate, three times a day, for improving healing, joint problems, and arthritis. Up to 3,000 mg per day has been used safely. These dosages were studied for periods of several months. Lower dosages, 25 to 500 mg per day, are found in products used for improving the structure of the body. Athletes typically use 500 to 1,500 mg per day during the preseason and season to promote healing and prevent injury. Glucosamine supplements are available in tablets, capsules, powdered drinks, and liquids. As individual needs vary, always check with your health care practitioner and follow the directions on the products you purchase for the safe use of glucosamine supplements.

Cofactors: Glucosamine supplements may contain other ingredients that are important to healing or that stimulate the growth of connective tissues, such as boron, chondroitin, shark cartilage, calcium, magnesium, vitamin C, vitamin E, flaxseed oil, SAM-e (S-adenosylmethionine), and bioflavonoids.

Concerns: Most people of any age can benefit from glucosamine intake to ensure proper growth and function of cartilage. Lower dosages are more suitable for prolonged use; higher dosages have been used in studies for several months and with no reported major side effects. While glucosamine has a good safety record in animal and human studies, gastrointestinal upset has been observed to occur in rare cases. Try taking glucosamine supplements with meals if this occurs. Because glucosamine may be derived from shellfish, there is a remote chance that it may be allergenic to people sensitive to shellfish.

Use Guidelines: Use glucosamine supplements on a regular basis, and high therapeutic dosages for periods of up to several months.

Glutamic acid (also L-glutamic acid)
Supplement Type: Amino acid
Overview: Glutamic acid is a nonessential amino acid with several important biological functions. It forms part of many proteins, is an intermediary in the Krebs cycle (which produces energy), helps remove the metabolic

waste product ammonia, and improves energy production from the branched-chain amino acids. Glutamic acid is a lesser-known dietary supplement amino acid. Its role in energy production and clearance of ammonia from the body is well documented.

Benefits: Glutamic acid promotes and maintains energy.

Ingredient Form: L-glutamic acid.

Effective Supplement Dosages: For period use for improving energy levels and exercise performance, take between 500 mg and 2,000 g of L-glutamic acid per day.

Cofactors: Vitamin B_6.

Concerns: Glutamic acid is not an essential nutrient because it is made in the body. It also occurs in plentiful amounts in the diet. Use of glutamic acid dietary supplements is popular among athletes, but no one should take megadoses of glutamic acid, because the adverse effects of such large amounts are not fully known; it may be toxic to your nervous system. For adult use only; not for use by children or by pregnant or lactating women. Persons sensitive to MSG may have a similar reaction to glutamic acid.

Use Guidelines: Use glutamic acid supplements periodically.

Glutamine (also L-glutamine)

Supplement Type: Amino acid

Overview: Glutamine is a nonessential amino acid found in proteins. It is formed from glutamic acid in the body. Glutamine supplements have been found to improve muscle growth, prevent muscle breakdown, stimulate the immune system, and induce healing of the gastrointestinal tract, including ulcers. Glutamine has recently gained in popularity among athletes for its muscle-binding effects. Glutamine is also thought to help suppress the catabolic hormone cortisol. Glutamine's gastrointestinal healing properties are well established, and use of glutamine supplements should be considered for nutritional treatment of gastrointestinal disorders.

Benefits: Glutamine promotes and maintains muscle mass, promotes gastrointestinal health, and stimulates the immune system.

Ingredient Form: L-glutamine.

Effective Supplement Dosages: Glutamine occurs in high amounts in whey protein, and can be supplied, along with other amino acids, by drinking a whey protein supplement with 15 to 30 g of whey protein per day. Glutamine is also available in its free form, and glutamine supplements are taken in a wide range of dosages depending upon the specific use. For general nutrition supplementation, a dosage ranging from 500 mg to 2,000 mg per day is beneficial. Higher dosages should be taken for short periods of time, and under a doctor's supervision if you are using glutamine as nutritional therapy for a disease condition.

Cofactors: Essential vitamins, minerals, and amino acids.

Concerns: Glutamine is not an essential nutrient. It is one of the most prevalent amino acids in the body. Some studies show that poor health is associated with reduced levels of the body's supply of glutamine. Glutamine is considered safe and effective when used properly. Do not take megadoses of glutamine supplements unless you are doing so for a specific medical condition and under a doctor's supervision. For adult use only; not for use by children or by pregnant or lactating women unless under a doctor's supervision. Short-term studies report beneficial effects from using glutamine supplements, but long-term studies are needed to verify its safety over extended periods. For safe and effective use of glutamine supplements, use for three to four months, discontinue use for two to three weeks, and repeat cycle as desired.

Use Guidelines: Use glutamine supplements periodically when needed.

Glutathione

Supplement Type: Metabolite

Overview: Glutathione is a tripeptide, consisting of glutamic acid, cysteine, and glycine. It is one of the body's best antioxidants, and is also a detoxifying agent, aids immune system functioning, and protects red blood cells. Natural glutathione production tends to decrease with age, making supplementation of glutathione and glutathione cofactors particularly important for mature adults.

Benefits: Glutathione provides antioxidant protection, promotes good health, promotes longevity, and supports liver health.

Ingredient Form: Glutathione.

Effective Supplement Dosages: For daily use as a dietary supplement, take glutathione in dosages of between 20 and 160 mg per day. Higher dosages have been used

safely in clinical studies, 500 mg to 1,500 mg per day, and may be indicated if you are using glutathione as supportive nutritional therapy for a disease condition.

Cofactors: Precursors and cofactors of glutathione are L-cysteine, N-acetyl-cysteine, glycine, L-glutamic acid, vitamin C, L-methionine, and selenium.

Concerns: Glutathione is not an essential nutrient but is beneficial to health. Its use as a dietary supplement is considered safe and effective by all ages and both sexes when used as directed.

Use Guidelines: Glutathione is an optional supplement for daily use.

Glycerol

Supplement Type: Carbohydrate

Overview: Glycerol is a three-carbon molecule that is the backbone of triglycerides and phospholipids. Glycerol, a liquid, is a common solvent in pharmaceutical preparations and herbal liquid extracts. Glycerol is used as an emollient in skin-care products. Researchers have recently found that as a dietary supplement, glycerol may help the body remain better hydrated under conditions of prolonged physical exertion. However, researchers are still trying to determine the best dosages for maintaining hydration and the exact benefits. The use of glycerol supplements to better improve and maintain hydration looks promising. Glycerol supplements may have unexplored benefits in clinical use as a medical food for patients who are at risk for dehydration. If you want to try using glycerol for athletic or exercise performance, start with lower dosages to see how your body responds. It may take two to three weeks for your body to adjust to glycerol supplements.

Benefits: Maintains hydration during long periods of physical exertion.

Ingredient Form: Glycerol.

Effective Supplement Dosages: Dosages of 10 to 40 g per day of glycerol, taken with water, should be used periodically when enhancement of hydration is desired.

Cofactors: Water, electrolytes, glucose, B vitamins.

Concerns: Glycerol is not an essential nutrient. Its use to improve hydration during athletic events is still under examination. Some side effects reported in research studies include bloating, nausea, and light-headedness. Glycerol supplements should be used by adults only, not by children or by pregnant or lactating women unless under a doctor's supervision.

Use Guidelines: Use glycerol supplements on a periodic basis.

Glycine

Supplement Type: Amino acid

Overview: Glycine is a nonessential amino acid; it is synthesized in the body from serine. Glycine is a sweet-tasting amino acid and is an important precursor of several substances, including protein, DNA, phospholipids, collagen, and creatine. It is necessary in nervous system function as an inhibitory neurotransmitter. Too much glycine can actually interfere with energy production and cause fatigue, while just the right amount of glycine can help improve energy production. Clinical studies have shown that glycine supplements can cause an increase in growth hormone levels in the bloodstream. Research on glycine also reports cellular protective effects. Although preliminary, this new research points to glycine as being a promising longevity nutrient.

Benefits: Glycine supports good health and stimulates growth hormone production.

Ingredient Form: Used in dietary supplements as glycine.

Effective Supplement Dosages: The primary reason glycine supplements are taken is for stimulation of growth hormone production, which requires a daily dosage of 5 to 8 g per day.

Cofactors: Other growth hormone–elevating amino acids, such as arginine, lysine, ornithine, and phenylalanine.

Concerns: Glycine is not an essential nutrient, but it is made in the body and required for many important functions. Use of glycine supplements should be restricted to short periods, two to three months at a time. For use by healthy adults; not for use by children or by pregnant or lactating women unless under a doctor's supervision. Under medical supervision, glycine and other growth hormone–stimulating amino acids may be indicated for children with slow or stunted growth due to low growth-hormone production.

Use Guidelines: Use glycine supplements on a periodic basis as required.

Goldenseal (also *Hydrastis canadensis*)

Supplement Type: Botanical

Overview: The primary active phyto-chemicals in goldenseal, hydrastine and berberine, have vasoconstrictive, antibacterial, spasmolytic, and sedative effects, and reduce inflammation of mucous membranes, stimulate peristalsis, and stimulate the uterine muscles. Goldenseal is one of the herbs I consider to be potentially harmful if used incorrectly. If you use it, alone or in combination with other herbs, use it only for short periods of time, and under a doctor's supervision. Dr. J. Zuess notes that, "Goldenseal has become threatened with extinction in the wild due to overharvesting. I never recommend it any longer. There are many other herbal immunostimulants."

Benefits: Goldenseal has no clear beneficial use in dietary supplements. It is sometimes included in digestive aid supplements and immune-stimulating supplements along with other herbs.

Ingredient Form: Dietary supplement products contain goldenseal root standardized extracts (10% alkaloids, or 5% hydrastine, or 2.5% berberine).

Effective Supplement Dosages: When taken as a phytomedicine, 125 to 250 mg per day of standardized goldenseal root is used. Do not use for extended periods (more than three weeks), unless otherwise instructed by your doctor.

Cofactors: Other herbs.

Concerns: Goldenseal is not an essential nutrient. While it has a history of use as a medicinal herb, the potential side effects and lack of clear scientifically determined benefits do not support the use of this herb in dietary supplements. Side effects include lowering of heart rate, rise in blood pressure, and central nervous system paralysis; it may induce spontaneous abortion at high dosages. Use of goldenseal should be avoided by pregnant or lactating women and by children.

Use Guidelines: Use of goldenseal supplements is optional; use with caution.

Gotu kola (also *Centella asiatica*)

Supplement Type: Botanical

Overview: Gotu kola contains a group of phytonutrients called asiaticosides, which are thought to stimulate tissue growth, in particular in the skin, connective tissues, and capillaries. Gotu kola is also used in topical preparations for promoting wound healing and healing of chronic skin lesions.

Benefits: Gotu kola is used in dietary supplements to maintain vascular health, improve circulation, and support the growth and repair of connective tissues and skin. Recent studies have reported on gotu kola's benefits for improving mental function in children and adults. Gotu kola improves skin appearance and may be used as nutritional support in the treatment of skin diseases and venous insufficiency.

Ingredient Form: Standardized gotu kola herb (8% to 10% triterpenes or asiaticosides).

Effective Supplement Dosages: Standardized gotu kola is used in dietary supplements in amounts ranging from 50 to 150 mg per day. Higher daily dosages may be used for therapeutic applications under a doctor's supervision.

Cofactors: Other circulatory health ingredients such as ginkgo, bioflavonoids, grape seed, Pycnogenol, and horse chestnut seed extract.

Concerns: Gotu kola is not an essential nutrient, but is beneficial as a dietary supplement. It has a long history of safe and effective use, and is considered nontoxic when used as directed. It is good for daily use. If you are using gotu kola as nutritional support for a skin disorder or other health condition, make sure you are getting proper medical supervision. Children or pregnant or lactating women should use gotu kola only under a doctor's supervision.

Use Guidelines: Gotu kola is becoming a popular supplement ingredient for daily use.

Grape seed extract, GSE (also *Vitis vinifera*)

Supplement Type: Botanical

Overview: The phytonutrients contained in grape seed extract have powerful antioxidant action; inhibit enzymes (collagenase and elastase) that break down and damage blood vessels, connective tissues, and skin; and maintain flexibility of blood vessels. Grape seed extract is a super botanical antioxidant and is increasingly used in dietary supplements. It should be included in your daily dietary supplement program; many comprehensive antioxidant formulas will contain it and other botanical antioxidants as well. Use of grape skin extract as a dietary supplement ingredient is also increasing, and it has similar benefits to grape seed extract. Grape seed extract contains phytonutrients similar to those contained in Pycnogenol, which is a proprietary pine bark extract used in supplements as a source of OPCs.

Benefits: Grape seed extract promotes health and well-being and stimulates, supports, and maintains circulatory system health. It also can be used as nutritional support for venous or circulatory system diseases.

Ingredient Form: Standardized grape seed extract (50% to 85% proanthocyanidins). Its standardized phytonutrients are also referred to as OPCs (oligometric proanthocyanidins) and polyphenols. OXI grape is a brand of grape seed extract used in supplement products.

Effective Supplement Dosages: Daily dosages of standardized GSE commonly used in dietary supplements range from 25 to 150 mg for nutritional purposes. Higher daily dosages (100 to 200 mg, three times per day), are used for nutritional support in circulatory disorders.

Cofactors: Other antioxidants, vitamins, and minerals.

Concerns: Grape seed extract is not an essential nutrient, but promotes good health. It is considered nontoxic. However, because of its potential blood thinning effects, people on anticoagulant therapy should use it under medical supervision. Rare allergic reactions may occur in people sensitive to grape products. Do not take megadoses of this supplement; higher dosages are not more beneficial. It is safe for all ages and both sexes.

Use Guidelines: Grape seed extract supplements can be taken every day.

Grape skin extract: *see* Grape seed extract

Greens Botanical Powders

Since the health food boom in the 1960s, botanicals such as spirulina and chlorella have been touted as Mother Nature's cure-alls. More recently, there has been a resurgence of these greens-type products in the health foods stores. These botanicals are essentially nutrient-dense foods. They are usually high in protein, enzymes, fiber, vitamins, minerals, nucleic acids, essential fatty acids, and phytonutrients. People taking them usually start to feel more energetic and healthier within a few days or weeks. The powders usually contain other ingredients, such as herbs and natural vitamin E.

If you are going to try a green product, look for one that has several ingredients, such as brown algae, barley, chlorella, and spirulina. Start slowly, because these products can really flush out your digestive tract. As you begin to tolerate them better, increase your dosage as recommended on the product's directions. Most quality products recommend taking several grams per day; however, many people report maintaining good results after a few months by cutting back to about half the recommended dosage.

Green tea (also *Camellia sinensis*)
Supplement Type: Botanical

Overview: Green tea contains phytonutrients with multiple health-promoting actions. It is high in polyphenols, which include bioflavonoids (in particular, catechins). The phytonutrients in green tea have been shown to exert powerful antioxidant activity, block cancer-causing nitrosamines from forming in the digestive system, slow down the digestion of carbohydrates, and lower serum cholesterol levels. Along with consumption of soy and a low-fat diet rich in vegetables, green tea is considered one of the main health treasures of Asia. Start consuming green tea beverages daily, and include green tea extract supplements in your dietary supplement program. Men and women alike will benefit from green tea consumption. Children can benefit from decaffeinated green tea products. There are many scientific studies to support the numerous health benefits of daily consumption of green tea; in one study, Japanese women who drank eight or more cups of green tea a day had a lesser risk of mortality from all causes of disease when compared to the national average.

Benefits: Green tea has various health effects, observed in populations where green tea is regularly consumed. These health effects include protection against free-radical damage, improvement of cardiovascular health, improved dental health, protection from developing gastrointestinal cancers, maintenance of blood sugar levels when taken with meals, and a reduction in the risk of degenerative disease. Green tea is an effective weight loss aid; it stimulates the metabolic rate.

Ingredient Form: Standardized green tea leaf extract (35% to 50% polyphenols or catechins). Also, regular consumption of green tea beverages.

Effective Supplement Dosages: For best results, take supplements containing 30 to 300 mg of standardized green tea leaf extract daily. Higher dosages can be used safely. Also, regular consumption of green tea as a beverage is recommended, three to five or more cups a day with supplements. Best taken with meals.

Cofactors: Other antioxidants.

Concerns: Green tea is not an essential nutrient, but is a beneficial source of health-promoting phytonutrients. It is nontoxic, safe, and effective for daily use. However, note that green tea extract and green tea contain caffeine. For persons who want to avoid caffeine in their diets, especially children and pregnant or lactating women, use decaffeinated green tea products.

Use Guidelines: Include a supplement containing green tea extract in your daily nutrition program.

Guar gum (also *Cyamopsis tetragonolobus*)

Supplement Type: Botanical

Overview: This is a dietary fiber that absorbs water and swells in the digestive system. It is used as a thickening agent in foods. In the 1970s and 1980s obesity researchers in the United Kingdom found that when they used guar gum supplements, patients had better appetite control and lost more weight. This was inspired by the discovery some people's stomachs empty quickly, regardless of what foods they eat. This causes them to be hungry frequently and overeat. When guar gum was given to these patients, it slowed down the rate at which the stomach emptied, and appetite control and weight loss were observed.

Benefits: Guar gum promotes a feeling of fullness and normal gastrointestinal function and lowers cholesterol levels and glucose and insulin blood levels. It is used by people who are on weight loss programs to help satisfy appetite and slow down the emptying of the stomach.

Ingredient Form: Guar gum is sold as a powder, intended for use as a beverage. Do not use guar gum in tablet, capsule, or other solid dose form.

Effective Supplement Dosages: Daily consumption will vary depending on the individual. Start ingesting small amounts per day, 2 to 8 g, to get your body used to ingesting guar gum. Then increase daily dosage as required, up to 8 to 16 g per day, in divided dosages. Higher dosages should be used only under medical supervision. Take with meals or as directed on product labels.

Cofactors: Other dietary fibers.

Concerns: Guar gum is not an essential nutrient. However, increasing fiber content in the diet has been shown to be beneficial. Because guar gum is a refined product, it should not be overconsumed. Guar gum has the ability to swell in the digestive system, and guar gum has been implicated in esophageal and bowel obstruction when taken in solid dose form, tablets or capsules. This is why you must use the drink form of guar gum. It may cause gastrointestinal cramping and gas. Keep well hydrated when taking guar gum. It is a common food additive, used as a thickener, and is nontoxic. Supplements are not for use by children unless under a doctor's supervision. Medical supervision is required when following a weight loss program.

Use Guidelines: Include a fiber supplement in your daily nutrition program.

Guarana (also *Paullinia cupana*)

Supplement Type: Botanical

Overview: Guarana contains caffeine and other related methylxanthines, such as theobromine and theophylline, which are central nervous system stimulants and have a mild diuretic effect. The methylxanthines also stimulate an increase in your fat-burning rate, and reduce appetite in some people. Guarana has a long history of safe use in South America. It is sold as beverages, similar to Coca-Cola, where it is used to stimulate mental and physical energy.

Benefits: Guarana is used in dietary supplements designed for stimulating mental alertness. It is also used in dietary supplement weight loss aids as part of a thermogenic herbal blend, to stimulate the metabolism of fats.

Ingredient Form: Standardized guarana extract (12% to 30% methylxanthines or caffeine).

Effective Supplement Dosages: Use as directed on product labels for best results, as use and dosages vary considerably among different products.

Cofactors: Other methylxanthine-containing herbs, such as yerba mate, tea, cocoa, and kola.

Concerns: Guarana is not an essential nutrient. Its regular daily use is not advised, and it is not for use by children or by pregnant or lactating women. As with all caffeine-containing products, nervousness and other side effects can occur. Do not use if you have heart problems or other medical conditions for which you have been advised to avoid caffeine. If taking a guarana-containing weight loss aid, do so under a doctor's supervision.

Use Guidelines: Periodic use of guarana to increase mental alertness, or as a weight loss aid, is optional.

Guggul (also *Commiphora mukul*)

Supplement Type: Botanical

Overview: Guggul contains guggulsterones, which have been shown to stimulate the liver to clear out the bad LDL cholesterol from the bloodstream. Guggul has been shown to be effective in lowering blood lipid levels in clinical studies. If you have a concern about cardiovascular health, have a history of cardiovascular illness in your family, or are suffering from cardiovascular illness, consider including guggul in your heart health dietary supplement program.

Benefits: Improves circulatory system health, lowers LDL cholesterol, and increases the good HDL cholesterol. A high level of LDL cholesterol is associated with formation of blood clots and other circulatory system disfunction; reducing LDL cholesterol may help reduce your risk of these disorders. Guggul is also reported to help with weight management.

Ingredient Form: Gugulipid is a proprietary standardized guggul extract (2.5% total guggulsterones).

Effective Supplement Dosages: As a dietary supplement to promote circulatory system health, take a dose of 500 to 1,000 mg of Gugulipid per day. Higher therapeutic dosages may be used under a doctor's supervision as nutritional support when being treated for cardiovascular disorders.

Cofactors: Other cardiovascular health ingredients, such as garlic.

Concerns: Guggul is not an essential nutrient, but is beneficial, especially for promoting healthy cholesterol levels. It has a history of use in Indian Ayurvedic medicine and is considered safe when used in recommended dosages. If you are taking guggul for a medical condition, do so under a doctor's supervision.

Use Guidelines: Include a guggul-containing supplement into your daily nutrition program if you are concerned about promoting and maintaining cardiovascular health.

Gymnema (also *Gymnema sylvestre*)

Supplement Type: Botanical

Overview: Gymnema has been shown to have hypoglycemic activity, that is, it lowers blood sugar levels by stimulating insulin secretion. The Western medical community is slowly but surely widening the range of nutritional therapies it uses for management of diabetes. If you are diabetic, encourage your doctor to explore some of these alternative-medicine practices. But start slowly, and do not discontinue use of medications until approved by your doctor. Gymnema is sometimes used in weight loss nutritional aid products for its insulin-boosting effects, in the belief that many overweight people have insulin secretion or function problems. If you are using gymnema products, be aware that the hypoglycemic effect may cause dizziness in some people.

Benefits: Used in traditional Indian Ayurvedic medicine in the management of blood sugar level disorders, it is reported to be beneficial to individuals with Type I diabetes as supportive therapy (in addition to standard medical treatment).

Ingredient Form: Standardized gymnema leaf extract (25% gymnemic acids); GS4 is one brand name.

Effective Supplement Dosages: For use in controlling blood sugar levels, through causing a hypoglycemic effect, use 500 to 750 mg of standardized gymnema extract per day, in divided dosages. Use as directed on the label. Gymnema's primary use as a dietary supplement is in supportive therapy of people with blood sugar problems, which should be treated under a doctor's supervision.

Cofactors: Other dietary supplement ingredients for blood sugar control, such as chromium, vanadium, fiber, and ginseng.

Concerns: Gymnema is not an essential nutrient, but can be beneficial for people with blood sugar level problems. While gymnema has a long history of use as an herbal medicine, its effectiveness in stimulating insulin and causing hypoglycemic effects has only been verified in animal studies. Gymnema should be used under a doctor's supervision in the treatment of medical conditions. Not for use by children or by pregnant or lactating women unless under medical supervision. It is considered nontoxic and safe when used as directed. Do not use if you are hypoglycemic.

Use Guidelines: Use gymnema supplements periodically for specific reasons.

Hawthorn (also *Crataegus laevigata*)
Supplement Type: Botanical

Overview: Hawthorn is rich in bioflavonoids and has been shown in clinical studies to dilate peripheral and heart blood vessels. Hawthorn is also used as a general cardiac tonic for promoting regular heartbeat and blood pressure. New medical research indicates that regular use of hawthorn supplements may also keep the circulatory system flexible, especially in the region around the heart, the aortic arch.

Benefits: Hawthorn improves blood supply to the heart and improves circulation. It is used in Europe as a phytomedicine to treat patients with mild cases of reduced heart function, including cardiac insufficiency. The bioflavonoids contained in Hawthorn increase coronary blood flow, heart rate, and cause vasodilation, which results in improved heart function.

Ingredient Form: Standardized hawthorn extract (5% vitexin). Also standardized for hyperoside.

Effective Supplement Dosages: For promotion of cardiovascular health, use dietary supplements containing 150 to 300 mg of standardized hawthorn extract per day. Higher dosages may be indicated for nutritional treatment of specific medical conditions, as determined by your doctor.

Cofactors: Sometimes used in combination dietary supplement formulas to promote heart health with coenzyme Q_{10}, carnitine, arginine, ginkgo, B vitamins, magnesium, and antioxidants.

Concerns: Hawthorn is not an essential nutrient, but contains phytonutrients essential for promotion of heart health and good circulation. Use under medical supervision if a medical condition exists. Considered safe when used as directed. In higher doses, it causes sedation and low blood pressure, which can lead to fainting. For adult use only; not for use by children or by pregnant or lactating women unless under a doctor's supervision.

Use Guidelines: Use hawthorn supplements on a regular basis if you have concerns about promoting and maintaining cardiac and circulatory system health.

Histidine (also L-histidine)
Supplement Type: Amino acid

Overview: Histidine is recognized as an essential amino acid for infants but not for adults. It is important in growth and repair of human tissues. Histidine also functions in the formation of white and red blood cells and has a history of use in the management of arthritis due to its anti-inflammatory properties. Histidine is a precursor of the neurotransmitter histamine. Histidine supplement use should be restricted to short periods of time, and under conditions of diagnosed low histidine blood status. There have been no reported benefits of taking histidine supplements by healthy people with normal histidine status. Keep in mind that people under stress and athletic people can benefit from increased dietary intake of essential and nonessential amino acids from a high-quality protein supplement drink or an amino acid supplement in tablet form.

Benefits: Histidine supplements help nutritionally support normal growth and development.

Ingredient Form: L-histidine.

Effective Supplement Dosages: Histidine has been used safely in clinical studies in dosages between 1,000 and 5,000 mg per day for a few months at a time.

Cofactors: None.

Concerns: Histidine is an essential nutrient. Its use has been indicated in clinical settings for people with low blood levels of histidine, in particular, individuals with arthritis. No major side effects have been reported from using histidine supplements. Do not take megadoses of histidine, or take histidine for prolonged periods of time. For adult use only; not for use by children or by pregnant or lactating women unless under a doctor's supervision. Use under medical supervision for health conditions.

Use Guidelines: Use histidine supplements periodically when you want to selectively increase your dietary histidine levels.

Honey

Supplement Type: Concentrate

Overview: Honey is a product of bees collecting and processing nectar from different types of flowers. After collection from beehives, honey is usually purified for commercial use. Honey is mainly composed of the simple sugars dextrose, levulose, and sucrose. Honey also contains some minerals, vitamins, and phytonutrients. There are several supplement companies that market "health from the hive products." While honey's claim to medical fame is based mostly on traditional medicinal use, I have encountered hundreds of people who believe that use of honey, bee propolis, and bee pollen restored their health, in particular, their gastrointestinal health. Honey is also used in skin care and hair care products due to its moisturizing and skin softening properties.

Benefits: Taken internally, honey is recognized for its soothing effects on the gastrointestinal system. It is also used as a natural sweetener in herbal products. Honey has a history of use as a topical healing aid and antibacterial substance. The antibacterial effects are thought to be due in part to the high sugar content, which literally sucks the water from the bacteria and creates an environment in which they cannot survive.

Ingredient Form: Purified honey.

Effective Supplement Dosages: One to two tablespoons added to teas and other beverages to soothe the throat and stomach. Honey is sometimes added to multinutrient dietary supplements in amounts ranging from 50 to 1,000 mg per daily dosage.

Cofactors: Honey provides the sweet base for soothing herbs, such as chamomile, or active phytomedicines in natural cough and sore throat remedies.

Concerns: Honey is not an essential nutrient. Its use as a health remedy dates back over four thousand years. Honey is considered a safe food product for adults and children, but not for infants one year or younger, because honey may contain spores of the bacterium *Clostridium botulinum,* which can grow in the intestines. While this does not cause problems in adults, health officials have attributed cases of botulism poisoning in infants to contaminated honey. Because of its high sugar content, honey should not be overconsumed by anyone.

Use Guidelines: Use honey on a daily basis when desired.

Hops (also *Humulus lupulus*)

Supplement Type: Botanical

Overview: Hops is recognized for its sedative and calming effects on the nervous system. Hops and other herbal products can promote sleep and relaxation. However, do not become dependent on these products. If irregular sleep patterns or nervousness persist, consult your doctor.

Benefits: Hops is used in dietary supplements designed for promoting sleep and calming.

Ingredient Form: Standardized hops fruit extract (4% to 6% bitter acids).

Effective Supplement Dosages: The daily dosage is 100 to 250 mg a day, before bedtime. Smaller amounts may be added to multiple-herb formulas, 25 to 100 mg per day.

Cofactors: Other relaxing or sleep-enhancing herbs, such as kava kava, passionflower, and valerian.

Concerns: Hops is not an essential nutrient, but has beneficial uses for promotion of sleep and relaxation. Not for use by children or by pregnant or lactating women unless under a doctor's supervision. Do not use for prolonged periods of time—over two weeks—in high dosages. Do not use if you are suffering from depression. Hops supplements can cause allergic reactions in some people. Do not use in conjunction with sleep or antianxiety medications.

Use Guidelines: Use hops-containing supplements to promote relaxation and a good night's rest.

Horse chestnut (also *Aesculus hippocastanum*)

Supplement Type: Botanical

Overview: Horse chestnut seed supplements are known for their vascular system tightening effects. These improvements in vascular system structure are thought to be due to horse chestnut seed's stabilizing effect on cell membranes and normalizing effect on capillary tone. For people with vascular problems, horse chestnut dietary supplements can be beneficial. Use as directed on the labels. The beneficial results from clinical studies and from patient use are impressive. It takes several weeks for the benefits of horse chestnut to be observed.

Benefits: Horse chestnut supports and promotes vein structure and function, and has been used in clinical studies to treat venous insufficiency, treat edema, and help reduce leg pain. Also, it can be beneficial in the treatment and management of hemorrhoids and varicose veins.

Ingredient Form: Standardized horse chestnut seed extract (13% to 24% aescin or triterpene glycosides).

Effective Supplement Dosages: Daily dosages of horse chestnut for use as a dietary supplement range from 25 to 150 mg of standardized extracts. In medically supervised clinical studies, 600 mg per day of horse chestnut extract was used safely for nineteen weeks and was found to be effective for treating chronic venous insufficiency.

Cofactors: Other herbs promoting circulatory system health such as grape seed extract, ginkgo, Pycnogenol, and gotu kola.

Concerns: Horse chestnut extract is not an essential nutrient. It has a history of use in Europe to treat vein disorders. It has recently been introduced into the United States for sale as a dietary supplement. It has been shown to be safe and effective in short-term studies lasting up to five months; the effects of long-term use have not been determined. If you are on anticoagulant drugs, do not use, or use with caution under a doctor's supervision. Not for use by children or by pregnant or lactating women unless under a doctor's supervision. Side effects can include gastrointestinal upset, headache, and dizziness. Severe side effects can develop with overdosage, such as vomiting, vision disorders, and reddening of the skin.

Use Guidelines: Give horse chestnut seed supplements a try if you have varicose veins, hemorrhoids, or related concerns about promoting or maintaining the structure and function of your veins.

Horsetail (also *Equisetum arvense*)

Supplement Type: Botanical

Overview: As a dietary supplement, horsetail is most notable for its silicon content. Horsetail is a plant you can find growing in weedy lots, along railroad tracks, and in similar places. Due to its silicon content, horsetail can be used as a sort of natural steel wool pad to help clean pots and pans when camping.

Benefits: Used as a source of silicon in dietary supplements.

Ingredient Form: Use horsetail that has been standardized to silicon content.

Effective Supplement Dosages: Dosages will vary depending upon how much silicon is being supplied from the horsetail. Refer to the silicon entry for information on dietary amounts.

Cofactors: Used in bone health formulas along with calcium, magnesium, boron, and other bone-health-enhancing nutrients.

Concerns: Horsetail is not an essential nutrient. It is used in small amounts in dietary supplements to supply silicon. As a traditional herbal medicine, horsetail is thought to be a mild diuretic. However, there is some concern about the safety of horsetail for this use at high dosages. It should therefore not be used in high dosages or as an herbal medicine. Its use in small amounts in dietary supplements as a source of silicon is considered safe. Not for use by children or by pregnant or lactating women unless under a doctor's supervision. Also, note that horsetail contains trace amounts of nicotine.

Use Guidelines: Small amounts of horsetail will be encountered in some supplements to supply silicon. However, do not take high amounts of horsetail supplements unless for a specific reason as prescribed by your health care practitioner.

Inosine

Supplement Type: Metabolite

Overview: Inosine is a naturally occurring substance found in all human tissues, particularly in skeletal muscles and the heart muscles. It is involved in the regeneration of ATP, promoting its synthesis and replenishment. It also stimulates the production of 2,3-diphosphoglycerate, which is one of the substances essential in the transport of oxygen molecules from red blood cells to muscle cells for energy production. Inosine's use in dietary supplements is popular among strength athletes; you will rarely encounter it in other products.

Benefits: Inosine promotes energy and performance in strength athletes.

Ingredient Form: The best supplement form of inosine is inosine hypoxanthine riboside (inosine HXR). Avoid using inosinic acid, which can contribute to uric acid formation.

Dosages: For use by strength athletes, 700 to 1,400 mg per day.

Cofactors: Creatine.

Concerns: Inosine is not an essential nutrient. Studies of its usefulness in increasing muscle performance in strength athletes have shown mixed results; some studies report an improvement and others do not. While there are no reports of adverse side effects, do not take megadoses of inosine, or take it for prolonged periods of time, over four months. People with gout should avoid inosine supplementation, as it contributes to the formation of uric acid and could aggravate this condition. For periodic use by healthy adults. Not for use by children or by pregnant or lactating women unless under a doctor's supervision.

Use Guidelines: Strength athletes can use inosine-containing supplements periodically to enhance performance.

Inositol (also Myoinositol, hexahydroxycyclohexane)

Supplement Type: Metabolite

Overview: Inositol is a vitamin-B-like metabolite that displays lipotropic action, that is, fatty acid metabolism in the liver. It also assists in carbohydrate metabolism and calcium functioning. The body makes inositol, but supplemental intake is thought to ensure an adequate supply. The exact benefits of taking inositol supplements have not been determined. Effectiveness as a weight loss aid is unconfirmed. Inositol may be useful, along with choline and other lipotropics, in the early stages of weight loss to help correct fatty liver condition, common to obese individuals. Consult your doctor when using inositol and other nutritional weight loss aids.

Benefits: Inositol supplements are commonly used along with other fat-metabolizing nutrients as dietary supplement weight loss aids. It may also be useful in the nutritional treatment of some skin disorders, including eczema.

Ingredient Form: Myoinositol, inositol hexanicotinate.

Effective Supplement Dosages: For daily nutritional support, supplements usually contain 10 to 150 mg per day. Weight loss products can contain 250 to 1,000 mg of inositol per day, but should not be taken for prolonged periods of time.

Cofactors: Choline and B vitamins.

Concerns: It is safe for all ages and both sexes when used in prescribed nutritional amounts. High dosages may cause gastrointestinal upset, nausea, diarrhea, and dizziness, and should not be used by children unless prescribed by a doctor. If mild gastrointestinal upset occurs, try reducing the daily dosage, and take with meals.

Use Guidelines: Inositol is a common ingredient in multinutrient dietary supplement products taken every day. High therapeutic dosages should be restricted to short periods of time.

Iodine

Supplement Type: Mineral

Overview: Iodine is an essential part of the thyroid hormones thyroxine and tri-iodothyronine, and is vital for proper thyroid gland functioning. The thyroid gland regulates normal metabolism, growth, and energy production. Most vitamin-mineral dietary supplements contain iodine, which has a history of safe use in such formulations. Some dietary supplement weight loss aids also contain iodine. If you are using multiple supplements, make sure that your total iodine intake is not too high. Up to 1,000 mcg per day from all dietary sources, food and dietary supplements, is considered to be safe.

Benefits: Daily supplement intake of iodine ensures maintenance of adequate dietary iodine intake. Iodine deficiency causes goiter, a condition in which the thyroid gland enlarges.

Ingredient Form: Supplements contain iodine; some contain iodine from kelp concentrate.

Effective Supplement Dosages: The adult RDI for iodine is 150 mcg. Iodine is found in most vitamin-mineral formulas in dosages of between 25 and 150 mcg per day.

Cofactors: Essential vitamins and minerals.

Concerns: Iodine deficiency is not as common as it once was. Iodized salt was introduced in the United States to help prevent iodine deficiency in areas of the country where the food supply is low in iodine. Excessive iodine intake can produce side effects such as thyroid gland dysfunction, a metallic taste in the mouth, rash, and headache. Never take megadoses of iodine.

Use Guidelines: Take an iodine-containing dietary supplement daily.

Iron

Supplement Type: Mineral

Overview: Iron is best known for its essential oxygen transport role as part of hemoglobin in the blood, and myoglobin in the muscles. Iron is found in a number of enzymes and is stored in bone marrow and liver and spleen tissues. While iron is one of the more potentially toxic of the mineral dietary supplement ingredients, iron supplements are safe and effective in maintaining good health when used properly.

Benefits: Daily dietary supplement intake of iron prevents iron deficiency anemia and impaired immune function.

Ingredient Form: Organic forms of iron, such as iron fumarate and iron glycinate, are preferred.

Effective Supplement Dosages: The adult RDI for iron is 18 mg. Iron is a standard ingredient in most vitamin-mineral supplements. Daily dosages typically range between 5 and 30 mg. Do not take megadoses of iron-containing dietary supplements, though

doctors may prescribe higher iron intake for certain medical conditions for short periods of time.

Cofactors: Other essential vitamins and minerals.

Concerns: Excessive intake of iron is harmful. Each year in the United States thousands of iron poisoning cases are reported, many involving children, with several deaths. Overdose of iron occurs when children have access to iron-containing supplements and ingest large quantities of such products. A lethal dosage for one- to two-year-old children is about 3,000 mg. For adults, the lethal dose ranges from 200 to 250 mg per kg (2.2 pounds) of body weight. Single oral dosages of 200 mg can cause abdominal cramping, diarrhea, nausea, and constipation. Contact a poison control center immediately if iron overdosing occurs.

Use Guidelines: Iron-containing dietary supplements can be taken safely on a daily basis at recommended levels.

Isoleucine (also L-isoleucine)

Supplement Type: Amino acid

Overview: Isoleucine is an essential amino acid, and along with leucine and valine is one of the branched-chain amino acids (BCAAs). Isoleucine is found in proteins, and because of its branched-chain structure is one of the amino acids that is used for energy, especially during periods of stress and intensive exercise. The BCAAs were first used in clinical settings in intravenous solution feedings for patients who are severely physically stressed, such as burn patients. When the body is stressed, it uses more BCAAs for energy, which makes them less available for vital growth needs. In hospital settings, BCAA administration has been shown to restore a positive nitrogen balance; a negative nitrogen balance indicates that the body's muscles are wasting, and a positive nitrogen balance can mean that the muscles are being maintained or built up. In clinical studies on athletes, BCAA administration improves athletic performance, muscle growth, and muscle recovery.

Benefits: Isoleucine helps reduce muscle protein breakdown. It increases mental alertness and exercise performance.

Ingredient Form: Used in dietary supplements as L-isoleucine.

Effective Supplement Dosages: As a dietary supplement for athletes, 800 to 3,000 mg per day during athletic season. Also can be taken by people undergoing mental or physical stress.

Cofactors: The other BCAAs, leucine and valine.

Concerns: Isoleucine is an essential nutrient, and adequate dietary intake is essential for good health. There are no reported side effects from using isoleucine supplements. For adult use only. Not for use by children or by pregnant or lactating women unless under a doctor's supervision.

Use Guidelines: Take isoleucine supplements as needed on a periodic basis.

Kava kava (also *Piper methysticum*)
Supplement Type: Botanical
Overview: Kava kava root extract has been shown to have calming, antianxiety, mild sedative, muscle relaxing, and local anesthetic effects. It also lowers the heart rate. Kava kava is one of my favorite herbs. I use it to clear away stress, reduce tension, relax my muscles, and promote a good night's sleep. It also helps stimulate better concentration. Kava kava can be beneficial for menopausal women. In a study of forty patients, kava kava extract reduced the severity of symptoms associated with menopause, including depression and anxiety. However, don't overuse or abuse kava kava. A few weeks at a time, up to three months, is good for most people. If you want to make sure that your kava kava product is standardized and potent, take some from the capsule or tablet and put it on your tongue. A good product will cause a slight tingling or numbing sensation, which is from the anesthetic actions of the kavalactones.

Benefits: Kava kava root extract has been examined in several clinical studies and shown to be effective in promoting relaxation and reducing nervousness, stress, and anxiety.

Ingredient Form: Standardized kava kava root extract (30% kavalactones).

Effective Supplement Dosages: A daily dosage of between 200 and 400 mg of standardized kava kava root extract has been found to be effective, yielding 60 to 120 mg of kavalactones per day. It is best taken at night. Results are usually seen within a few hours; antianxiety effects take 1–3 weeks.

Cofactors: Other calming herbs, such as chamomile, hops, St. John's wort, and valerian.

Concerns: Kava kava is not an essential nutrient, but is beneficial for relieving anxiety and feelings of stress. Kava kava has a long history of safe use when used in moderation. Kava kava can impair motor reflexes and ability to drive and operate heavy machinery in some people. Not to be used by children or by pregnant or lactating women, unless under a doctor's supervision. It may temporarily worsen Parkinson's disease as well. Do not take for more than three months at a time. Medical supervision is recommended for people using kava kava for self-treatment of severe anxiety or sleep disorders. Heavy daily use of kava kava beverages or kava kava dietary supplements has been associated with developing a yellow, scaly skin rash. This rash is reported to disappear quickly when kava kava use is discontinued. You should avoid drinking alcoholic beverages or using any sedative drugs while taking kava kava. Consult your doctor before using kava kava dietary supplements if you are taking any medications.

Use Guidelines: Use kava kava supplements periodically when needed.

Kelp: *see* Iodine

Klamath blue-green algae: *see* Greens Powders

Kola, Cola (also *Cola acuminanta, Cola nitida*)

Supplement Type: Botanical

Overview: Kola is the nut of a tropical tree. It contains caffeine, bioflavonoids, and other phytonutrients. Its main use is for its central-nervous-system-stimulating effects from the caffeine it contains. Also, antioxidant activity is expected from the bioflavonoid content. Kola has a long history of use in foods and beverages. Its use in dietary supplements is well established. More recently, kola extract has been included in nutritional weight loss aids for its metabolic and energy-stimulating effects, which seem to provide dieters with more energy, appetite control, motivation, and an increased rate of fat loss. However, make sure not to overdose on kola or become dependent upon it for long periods of time.

Benefits: The primary benefit of kola is promoting mental alertness. It is a mild diuretic, and also promotes feelings of energy.

Ingredient Form: Standardized kola nut extract (7% to 15% caffeine).

Effective Supplement Dosages: Take 300 to 900 mg a day when you need a mental energy boost. Smaller daily dosages intended for long-term use, may be found in multinutrient products formulated to increase mental alertness and energy.

Cofactors: Kola nut is sometimes found with other stimulating herbs, such as guarana and yerba mate.

Concerns: Kola is not an essential nutrient. Its use as a dietary supplement product for stimulating mental alertness should be limited to periods of only a few days. See caffeine entry for more concerns and cautions associated with caffeine intake. For adult use only; not for use by children or by pregnant or lactating women unless under a doctor's supervision.

Use Guidelines: Take kola-containing supplements on a short-term basis only.

Lactobacillus: *see* Probiotics

Lecithin (also Phosphatidylcholine)

Supplement Type: Lipid constituent

Overview: Lecithin is a type of phospholipid that has a molecule of choline attached to the phosphate molecule. Lecithin supplies the body with the essential nutrient choline and is involved in important biological functions, including brain development, learning, and fertility. It can help lower serum cholesterol, improve short-term memory, improve endurance, serve as a precursor of the important neurotransmitter acetylcholine, and prevent fatty liver. Lecithin supplements have been much used in the last fifty years. Clinical studies have verified that blood levels of choline are maintained at a higher level for a longer time when derived from lecithin than from choline chloride. Lecithin occurs in high amounts in beef liver and egg yolks.

Benefits: Lecithin promotes brain function and wellness and heart and circulatory system wellness. It improves memory, maintains liver health, and improves physical performance.

Ingredient Form: The lecithin used most in supplements is extracted from soybeans.

Effective Supplement Dosages: Dietary supplement dosages of lecithin typically range between 500 and 2,000 mg per day, for general nutritional purposes. Higher amounts are sometimes used, especially in the management of blood lipids and degenerative nervous system cases.

Cofactors: Essential vitamins and minerals.

Concerns: Lecithin is not an essential nutrient, but it contains the essential nutrient choline and contains the essential fatty acid linoleic acid; soy lecithin also contains linolenic acid. Lecithin is a very safe and effective dietary supplement ingredient that can be used by both adults and children.

Use Guidelines: Use lecithin-containing supplements on a regular basis.

Leucine (also L-leucine)

Supplement Type: Amino acid

Overview: Leucine is one of the branched-chain amino acids (BCAAs), and an essential amino acid. It is found in proteins and is an important source of muscle energy during exercise. Leucine is used at a higher rate for energy than the other BCAAs, isoleucine and valine. L-leucine is very beneficial for athletes, especially in preseason training and during the season. It helps maintain and build muscle mass, and provides energy as well.

Benefits: Leucine is required for growth and maintenance of good health. Leucine promotes energy and endurance.

Ingredient Form: L-leucine.

Effective Supplement Dosages: In addition to leucine derived from dietary protein intake, take 1.5 to 6 g per day of leucine supplements for athletic performance.

Cofactors: The other BCAAs, isoleucine and valine.

Concerns: L-leucine is an essential nutrient. Adequate protein intake is required to prevent leucine deficiencies. Use of supplements should be restricted to periods of increased physical activity. Leucine supplements are for use by healthy adults and are not for use by children or by pregnant or lactating women unless under a doctor's supervision.

Use Guidelines: Take leucine supplements periodically when needed.

Licorice (also *Glycyrrhiza glabra*)

Supplement Type: Botanical

Overview: Licorice root contains a phytoactive substance called glycyrrhizin (a triterpene glycoside) as well as several bioflavonoids. Glycyrrhizin is reported to promote healing of ulcers. Licorice root has a long history of safe use as a food and as an herbal medicine when used properly. However, caution should be exercised, as discussed below, when using high dosages of standardized licorice root extract for supportive treatment of gastrointestinal ulcers. Licorice root is also used as an ingredient in herbal expectorant products, but its effectiveness for this purpose has not been conclusively verified in clinical studies.

Benefits: Licorice root supports gastrointestinal health. It promotes natural secretions of the stomach wall mucosa, which provide protection to the stomach lining.

Ingredient Form: Standardized licorice root extract (2% to 4% glycyrrhizin).

Effective Supplement Dosages: Licorice root extract is taken for short periods of time, up to six weeks, 500 to 1,000 mg, three times per day, before meals. Higher dosages may be prescribed under a doctor's supervision or when using unstandardized powdered forms. Small amounts of licorice root are sometimes used in digestive health formulas. Glycyrrhizin is also used as a flavoring agent, and is considered safe when used in small quantities in food products.

Cofactors: Ginger, chamomile, aloe gel.

Concerns: Licorice root is not an essential nutrient. It can be used safely and effectively for promotion of stomach health, and as a medicinal herb in supportive treatment of gastric and duodenal ulcers. However, there are potential side effects with long-term use of therapeutic dosages of licorice root. When glycyrrhizin is metabolized in the body, one of its breakdown products has a mineralocorticoid effect on the body. Mineralocorticoids help control the body's water and mineral balance, but prolonged use or high dosages of licorice root may cause sodium retention and water retention and potassium loss in some people. This can lead to development of hypertension, edema, and related conditions. Maintaining adequate potassium intake while using licorice root supplements may help to offset these effects. Licorice root should not be used by children, by pregnant or lactating women, or by people with liver disorders, kidney insufficiency, hypokalemia (potassium deficiency), heart problems, or high blood pressure. Do not use longer than six weeks at a time. It is best used under a doctor's supervision for nutritional supportive treatment of stomach and duodenal ulcers.

Use Guidelines: Use licorice root supplements periodically when needed.

Linoleic acid

Supplement Type: Essential fatty acid

Overview: Linoleic acid is the primary essential fatty acid required by the body, and is needed in the manufacture of other fatty acids and fatty-acid-derived biochemicals. See essential fatty acids box for more details on linoleic acid and other fatty acids. Most diets are too high in linoleic acid and too low in alpha-linolenic acid. Make an effort to keep your fat intake below 25 percent of total daily calories, reduce saturated fatty acid intake, and reduce cholesterol intake to promote health.

Benefits: Required for growth, development, and maintenance of proper health.

Ingredient Form: Linoleic acid.

Effective Supplement Dosages: Linoleic acid is usually plentiful in the diet, but people on low-fat diets or on weight loss diets may benefit from linoleic acid supplements, 500 to 3,000 mg per day.

Cofactors: Other healthy fatty acids, such as alpha-linolenic acid, DHA, and EPA.

Concerns: Linoleic acid is an essential nutrient. Deficiencies are rare but do occur in infants and individuals with malnutrition. Linoleic acid supplements are safe and effective for all ages and both sexes.

Use Guidelines: Use linoleic supplements on a regular basis as part of your daily nutrition program.

Linolenic acid (also Alpha-linolenic acid)

Supplement Type: Essential fatty acid

Overview: Linolenic acid is an essential polyunsaturated fatty acid that is used in many important biochemical reactions and as part of cell membranes and other structures. It is required for proper growth and is needed to make other important fatty acids, including EPA and DHA. In a recent study Harvard researchers determined that regular consumption of oil-based salad dressings may protect against fatal heart attacks, due to the beneficial effects of linolenic acid. Balancing dietary lipids should be a major concern in your dietary planning. Essential fatty acids can have wonderful health-promoting effects, but you must watch out for overeating, or eating too many of the wrong lipids, such as saturated fats and cholesterol.

Benefits: Linolenic acid is essential for growth, development, and good health. It promotes heart health and helps maintain a healthy nervous system. Linolenic acid promotes radiant skin.

Ingredient Form: Alpha-linolenic acid is supplied mostly as a component of plant oils, in particular flaxseed oil.

Effective Supplement Dosages: As a dietary supplement, 500 to 2,000 mg per day can be taken as part of a healthy, low-fat diet.

Cofactors: EPA, DHA, GLA, and linoleic acid.

Concerns: Alpha-linolenic acid is an essential nutrient. While deficiencies are rarely reported, nutritionists believe that the typical American diet is too low in linolenic acid and too high in linoleic acid, creating an imbalance. Linolenic acid is safe but should not be overconsumed because it is a source of calories. It is safe for use by individuals of all ages and both sexes.

Use Guidelines: Include a supplement containing alpha-linolenic acid in your daily nutrition program.

Lipoic acid (also α-lipoic acid, alpha-lipoic acid, thioctic acid)

Supplement Type: Metabolite

Overview: Lipoic acid is called the "universal antioxidant" because it functions in almost all parts of the body. It also functions to regenerate other antioxidants, in particular vitamin C, glutathione, and coenzyme Q_{10}, thereby improving their function as well. Lipoic acid is also involved in energy metabolism. Lipoic acid is gaining a reputation as a brain and eye wellness antioxidant, due to its ability to enter into and function in these tissues.

Benefits: Lipoic acid has only recently begun to appear in dietary supplements. It is reported to display excellent antioxidant activity and protects against free-radical damage, especially in nervous system tissues and the lens of the eyes.

Ingredient Form: Alpha-lipoic acid; one brand is Lipotec.

Effective Supplement Dosages: Nutritional dosages in antioxidant formulas and comprehensive vitamin-mineral formulas range from 15 to 125 mg per day. Higher dosages, up to 600 mg per day, have been safely used under medical supervision for short periods of therapeutic use.

Cofactors: The other antioxidants, such as vitamin C, vitamin E, coenzyme Q_{10}, and glutathione.

Concerns: While this is a relatively new dietary supplement ingredient, no harmful effects have been reported from regular use at nutritional dosages. For adults only; not for children or for pregnant or lactating women unless under medical supervision.

Use Guidelines: Mature adults especially should include lipoic acid in their daily supplement program.

Liposerine: *see* Lecithin

Liver extracts: *see* Glandulars

Lutein: *see* Beta carotene and Carotenoids

Lysine (also L-lysine)

Supplement Type: Amino acid

Overview: Lysine is an essential amino acid. It is part of proteins, and is found in large quantities in muscle tissue. It is needed for proper growth and bone development, and it aids in calcium absorption. Lysine supplementation has been shown to nutritionally fight cold sores and herpes viruses. It is required for the formation of collagen, enzymes, antibodies, and carnitine. Lysine can become depleted in the brain by excess intake of arginine and ornithine. Supplemental intake may be required under certain situations, such as to fight off cold sores, or if you are taking supplemental amounts of arginine and ornithine.

Benefits: Lysine is required for maintenance of good health.

Ingredient Form: L-lysine, as part of a full-spectrum amino acid complex from protein, or in amino acid pills.

Effective Supplement Dosages: Ideally, adequate lysine intake should be derived from the diet. If lysine supplements are indicated for a particular nutritional or therapeutic reason, consult with your health care professional. For warding off cold sores, use a topical lysine ointment and daily lysine supplement intake of between 2 and 3 g for a few weeks.

Cofactors: The other essential amino acids.

Concerns: Lysine is an essential nutrient. Adequate intake is required for maintenance of good health. Do not take megadoses of lysine. It should be used by adults only, and not by pregnant or lactating women unless under a doctor's supervision. While lysine as part of dietary proteins is very safe, the exact effects of long-term use of lysine supplements are not known. Use lysine supplements for short intervals of time, or as otherwise directed by your doctor.

Use Guidelines: Take lysine supplements on a periodic basis when needed.

Lycopene: *see* Beta carotene

Magnesium

Supplement Type: Mineral

Overview: Magnesium is an important structural component of bone and is involved in many metabolic reactions, including energy production and synthesis of proteins and nucleic acids. It plays a role in the relaxation of muscle tissues and the maintenance of heart health and function. Improvements in athletic performance have recently been reported among athletes taking magnesium supplements.

Benefits: It is important to maintain adequate intake of magnesium for general health. Magnesium supplementation has been used to improve physical performance, alleviate PMS discomfort, increase the rate of fat loss in exercising women, reduce the occurrence of muscle spasms due to magnesium deficiency, and improve heart and circulatory system health.

Ingredient Forms: Magnesium oxide, magnesium carbonate, magnesium glycinate, magnesium citrate, magnesium malate.

Effective Supplement Dosages: The adult RDI for magnesium is 400 mg. Daily dosage from magnesium can range from 50 to 400 mg per day for nutritional uses. Intake of 400 mg per day has been shown to help reduce abdominal pain associated with PMS, and to help increase weight loss in women along with diet and exercise.

Cofactors: Magnesium supplement intake should be balanced with calcium in a 1:2 magnesium-calcium ratio. For example, if you are taking 300 mg of magnesium, take at least 600 mg of calcium.

Concerns: Magnesium toxicity is rare. Symptoms include muscle weakness, irritability, nausea, and depression. Excessive intake has a laxative effect, and can cause abnormal kidney function, nausea, vomiting, and low blood pressure. It is safe for all ages and both sexes when used properly.

Use Guidelines: Include magnesium supplements as part of your daily supplement program.

Magnesium stearic acid: *see* Excipients

Maitake mushroom (also *Grifola frondosa*)
Supplement Type: Botanical
Overview: Maitake mushroom contains phytonutrients called polysaccharides, which stimulate immune system function. Maitake mushroom supplements have been studied in China and Japan as supportive therapy in cancer treatment. In addition to the polysaccharide content stimulating the immune system, medical researchers think it also stimulates production of antitumor substances. It also

has reported uses for treating diabetes and high cholesterol. However, more research is needed to determine maitake's exact beneficial effects for these disorders.

Benefits: Maitake mushroom promotes immune system function.

Ingredient Form: Standardized maitake mushroom powder, with standardized polysaccharide content.

Dosages: Depending on the specific standardized maitake mushroom powder product, daily dosages can typically range between 50 and 500 mg. Use for two to three months at a time, so as to not overstimulate the immune system.

Cofactors: Other immune-stimulating herbs, such as echinacea.

Concerns: Maitake mushroom is not an essential nutrient. It has a long history of use in Asia as a food and in herbal medicines. As a dietary supplement, clinical studies report no major side effects. For adult use only; not for use by children or by pregnant or lactating women, unless under a doctor's supervision. Use under medical supervision if you are taking immune-stimulating botanicals for a disease condition.

Use Guidelines: Take maitake supplements on a periodic basis when needed.

Manganese
Supplement Type: Mineral
Overview: Manganese is an essential trace mineral required for energy production. It is a component of enzymes and the anti-

oxidant superoxide dismutase (SOD). Manganese aids in bone and connective tissue formation. Manganese is one of the key trace minerals essential for health and well-being.

Benefits: Maintains bones, connective tissues, and overall health.

Ingredient Forms: Manganese glycinate, manganese arginate, manganese gluconate, magnesium carbonate, magnesium sulfate.

Effective Supplement Dosages: The adult RDI for manganese is 2 mg. Manganese is a common ingredient in dietary supplement formulas. Typical dosages range from 1 to 6 mg per day.

Cofactors: The other essential vitamins and minerals.

Concerns: Manganese toxicity is rarely reported and manganese deficiency is infrequent. Manganese-containing supplements are safe for all ages and both sexes when used correctly.

Use Guidelines: Take manganese-containing supplements each day as part of your nutrition program.

Medium-chain triglycerides (MCTs)

Supplement Type: Nonessential fatty acids

Overview: MCTs contain saturated fatty acids, usually derived from coconut oil and palm oil. MCT dietary supplement products are usually high in caprylic and capric acids and are routinely used as medical foods for people who have problems digesting long-chain fatty acids. MCTs behave differently in the digestive system than long-chain fatty acids and are able to pass from the intestines directly to the bloodstream instead of first traveling through the lymph system. MCTs are reported to be metabolized more quickly for energy than long-chain fatty acids. They can also increase metabolic rate under certain conditions. Bodybuilders use MCTs during their contest preparation training, and long-distance runners use them as a source of energy, but the exact benefits of MCT supplementation in healthy people are yet to be determined. It is also important to remember that MCTs are loaded with saturated fatty acids, which may have long-term adverse effects. MCT dietary supplements do not have any health-enhancing uses for healthy people.

Benefits: A dietary source of nonessential fatty acids. May promote thermogenesis.

Ingredient Form: Purified liquid MCT oil, from plant oils.

Effective Supplement Dosages: Typical dosages of MCTs range from 1 to 4 tablespoons per day.

Cofactors: A balanced diet.

Concerns: MCTs are not essential nutrients. Eating too many nonessential lipids can lead to obesity, cancer, and coronary heart disease. If used as a diet aid, make sure all the essential nutrients are being supplied as well, as part of a balanced diet. While MCTs are considered nontoxic, their use should be restricted to adults only, for specific reasons. Not for use by children or by pregnant or lactating women, unless under a doctor's supervision. Regular daily consumption is not recommended unless you are being treated for a medical disorder. Reported side effects include gastrointestinal upset, abdominal cramping, and diarrhea.

Use Guidelines: MCT supplement use on a periodic basis is optional.

Melatonin

Supplement Type: Metabolite

Overview: Melatonin is actually a hormone produced by the pineal gland. With aging, or under conditions of stress or long exposure to light, melatonin levels may be reduced in the body. Melatonin regulates the body's sleep-wake cycle, with levels of the hormone rising during darkness to promote a good night's sleep. Dysfunctional melatonin secretion can lead to poor sleep patterns. Clinical studies have proven that melatonin supplements can help you get to sleep more quickly and stay asleep longer. Melatonin is an interesting hormone. In addition to regulating the sleep-wake cycle, there is some experimental evidence that melatonin has antioxidant activity. It also can help prevent or recover from jet lag. There is additional evidence in test-tube studies that melatonin has inhibitory effects on tumor growth. It is interesting to note that melatonin levels increase during deep meditation, and natural-healing practitioners believe that this increased melatonin production helps prevent disease. Future research will determine how melatonin might fit into a daily antiaging supplement program. There is also research under way examining the probable role melatonin plays in preventing and/or fighting cancer.

Benefits: Melatonin promotes normal and restful sleep.

Ingredient Form: Found in dietary supplements as melatonin.

Effective Supplement Dosages: While there are no officially established dosages for melatonin, daily dosages between 500 and 3,000 mcg have been shown to be safe and effective for promoting good sleep. Many brands of melatonin contain doses that are too high; 500 to 1,000 mcg (½ to 1 mg) is ample for most people.

Cofactors: Other sleep-promoting dietary supplement ingredients, such as valerian.

Concerns: Melatonin is not an essential nutrient. It is a hormone, so technically, taking melatonin supplements is a type of hormone replacement therapy. If you plan to use melatonin regularly, inform your doctor. Since 1994 millions of Americans have been taking melatonin supplements with no major side effects being reported. For adult use only; not for use by children or by pregnant or lactating women unless under a doctor's supervision.

Use Guidelines: Use melatonin supplements periodically when needed.

Methionine (also DL-methionine, L-methionine)

Supplement Type: Amino acid

Overview: Methionine is an essential sulfur-bearing amino acid. It is involved in the manufacture of many substances in the body, including choline, creatine, melatonin, and

DNA. Methionine is recognized for its removal of metabolic waste products from the liver, its role in the breakdown of fats, and its ability to help prevent fatty buildup in the liver and arteries. Methionine's role in the manufacture of other biochemicals is very important. Some research indicates that methionine affects the production of neurotransmitters, and may be useful in the treatment of depression.

Benefits: Methionine is a liptropoic nutrient, important in fat metabolism, and is required for health. It promotes cardiovascular health.

Ingredient Form: DL-methionine is commonly added to meal-replacement drinks and protein beverages for fortification of low-quality plant proteins. L-methionine is commonly used in dietary supplement formulas.

Effective Supplement Dosages: Methionine is sometimes found in dietary supplements in amounts ranging from 500 to 2,000 mg per daily serving. Smaller amounts are also used, in particular in liver health dietary supplement formulas, along with other ingredients.

Cofactors: The other lipotropics.

Concerns: Methionine is an essential nutrient. Vegetarians can become deficient in it, since most plant proteins are low in methionine. Dietary supplements are sometimes used to help with fat loss programs. Methionine dietary supplements are considered safe when used in the recommended dosages. For adults only; not for children or for pregnant or lactating women, unless under a doctor's supervision.

Use Guidelines: Use methionine supplements on a regular basis when needed.

Microcrystalline cellulose (Emcocel): *see* Excipients

Milk thistle (also *Silybum marianum*)
Supplement Type: Botanical
Overview: Milk thistle seed extract is composed mainly of a bioflavonoid complex called silymarin. Silymarin is actually a group of related compounds (called flavonolignans), consisting primarily of silibinin, silydianin, and silycristin. The combined actions of the silymarin compounds result in three main functions, with primary actions on the liver: (1) they protect the outer liver cell membranes from chemical damage; (2) they exert potent antioxidant activity, which also protects liver cells from chemical and free-radical damage; and (3) they stimulate regeneration and growth of damaged liver cells. Milk thistle is one dietary supplement ingredient that should be included in your daily supplement program. The liver is the body's central detoxifying organ. After digestion, all substances absorbed into the body are transported to the liver. Once in the liver, substances, including nutrients, can be altered, stored in the liver, or passed on to the circulatory system to be transported to the rest of the body. A properly functioning liver is essential to optimal health. Milk thistle's liver protection effects are so powerful that it has been shown in clinical studies to reduce the harmful effects of death cap mushroom

(*Amanita phalloides*) poisoning, reduce liver damage from long treatment with butyrophenone and phenothiazine drug therapies, protect against the harmful effects of excessive ingestion of acetaminophen, and reduce liver damage from anesthesia used during surgery. Therefore, milk thistle supplement use should be considered when taking drugs that may be harmful to the liver.

Benefits: As a dietary supplement, milk thistle promotes, restores, stimulates, and maintains liver health. It helps protect liver cells against toxic chemicals and promotes normal liver functioning. Used therapeutically, milk thistle helps restore liver function due to liver damage from alcohol, drugs, and other substances that can damage the liver. It is also used for supportive treatment in chronic liver inflammatory diseases, liver cirrhosis, and hepatitis. Milk thistle can help prevent gallstone formation, and it has a role in liver detoxification programs.

Ingredient Form: Standardized milk thistle seed extract (70% to 80% silymarin).

Effective Supplement Dosages: As a dietary supplement to improve liver health, take 420 to 800 mg per day of standardized milk thistle seed extract, in divided dosages. Clinical studies report that improvements in liver function occur within two to eight weeks. Lower daily dosages of milk thistle, 100 to 400 mg per day, are also used in dietary supplements to support the health of the liver on a regular basis.

Cofactors: Curcumin, dandelion, NAC (N-acetyl-cysteine), and lipoic acid.

Concerns: Milk thistle seed extract is not an essential nutrient, but it is a very beneficial botanical dietary supplement ingredient. More than a hundred clinical studies have shown it can help cure liver problems and support the health and function of the liver. Side effects with high dosages include occasional temporary diarrhea. If used for supportive treatment of liver disease, seek proper medical treatment. Milk thistle has a reported history of safe use that spans over two thousand years. For adult use only; not for use by children or by pregnant or lactating women, unless under a doctor's supervision.

Use Guidelines: Use milk thistle supplements on a regular basis, especially if you are concerned about promoting and maintaining liver health.

Molybdenum

Supplement Type: Mineral

Overview: Molybdenum is an essential trace mineral found in the body in small amounts. It is present in enzymes that are involved in energy production, uric acid formation, and nitrogen metabolism, such as sulfite oxidase, aldehyde oxidase, and xanthine oxidase. Molybdenum intake has been determined to be essential for good health.

Benefits: Essential nutrient required for maintenance of health.

Ingredient Form: Sodium molybdate, molybdenum chelates.

Effective Supplement Dosages: The adult RDI for molybdenum is 75 mcg. Common molybdenum daily dietary supplement dosages range from 25 to 150 mcg. Molybdenum is a common ingredient in many vitamin-mineral formulations intended to be taken daily.

Cofactors: Essential vitamins and minerals.

Concerns: Excessive molybdenum intake may result in goutlike symptoms, growth disorders, and copper deficiency. Safe for use by all ages and both sexes when used properly. Never take megadoses of molybdenum.

Use Guidelines: Take molybdenum-containing dietary supplements as part of your daily nutrition program.

N-acetyl-L-carnitine: *see* Carnitine

N-acetyl-cysteine: *see* Cysteine

N-acetyl-glucosamine: *see* Glucosamine

MSM (also Methylsulfonylmethane)

Supplement Type: Metabolite

Overview: MSM is a sulfur-containing substance that occurs naturally in plants and animals. MSM serves as a supply of biologically accessible sulfur, to be used in structural proteins and enzymes. MSM's most noted use as a dietary supplement is in the nutritional treatment of connective tissue disorders. Studies have shown that MSM stimulates collagen formation. MSM also plays a role in promoting immune system function by supplying the sulfur needed in the formation of IgG, an important immunoglobulin. Research also indicates that MSM supplements help build up and maintain the linings of the gastrointestinal tract and respiratory tract. While some clinical research on MSM was done a number of years ago and reported beneficial results, this supplement has just begun to increase in popularity. As researchers discover new insights into degenerative processes and diseases, they learn more about the role played by nutrient deficiencies. Poor body sulfur status is associated with a state of poor health, and use of MSM in these individuals has been reported to show beneficial health effects. However, more research is needed to conclusively determine the long-term safety of using MSM supplements, best dosages, and cofactors.

Benefits: MSM supplements promote the growth and maintenance of connective tissues, resulting in improvements in joints, skin, hair, and other tissues. MSM also supports the proper structure and function of the gastrointestinal and respiratory system tracts, as well as immune system function.

Ingredient Form: Found in supplements as methylsulfonylmethane.

Effective Supplement Dosages: MSM is typically taken periodically at dosages ranging from 250 to 1,500 mg a day, mostly as part of nutritional therapy to improve connective tissues, immune system function, and gastrointestinal and respiratory system health. You will also encounter MSM added to multi-nutrient formulas, usually in smaller amounts, 50 to 200 mg per day.

Cofactors: Vitamins and minerals.

Concerns: MSM contains the essential nutrient sulfur, which is important to good health but for which no official dietary intake guidelines have been established. Because

MSM is a relatively new dietary supplement ingredient, caution should be exercised when using it. There have been no major side effects reported from people using MSM. For adult use only; not for use by children or by pregnant or lactating women unless under a doctor's supervision.

Use Guideline: The major current use of MSM supplements is for people who are experiencing pain and inflammation from connective tissue disorders, allergies, or gastrointestinal concerns, or who are just feeling run down. Use high therapeutic dosages periodically. Lower dosages can be included in your daily supplement program if you are looking to prevent or nutritionally manage the aforementioned conditions.

Nettle (also *Urtica dioica*)

Supplement Type: Botanical

Overview: Nettle contains phytonutrients that have beneficial effects on the prostate. It is used in Europe as an effective treatment for urinary difficulties arising from the onset of benign prostatic hyperplasia (BPH). Nettle root extract is high in beta-sitosterol, which is thought to be active in normalizing prostate function, achieving hormonal balance, and reducing inflammation. Nettle root is an herb with more therapeutic uses than nutritional uses. It is also considered a mild diuretic.

Benefits: Promotes and maintains prostate and urinary tract health in men. It's also beneficial in relieving symptoms of hay fever (leaf extract).

Ingredient Form: Standardized nettle root extract (0.8% to 2% phytosterols or beta-sitosterol).

Effective Supplement Dosages: For occasional use as a dietary supplement, 400 to 800 mg per day of nettle root extract. The dose of the leaf extract for use in hay fever is one or two capsules, every four hours.

Cofactors: If you are concerned about prostate health, include nettle in your dietary supplement program with other prostate health ingredients such as zinc, saw palmetto berry extract, pygeum, lycopene, selenium, copper, and beta-sitosterol.

Concerns: Nettle is not an essential nutrient. It can be beneficial to prostate and urinary system health. It is generally considered a safe botanical, but it may cause an allergic effect in some people, and it should not be used for extended periods of time (more than four months) until long-term studies verify its safety and effectiveness. For use by adult males only; not for children or women. Women may safely use the leaf extract. Always consult your doctor for medical supervision when treating prostate and hay fever health problems.

Use Guidelines: Males who are concerned about promoting or maintaining prostate health should take nettle root extract supplements periodically, in three- to five-month cycles.

Octacosanol

Supplement Type: Botanical isolate

Overview: Octacosanol is a component of wheat-germ oil. Octacosanol has been shown in clinical studies to benefit athletic performance by increasing endurance and improving reaction time. The exact details of how octacosanol does this are under investigation. Octacosanol may also help improve performance in the workplace by enhancing stamina and improving neuromuscular functioning.

Benefits: Octacosanol improves endurance, stamina, and reaction time in athletes.

Ingredient Form: Octacosanol is derived from rice bran or wheat germ oil.

Effective Supplement Dosages: Dosages of octacosanol of 1 to 2 mg per day have been shown in clinical studies to be safe and effective.

Cofactors: None.

Concerns: Octacosanol is not an essential nutrient. Octacosanol is considered nontoxic when taken in recommended dosages. Do not take megadoses of octacosanol. For healthy adults only; not for use by children or by pregnant or lactating women unless under a doctor's supervision.

Use Guidelines: Octacosanol can be taken as part of your daily supplement program. Use it if you want to maintain or promote good energy levels.

Oligomeric proanthocyanidins (OPCs):
see Bioflavonoids, Grape seed extract

Olive leaf (also *Olea europa*)

Supplement Type: Botanical

Overview: Olive leaf contains a phytochemical that has antimicrobial action. One way it functions is to interfere with microbe protein synthesis, which essentially prevents microbes from reproducing. Olive leaf has been used against pathological microbes—bacteria, fungi, protozoa, and viruses—and in the treatment of ulcers, respiratory diseases, skin problems; it has also been used to strengthen immune function. However, until more studies are conducted to confirm its long-term safety, it is wise to use olive leaf only periodically, as with other immune system–stimulating botanicals.

Benefits: As a dietary supplement, olive leaf promotes immune system function. As a phytomedicine, olive leaf is an antimicrobial agent.

Ingredient Form: Standardized olive leaf extract (15% to 17% oleuropein).

Dosages: Olive leaf extract is a relatively new dietary supplement ingredient. For immune system support during stressful periods, 500 mg per day of standardized extract, up to four times a day, is generally the recommended dose regimen. Use for two to four weeks at a time, as required, for supportive therapy in treating mild ailments. As a daily dietary supplement, lower dosages are sometimes found in immune system–enhancing formulas. For adult use only; not for use by children or by pregnant or lactating women, unless under a doctor's supervision.

Cofactors: Immune system–stimulating botanicals, such as echinacea, cat's claw, or goldenseal.

Concerns: Olive leaf is not an essential nutrient. Its use in nutritional therapy for diseases should be undertaken only with medical supervision. For adults only; not for children or for pregnant or lactating women. Restrict use to two to four weeks unless otherwise advised by your doctor. It can cause allergic reactions, in particular during the first days of use; these are usually temporary. It can also cause fatigue, headache, nausea, and respiratory symptoms. Part of the symptoms are attributed to the body's having to cleanse itself of dead microbes.

Use Guidelines: Use olive leaf extracts only periodically, and under medical supervision when used as nutritional support during treatment of illness.

OPC-85: *see* Grape seed extract

OptiZinc: *see* Zinc

Ornithine (also L-ornithine)
   Supplement Type: Amino acid
   Overview: Ornithine is a nonessential amino acid that does not occur in proteins. Its primary metabolic role is in the urea cycle, which makes ornithine important in the removal of the metabolic waste product ammonia. Ornithine is formed from arginine, and like arginine, ornithine has been shown to increase blood serum levels of growth hormone. In bodybuilding circles, a complex form of ornithine, called OKG or ornithine alphaketoglutarate, is a common ingredient found in sports nutrition products. OKG has a history of clinical use as part of nutritional therapy for burn victims, for severe malnutrition, and to aid in postsurgical

healing. OKG consists of two ornithine molecules and one alphaketoglutarate molecule. OKG seems to work by stimulating a variety of metabolic functions: It acts as an ammonia scavenger, increases the glutamine supply in muscle tissue, reduces catabolism, elevates growth hormone levels, increases protein synthesis, and increases insulin secretion. OKG dosages of 2 to 4 g per day have been shown to be safe and effective. The use of ornithine and other amino acid "growth hormone stimulators" has risen tremendously among middle-aged people who are using supplements for antiaging purposes. The reasoning is that if mature people prevent their growth hormone levels from falling off with age, they will ultimately stay younger for a longer period of time.

   Benefits: Ornithine promotes increases in growth hormone levels and reduces ammonia blood levels.

   Ingredient Form: L-ornithine HCl.

   Effective Supplement Dosages: Dietary supplement use of L-ornithine ranges from 250 to 1,000 mg per day for nutritional use, and 1 to 4 g per day for therapeutic uses.

   Cofactors: Arginine, lysine, glycine, DL-phenylalanine.

   Concerns: Ornithine can have a beneficial effect on maintaining or elevating the body's levels of growth hormone. For use by adults only; not for use by those with liver or kidney problems, or by children or by pregnant or lactating women, unless under a doctor's supervision. Most of the research on ornithine supplementation was short-term in duration. Use ornithine for short intervals, three to four months, with three to four weeks off, then repeat cycle as needed.

Use Guidelines: Use moderate dosages of ornithine on a regular basis, and higher dosages periodically when needed.

Ornithine alphaketoglutarate (OKG): *see* Ornithine

OXI-Grape: *see* Grape seed extract

OXI-Pine: *see* Pycnogenol

Pancreatic extracts: *see* Glandulars

Passionflower (also *Passiflora incarnata*)
Supplement Type: Botanical
Overview: Passionflower contains phytonutrients, which promote an overall sedative effect on the central nervous system. Passionflower is widely used in Europe for its sedative and calming effects.

Benefits: Passionflower promotes relaxation, calming, and sleep.

Ingredient Form: Standardized passionflower extract (2% to 5% isovitexin).

Effective Supplement Dosages: As a dietary supplement, take before bedtime 100 to 300 mg.

Cofactors: Other relaxing herbs, such as kava kava and valerian.

Concerns: Passionflower is not an essential nutrient. Its use should be restricted to specific purposes. It is considered safe and effective when used properly. Do not over-

dose; the depressant action of this botanical can have serious side effects if it is taken in excess. For adult use only; not for use by children or by pregnant or lactating women unless under a doctor's supervision. Use under medical supervision for sleep disorders or other medical conditions.

Use Guidelines: Use passionflower-containing supplements periodically to promote stress reduction and sleep.

Pau d'arco (also *Tabebuia heptaphylla*)
Supplement Type: Botanical
Overview: Pau d'arco is native to Central and South America, where it is used as a traditional cure-all. Some experiments have detected antimicrobial action in pau d'arco extract, but more research is needed to make conclusive recommendations. Pau d'arco is one of the herbs that fits into the might-be-effective category, based on a long history of use as a traditional medicine. It also has a reputation as an antitumor agent based on test-tube studies that have not been verified in clinical studies.

Benefits: Supports immune function.

Best Ingredient Form: Standardized pau d'arco bark.

Dosages: Refer to product labels.

Cofactors: Other immune system stimulants and adaptogens.

Concerns: Pau d'arco is not an essential nutrient. Its use as a curing herb is based primarily on tradition. More clinical research is needed to verify the exact effectiveness.

When used as directed, pau d'arco is considered safe. For adult use only; not for use by children or by pregnant or lactating women.

Use Guidelines: Use supplements containing pau d'arco periodically when needed to stimulate your immune system.

Peptide FM (also Bioactive oligopeptides)

Supplement Type: Metabolite

Overview: Peptide FM is a group of oligopeptides (short chains of amino acids) extracted from food-grade bovine globin (blood) protein, wheat protein, and casein. Peptide FM plays a role in the metabolism of fat; it inhibits digestion and absorption of fatty acids. In clinical and animal studies, ingestion of Peptide FM with meals has been shown to reduce body fat, which is thought to occur by reducing the absorption of fats into the body. Peptide FM also lowers blood triglyceride levels. During a three-month clinical study, using 0.6 to 1.2 g per day of Peptide FM effectively decreased body fat.

Benefits: Peptide FM reduces blood triglyceride levels and promotes a healthy cardiovascular system. It promotes the reduction of body fat accumulation, and stimulates weight loss.

Ingredient Form: Peptide FM is a unique branded ingredient made by DMV International and supplied to dietary supplement companies to use in their products.

Effective Supplement Dosages: The effective dosage range is 0.6 to 2 g per day of Peptide FM, taken with meals.

Cofactors: Other nutritional weight loss aids, fiber, lipotropics, and so on.

Concerns: Peptide FM is not an essential nutrient. It has a history of use in Japan and other countries in food products and as a dietary supplement. It is considered a generally-recognized-as-safe natural food ingredient in the United States. Short-term studies have verified its safety, during a three-month period of use, but its long-term effects have not been determined. For adults only; not for use by children or by pregnant or lactating women unless under a doctor's supervision. Consult your doctor when on a weight loss program.

Use Guidelines: Use supplements containing Peptide FM periodically as part of your weight management program.

Phenylalanine (also L-phenylalanine, D-phenylalanine, and DL-phenylalanine, which is a mixture of the D and L forms.)

Supplement Type: Amino acid

Overview: Phenylalanine is an essential amino acid and precursor of the nonessential amino acid tyrosine. Phenylalanine has many functions in the body and is a precursor of several important metabolites, such as the skin pigment melanin and several catecholamine neurotransmitters, including epinephrine and norepinephrine. The catecholamines are important in memory, learning, locomotion, sex drive, tissue growth and repair, immune system function, and appetite control. Phenylalanine is also used for combating pain, which can be useful for people with chronic pain disorders.

Studies have reported the D and L forms taken together work best. Phenylalanine increases growth hormone levels. Phenylalanine is backed by clinical research and has a history of safe and effective use as a dietary supplement.

Benefits: Supports brain function. Maintains appetite control. Improves learning and memory. Promotes maintenance of good health.

Ingredient Form: For pain control, DL-phenylalanine. For other uses, L-phenylalanine.

Effective Supplement Dosages: Phenylalanine is taken in dosages ranging from 100 to 500 mg once or twice a day. Higher daily dosages are also commonly used for short periods of time, 1,500 to 3,000 mg.

Cofactors: For growth hormone stimulation: ornithine, arginine, glycine.

Concerns: Phenylalanine is an essential nutrient, required for maintenance of good health. Its use as a dietary supplement has been demonstrated to be safe and effective. For adults only; not for use by children or by pregnant or lactating women unless under a doctor's supervision. Don't take phenylalanine if you have high blood pressure, or are taking an MAOI drug or St. John's wort. People with liver or kidney disease should also avoid it. Caution: The artificial sweetener aspartame is a dipeptide made up of phenylalanine and aspartic acid. Soft drinks containing aspartame carry warnings for people with a condition called phenylketonuria (PKU). This is a disease in which phenylalanine is not properly metabolized and can be very damaging.

Therefore people with PKU should not take phenylalanine supplements without the approval of their doctor.

Use Guidelines: Use phenylalanine supplements on a regular basis when seeking the desired results.

Phosphatidylserine (PS)

Supplement Type: Botanical isolate

Overview: PS is a nutrient that is essential to the functioning of all cells, with special activity in the brain, where it is involved in a variety of nerve cell functions, such as nerve transmission. PS has been shown in more than thirty clinical studies to be safe and effective in improving brain function, benefiting memory, reducing stress hormone production, improving mood, and benefiting learning. PS is derived from soy. Phosphatidylserine has been tested in more than sixteen clinical studies, using over 1,200 people, that verified its safety and effectiveness. In one interesting study, PS was shown to support nerve cell function. Using a special brain activity imaging technique, the brain activity of a fifty-nine-year-old female was shown to significantly increase after just three weeks of taking PS.

Benefits: Phosphatidylserine promotes brain wellness and increases memory, concentration, and learning ability.

Ingredient Form: Phosphatidylserine, Leci-PS is an exclusive brand of phosphatidylserine produced by Lucas Meyer, Inc., and sold to dietary supplement companies to be used in their products.

Dosages: Safe and effective dosages used in clinical studies range from 100 to 300 mg per day. Higher dosages, up to 800 mg per day, have also been used safely.

Cofactors: Other brain wellness supplement ingredients, such as Acetyl-L-carnitine, ginkgo, gotu kola, lipoic acid, and so on.

Concerns: Phosphatidylserine is not an essential nutrient. Researchers have determined that the number of brain cells decreases and the level of neurotransmitters declines during the aging process; phosphatidylserine can restore brain wellness. It is considered very safe. For adult use only; not for use by children or by pregnant or lactating women unless under a doctor's supervision.

Use Guidelines: Use phosphatidylserine supplements on a regular basis if you are concerned about maintaining or improving your brain wellness.

Phosphorus

Supplement Type: Mineral

Overview: Phosphorus is an important part of bone and is also found in lipids, cell membranes, nucleic acids, and proteins. It is present in all cells and occurs as phosphate or combined to other elements in body fluids such as sodium phosphate or dyhyrogen phosphate. It is part of the body's primary energy molecule, ATP (adenosine triphosphate). People who are at risk for phosphorus deficiency should make sure they are getting enough in their diets; this category includes athletes, the elderly, and individuals who are experiencing malnutrition from illness or drug therapy.

Benefits: Phosphorus is required for health, and for maintenance of structure and function of the body.

Ingredient Form: Phosphorus.

Effective Supplement Dosages: The adult RDI for phosphorus is 1,000 mg. Because phosphorus is usually plentiful in the diet, most dietary supplements do not contain it as an ingredient. When they do, it is typically supplied in the range of 50 to 200 mg per day.

Cofactors: Essential vitamins and minerals.

Concerns: Phosphorus is an essential nutrient and is required for optimal health. Symptoms of long-term phosphorus deficiency include poor bone formation, weakness, growth disorders, anorexia, and malaise. Excessive intake can cause gastrointestinal distress and adversely affect calcium metabolism. It is safe for use by all ages and both sexes when used correctly.

Use Guidelines: Use phosphorus-containing supplements and food products each day as part of your nutrition program.

Pine bark extract: *see* Pycnogenol

Plant Oils

You will commonly encounter plant oils contained in dietary supplement products. Plant oils contain fatty acids and are important sources of the essential fatty acids linoleic and linolenic. Some plant oils are high in GLA (gamma-linolenic acid) as well, such as borage, black currant, hemp, and evening primrose. Many scientific discoveries made during the 20th century support including more plant oils in your diet and reducing consumption of saturated animal fats and cholesterol. However, you must make sure not to overconsume plant oils, keeping in mind that 1 tablespoon contains 130 calories. You must also make sure to maintain a healthy body weight and a program of daily physical activity. Some other plant oils you will find in supplement products include flax, soy bean, pumpkin, walnut, sunflower, grape, canola, wheat germ, rice bran, olive, and sesame. To learn about the health benefits of the essential fatty acids contained in these plant oils, consult the specific entries on Linoleic, Linolenic, and GLA.

Potassium

Supplement Type: Mineral

Overview: Potassium is an essential mineral and a major component of all cells. It helps maintain fluid balance in the body, and functions in nerve transmissions, regulation of heartbeat, muscle contractions, and glycogen formation. Contemporary diets are usually too high in sodium and too low in potassium. Increase potassium intake by selecting foods high in potassium, such as fruits and vegetables. If you are taking liquid potassium supplements, be careful not to overconsume them. Many of them are very concentrated and deliver a potent amount of potassium in a small serving. Read the labels carefully.

Benefits: Adequate potassium intake maintains health and improves physical performance.

Ingredient Form: Potassium chloride, potassium ascorbate, potassium–amino acid complexes.

Effective Supplement Dosages: The adult Daily Reference Value (DRV) for potassium is 3,500 mg. Potassium is sometimes contained in dietary supplements, ranging in amounts from 50 to 400 mg.

Cofactors: Essential vitamins and minerals.

Concerns: Potassium is an essential nutrient and one of the body's electrolyte minerals; deficiency can occur under conditions of dehydration or malnutrition and during weight loss programs. Deficiency symptoms include drowsiness, weakness, low energy, nausea, anorexia, and cardiac dysrhythmia. Problems due to excessive potassium rarely occur but can be severe and cause hyperkalemia, which can result in cardiac arrest. It is safe for all ages and both sexes when used correctly.

Use Guidelines: Take potassium-containing supplements each day as part of your nutritional health program.

Pregnenolone (also 3-hydroxypregn-5-en-20-one)

Supplement Type: Metabolite

Overview: Pregnenolone is made by the body and is classified as a steroid hormone. It is used to make other hormones, such as DHEA and progesterone. Because of this, research indicates that taking pregnenolone can have the same effects as taking DHEA and other steroid hormones. Clinical research using pregnenolone supplements is limited, but has shown a general improvement in well-being.

Pregnenolone is another one of the metabolite hormone dietary supplement ingredients allowed under the new dietary supplement regulations. It is touted as one of the "youth" ingredients, like DHEA. There has been only limited research conducted on pregnenolone to determine its long-term safety and effects. At this time it is considered safe and effective in recommended dosages for short periods of time.

Benefits: Improves well-being and mood.

Ingredient Form: Pregnenolone.

Effective Supplement Dosages: Clinical studies have used pregnenolone in dosages of 25 to 100 mg per day. It is for short-term use only, one to four months. Use under a doctor's supervision. Lower dosages are also found in dietary supplement formulas, ranging from 1 to 15 mg per day.

Cofactors: None.

Concerns: Pregnenolone is not an essential nutrient. It is made by the body, and is a hormone. Research has determined that as a person ages, levels of pregnenolone and other hormones decrease. Individuals over forty may benefit from periodic use of pregnenolone as a form of hormone replacement therapy. Medical supervision is required. For adults only; not for use by children or by pregnant or lactating women unless under a doctor's supervision. Not for long-term use; use for only one to four months at a time. Use of pregnenolone supplements may cause skin rash.

Use Guidelines: Optional use as a dietary supplement.

Probiotics (also *Lactobacillus acidophilus, L. bulgaricus, L. sporogenes, Bifidobacterium bifidum, B. longum, Streptococcus thermophilus*)

Supplement Type: Microflora

Overview: Probiotics are supplements containing the beneficial microflora (bacteria) that normally inhabit a health digestive system. Under certain conditions—taking antibiotic drugs, stress, traveling, frequently eating out, ingesting chemicals in your food—the population of good microflora in your digestive tract can be reduced. An inadequate amount of the beneficial microflora can lead to gastrointestinal problems, and can ultimately compromise your health. This is mainly due to the fact that you are not experiencing the microflora's health-promoting effects, though you *are* feeling the adverse effects of higher populations of undesirable microflora. The relationship between consumption of cultured milk products such as yogurt and superior health led scientists to look at the how and why. Now, slowly but surely, probiotic supplements containing beneficial microflora have been coming onto the market. And it is no surprise that there are many scientific studies supporting the beneficial effects of using probiotic supplements: maintenance of normal digestive system function, restoration and balance of intestinal microflora, detoxification of harmful substances, improvement in immune system function, improved digestibility of food, control of lactose intolerance in some people, promotion of regularity, and maintenance of healthy cholesterol levels by reducing the amount of cholesterol absorbed from the intestines into the bloodstream. Maintaining proper digestive system function is vital. When you give it some thought, it is easy to understand that if your digestive system is high in harmful bacteria and low in benefical bacteria, this condition will adversely affect your total health and feelings of well-being. Focus on eating wholesome, healthy foods, rich in nutrients, low in fat and sugars, to help promote digestive system health, along with taking a probiotic-containing supplement.

Benefits: Promotes digestive system health and normal function. Can also be used to correct both constipation and diarrhea.

Ingredient Form: Choose probiotic supplements containing one or more types of microflora, including at the very least the lactobacillus and bifidobacterium types. Keep in mind that probiotic supplements contain live cultures; make sure the brand you choose guarantees potency and stability. Most probiotic formulas need to be refrigerated. Some innovative companies, such as ConAgra, have developed special strains of probiotic microflora (Lactobacillus GG, in the patented product Culturelle) and proven their effectiveness with clinical studies. Another brand of probiotic is Lactospore. The great thing about taking probiotics is that you will notice if they are effective or not within twenty-four to forty-eight hours. If you do not notice improvements in your intestinal function, then try another brand until you do. Finally, because stomach acid may kill the organisms, some formulas

contain special types of probiotics proven to be able to survive their trip through the harsh stomach environment, or are enterically coated, which means that they will resist digestion in the stomach and be digested only in the intestines.

Effective Supplement Dosages: Generally, you will encounter two categories of probiotic supplement ranges. Products sold as probiotic formulas will typically contain from 2 billion to 12 billion cells per daily dosage. In multinutrient formulas, the cell content is usually lower, 250 million to 2 billion probiotic cells.

Cofactors: Fructooligosaccarides (FOS), which are the preferred food for promoting and maintaining good microflora populations in your digestive system.

Concerns: Probiotics are not essential nutrients but are vital to good health. They are safe for all ages and both sexes. However, to ensure safe use by children, it is best to consult your doctor, and contact the company to make sure that its product is suitable for use by children. There are now probiotic supplements designed specifically for children; some come in chewable forms.

Use Guidelines: Use probiotic-containing formulas on a regular basis to promote digestive system health. Increase your daily dosage accordingly during periods of increased stress; before, during, and after traveling; and when taking antibiotics (which kill your good microflora as a side effect of killing the disease-causing bacteria).

Proline (also L-proline)

Supplement Type: Amino acid

Overview: Proline is a nonessential amino acid. It occurs in high amounts in connective tissues. It can be made in the body from the amino acids ornithine and glutamic acid. Hydroxyproline, which is another amino acid abundant in connective tissues, is made from proline. Proline is important in the growth, repair, and maintenance of connective tissues, such as tendons and cartilage as well as skin, hair, and nails. Knox is a national brand that contains proline and is reported to help build strong hair and nails.

Benefits: Proline supports joint health and promotes healthy skin, hair, and nails.

Ingredient Form: L-proline is found in supplements, usually as part of hydrolyzed gelatin.

Effective Supplement Dosages: As a dietary supplement, 500 to 2,000 mg per day.

Cofactors: Hydroxyproline.

Concerns: Proline is not an essential nutrient. Clinical studies have shown that supplemental proline in particular, as part of hydrolyzed gelatin, increases the thickness of connective tissues. It is considered safe when used as directed. For adults only; not for use by children or by pregnant or lactating women unless under a doctor's supervision. Not for those with liver or kidney disease.

Use Guidelines: Use proline-containing supplements on a regular basis to promote strong and healthy connective tissues.

Pycnogenol (also *Pinus pinaster*)

Supplement Type: Botanical

Overview: Pycnogenol is a trade name for the botanical extract of natural antioxidants from the French maritime pine tree *(Pinus pinaster)*. The extract is prepared from cultivated trees, using only the bark. It contains a variety of plant compounds, including bioflavonoids, proanthocyanidins, procyanidin oligomers (PCO's), caffeic acid, gallic acid, and ferulic acid. Pycnogenol is standardized and has been proven in clinical studies to have cardiovascular benefits, to stimulate the immune system, to improve the appearance of the skin, to treat varicose veins, to relieve the pain of arthritis, and to reduce inflammation. Pycnogenol is considered the gold standard of procyanidin oligomer botanicals, due to the clinical research confirming its absorption, safety, and effectiveness. However, note that procyanidins and other phytonutrients found in Pycnogenol are also found in other botanical extracts.

Benefits: Pycnogenol improves circulatory system structure and function, stimulates immune system function, and reduces inflammation.

Ingredient Form: Pycnogenol is a brand of standardized *Pinus pinaster* bark extract, used in dietary supplements. OXI Pine is another brand of pine bark extract similar to Pycnogenol.

Effective Supplement Dosages: As a dietary supplement antioxidant, 25 to 100 mg per day. Dosages between 200 and 400 mg per day may be needed for nutritional treatment of varicose veins and inflammation under medical supervision.

Cofactors: Other antioxidants.

Concerns: Pycnogenol is not an essential nutrient, but has been shown in clinical studies to have beneficial effects. Research has shown that Pycnogenol is well tolerated and nontoxic when used as directed. It is safe for use by all ages and both sexes when used correctly. An allergic reaction may occur in sensitive individuals.

Use Guidelines: Take Pycnogenol-containing supplements on a daily basis as part of your daily nutritional health program.

Pygeum (also *Pygeum africanum*)

Supplement Type: Botanical

Overview: Pygeum contains phytosterols, including beta-sitosterol. It has been shown in clinical studies to be an effective treatment for benign prostatic hyperplasia. Pygeum is also reported to improve male sexual function and fertility. Pygeum is widely used in Europe to relieve prostate disorders. It is interesting to note that, like saw palmetto, Pygeum is also high in beta-sitosterol; this is most likely a main active component of these botanical supplements.

Benefits: Pygeum promotes prostate health and improves male sexual function.

Ingredient Form: Standardized pygeum bark extract (10% to 13% phytosterols).

Dosages: As a dietary supplement, 100 to 200 mg per day for eight- to twelve-week periods.

Cofactors: Saw palmetto berry extract and nettle root extract.

Concerns: Pygeum is not an essential nutrient. It is considered safe and effective when used as directed for short periods. It is for use only by adult males concerned about restoring or promoting prostate function. It is best used under a doctor's supervision when a prostate disorder exists. It may cause temporary gastrointestinal upset. Not for use by children or women.

Use Guidelines: Use pygeum-containing supplements periodically to promote prostate health and function.

Pyruvate

Supplement Type: Metabolite

Overview: Pyruvate is a three-carbon molecule that is made in the body by splitting glucose in half. It is also found in the diet. Pyruvate has been used in clinical studies as a source of energy and has been shown to improve endurance by enhancing the transport of glucose into the muscles. Clinical studies using pyruvate supplements have resulted in a greater reduction in body fat than when compared to dieting without pyruvate; however, 25 g or more per day of pyruvate were used. While clinical studies report beneficial effects, more studies are needed to confirm pyruvate's safety and effectiveness.

Benefits: Pyruvate supplements improve endurance and increase the rate of fat loss.

Ingredient Form: Pyruvate is found in dietary supplements as sodium pyruvate.

Dosages: While clinical studies have used higher dosages, most dietary supplements recommend a daily dosage ranging from 5 to 10 g per day. Take with meals.

Cofactors: None.

Concerns: Pyruvate is not an essential nutrient. Short-term studies have reported various mild side effects including gastrointestinal upset, gas, bloating, loose stools, and diarrhea. This is perhaps due in part to the sodium content, which may cause intestinal fluid balance problems. The sodium content is of concern for people who are sensitive to high-sodium diets. Pyruvate's exact benefits as a dietary supplement need more research. For adults only; not for use by children or by pregnant or lactating women. Always consult your doctor when on a weight loss program. Do not use pyruvate for long periods of time.

Use Guidelines: Use of pyruvate supplements is optional.

Quercetin

Supplement Type: Botanical

Overview: Quercetin is a common bioflavonoid found in plants, and it is supplied in the diet from food and dietary supplement sources. Quercetin has antioxidant activity and is beneficial as an antiaging phytonutrient and a nutritional agent for preventing diet-related diseases such as diabetes, arteriosclerosis, and cataracts. Naturopathic doctors commonly use quercetin as part of nutritional therapy for allergies, due to its antihistamine action. Quercetin is also useful in some inflammatory conditions, as it has been shown to inhibit proinflammatory compounds related to arachidonic acid. Additionally, quercetin has been shown to inhibit the ulcer-causing bacterium *Helicobacter pylori*, and it is useful as part of ulcer treatment also because of its anti-inflammatory action. Quercetin and other bioflavonoids are relatively new health-promoting nutrients. Eating plenty of vegetables and fruits is a natural way to get bioflavonoids in your diet.

Benefits: Quercetin promotes health and well-being, is an antioxidant, and promotes cardiovascular wellness. Quercetin helps support treatment of inflammatory diseases and allergies. It promotes gastrointestinal health.

Ingredient Forms: Quercetin, quercetin dihydrate, quercitin chalcone.

Effective Supplement Dosages: As a dietary supplement for nutrition benefits, 15 to 60 mg per day. For nutritional therapy for allergies and inflammatory conditions, 250 to 500 mg, two to three times per day is commonly used for short periods of time under a doctor's supervision.

Cofactors: Other bioflavonoids; bromelain for inflammatory conditions.

Concerns: Quercetin is a semiessential nutrient. Bioflavonoids have numerous beneficial health effects, and diets high in quercetin and other bioflavonoids are related to a lower incidence of diseases. It is safe for all ages and both sexes when used as directed. Consult a physician if you are using quercetin supplements as supportive therapy for disease treatment.

Use Guidelines: Include quercetin-containing supplements as part of your daily nutrition program.

Red yeast rice (also *Monascus purpureus*)
Supplement Type: Botanical

Overview: Originating in China, red yeast rice is a type of yeast that when fermented on rice results in the production of natural statin-type chemicals, similar to the drug Lovastatin. Several clinical studies conducted in China report that taking as little as 1,200 mg of standardized red yeast rice supplements significantly lowered blood cholesterol levels within eight weeks, with no side effects. A recent clinical study conducted in the United States using 2,400 mg of standardized red yeast rice confirmed these results. Red yeast rice's statinlike substances block the formation of cholesterol in the liver. Biochemically, these statins exhibit 3-hydroxy-3-methylglutaryl coenzyme A (HMG-CoA) reductase inhibiting activity. When the statins stop this enzyme from functioning, cholesterol production in the liver drops. Interestingly, statins have also recently been shown to be beneficial in osteoporosis. Although red yeast rice is new to the United States, attention has turned nationwide to these supplements as economical alternatives to the statin drugs, such as Lovastatin. However, during the writing of this book, the FDA and red yeast rice supplement manufacturers were involved in a court battle to resolve whether or not red yeast rice supplements should be classified as drugs and no longer sold over the counter.

Benefits: Promotes healthy cholesterol blood levels and cardiovascular health.

Ingredient Form: Standardized red yeast rice (0.4% statins or Lovastatin). This means that 1,200 mg of 0.4% statin standardized red yeast rice contains 4.8 mg of HMG-CoA reductase inhibiting statins and 2,400 mg of 0.4% statin standardized red yeast rice contains 9.6 mg of statins.

Effective Supplement Dosages: A daily intake ranging from 1,200 to 2,400 mg per day of standardized red yeast rice lowered blood levels of total cholesterol and fatty acids.

Cofactors: Standardized garlic, folate, vitamin B_6 and vitamin B_{12}, vitamin E, vitamin C, beta-carotene, coenzyme Q_{10}.

Concerns: Red yeast rice is not an essential nutrient. In the short term, its use has been shown to be safe and effective for lowering cholesterol levels. For adult use only; not for use by children or by pregnant or lactating women unless under strict medical supervision. As with all statin compounds, reversible adverse effects may occur in the liver, and should be monitored by liver function blood tests. Discontinue use immediately if liver dysfunction is detected. Also, blocking cholesterol formation in the liver also blocks coenzyme Q_{10} production in the liver; the two use the same biosynthetic pathway. This means that use of statin-containing supplements or drugs can reduce your bloodstream levels of coenzyme Q_{10} and ironically promote a cardiovascular risk factor. To counteract this, take a daily supplement containing 60 to 120 mg of coenzyme Q_{10}.

Use Guidelines: Use supplements containing red yeast rice as part of your cholesterol health program. Best used under a doctor's supervision.

Reishi mushroom (also *Ganoderma lucidum*)

Supplement Type: Botanical

Overview: Like other medicinal and health-enhancing mushrooms, reishi mushroom contains polysaccharides that stimulate the immune system and have adaptogenic effects (enhancing the body's health by normalizing its functions and promoting balance and resistance to stress). Reishi also contains phytonutrients found to provide antiallergy effects. The appearance of medicinal mushrooms in dietary supplement products has been increasing. Most of them have a long history of safe and effective use in Asia. More research needs to be conducted on the various health-promoting effects of reishi mushrooms.

Benefits: Reishi mushroom is adaptogenic, promotes health and resistance to stress, and supports immune system function.

Ingredient Form: Reishi mushroom extracts.

Effective Supplement Dosages: Use as directed by the manufacturer. Also taken as a tea.

Cofactors: Other adaptogenic and immune-stimulating botanicals.

Concerns: Reishi mushroom is not an essential nutrient. Adaptogenic and immune system botanicals should be taken in cycles of several weeks. For adult use only; not for use by children or by pregnant or lactating women unless under a doctor's supervision. Only use as directed.

Use Guidelines: Use periodically when needed.

Royal jelly

Supplement Type: Concentrate

Overview: Royal jelly is a substance made by worker honeybees. It is fed to all bee larvae for a limited time, but is mainly fed to the queen bee. Queen bees grow larger and live longer than other bees, which led early health practitioners to believe that chemicals in royal jelly were responsible for these longevity effects. While royal jelly has a long history of use, clinical studies need to be conducted to verify its exact health effects. Royal jelly is mostly used in energy formulas. Royal jelly also contains protein, vitamins, minerals, and other substances. Royal jelly is also used in skin care products. Its use as an energy enhancer is intriguing, but clinical research is currently lacking to confirm royal jelly's exact benefits as a dietary supplement.

Benefits: Supports energy levels and a feeling of well-being.

Ingredient Form: Royal jelly standardized to 6% to 10% 10-hydroxy-2-decenoic acid (HDA).

Dosages: Dietary supplements contain a wide range of dosages of royal jelly, depending on its concentration of HDA. From 50 to 300 mg per day is most common; up to 1,000 mg can be found in health food store products.

Cofactors: Royal jelly is sometimes used in combination with other bee-related ingredients, such as bee pollen, bee propolis, and honey. A traditional Chinese combination of *Panax ginseng* and royal jelly is available as a concentrated drink (usually in small vials) or in tablets, capsules, or softgels.

Concerns: Royal jelly is not an essential nutrient. Its use in dietary supplements is based on a long history of traditional use. For adults only; not for use by children or by pregnant or lactating women unless under a doctor's supervision. Royal jelly may cause allergic reactions in some individuals.

Use Guidelines: Use royal jelly on a regular basis as part of your nutrition program.

SAM-e (also S-adenosylmethionine)

Supplement Type: Metabolite

Overview: SAM-e is made in your body from the amino acid methionine. Research indicates that as some individuals age, their production of SAM-e is reduced, which leads to the development of degenerative conditions, mainly arthritis and depression. Clinical studies have shown that SAM-e supplementation relieves depression as well as symptoms associated with rheumatoid arthritis, osteoarthritis, and fibromyalgia. The dual action of SAM-e is interesting, in that it both helps heal arthritic connective tissues and treats depression, which is common among people with arthritis.

Benefits: SAM-e promotes connective tissue health and joint function and promotes a positive mood.

Ingredient Form: Supplied in supplements as S-adenosylmethionine.

Effective Supplement Dosages: SAM-e has been used safely in clinical studies in dosages ranging from 400 to 1,600 mg per day, under a doctor's supervision.

Cofactors: Glucosamine, milk thistle.

Concerns: SAM-e is not an essential nutrient. It has biological activity that can be beneficial for individuals who cannot make proper amounts of SAM-e. For use by adults only; not for use by children or by pregnant or lactating women, unless under a doctor's supervision. In clinical studies lasting up to two years, SAM-e has been shown to be safe and effective, with minor occasional side effects such as gastrointestinal distress. Best used under medical supervision. SAM-e is expensive—the full antidepressant dose (1,600 mg/day) costs $240 a month.

Use Guidelines: Use SAM-e supplements periodically as needed.

Saw palmetto (also *Serenoa repens*)

Supplement Type: Botanical

Overview: In over twenty-two clinical studies saw palmetto extract has been shown to promote the health and function of the prostate in adult males. Saw palmetto extract has been reported in clinical studies to be an effective treatment for nonmalignant prostate conditions such as benign prostatic hyperplasia (BPH). In studies of BPH, saw palmetto extract was shown to improve urine flow, decrease prostate size, reduce inflammation, reduce frequency of urination at night, improve duration of bladder voiding, and reduce postmicturitional dribbling. Results are seen in four to six weeks, with progressive improvements with continued use. Use of saw palmetto is a must for anyone with BPH. Regular use of saw palmetto extract by middle-aged men may reduce their chances of developing BPH and other prostate problems later in life. When dealing with treatment of BPH, communicate to your doctor that there are a few pharmacological effects thought to be responsible for saw palmetto's actions: 5-alpha-reductase inhibition, antagonism of DHT (dihydrotestosterone) binding to prostatic receptors, inhibition of cyclooxygenase and lipoxygenase pathways, and inhibition of the arachidonic acid pathway. This information may be important in guiding your doctor's decision to use or not to use other medications.

Benefits: Saw palmetto berry supplements promote and maintain prostate health. They have antiandrogenic, antiedemic, and anti-inflammatory effects on the prostate gland.

Ingredient Form: Standardized saw palmetto fruit extract (80% to 95% phytosterols and fatty acids). Sabaltone is a brand of saw palmetto fruit extract used in some supplements.

Effective Supplement Dosages: As a dietary supplement, 160 to 320 mg per day of standardized saw palmetto extract. Higher dosages may be used for treatment of BPH, but remember that 320 mg per day has been shown to be effective, so going higher than this amount may not produce additional benefits. Most products will suggest using higher dosages for the first three to four months, then taking 160 mg per day as a maintenance dosage. Some dietary supplement products designed to support prostate health may contain smaller daily dosages of saw palmetto extract, along with other ingredients.

Cofactors: Pygeum, nettle root extract, and beta-sitosterol.

Concerns: Saw palmetto extract is not an essential nutrient but is beneficial for the promotion of prostate health. It is considered safe and effective for treatment of urinary and prostate problems due to benign prostatic hyperplasia (BPH). Saw palmetto has been shown to be safe and effective in clinical studies, and is considered nontoxic when used as directed. Some side effects observed in the studies include stomach upset and headaches. For use by male adults only. Not for use by children or women. If using it as a nutritional treatment for BPH, do so only under constant supervision by your doctor to ensure proper treatment and surveillance of potential prostate disease complications. Most clinical studies have been conducted for several weeks, up to one year. Safety of longer-term use of saw palmetto is therefore not established.

Use Guidelines: For use by males on a regular or periodic basis to promote and maintain prostate gland health.

Schisandra (also *Schisandra chinensis*)

Supplement Type: Botanical

Overview: Schisandra is a botanical with ancient Chinese origins, traditionally used for treating coughs, for its stimulatory and adaptogenic effects, and for liver protection. Modern science has confirmed these effects and observed improvements in mental function as well. Schisandra is one of the Chinese botanicals you will be encountering more frequently in adaptogenic and liver health dietary supplement formulas.

Benefits: Promotes liver health. Schisandra is an adaptogenic botanical that stimulates well-being and improved resistance. It also promotes brain wellness.

Ingredient Form: Standardized schisandra fruit extract (1% schisandrins).

Effective Supplement Dosages: Dietary supplements typically contain 40 to 200 mg per day.

Cofactors: Milk thistle for liver protection, and other adaptogenic botanicals for improved well-being and resistance during periods of stress.

Concerns: Schisandra is not an essential nutrient. It has a long history of use in traditional Chinese medicine. For adults only; not for use by children or by pregnant or lactating women unless under a doctor's supervision. Schisandra can produce central nervous system depression. Limit periods of use to a few months at a time.

Use Guidelines: Use schisandra-containing supplements on a periodic basis when needed.

Selenium

Supplement Type: Mineral

Overview: Selenium is an essential nutrient. It is a component of one of the body's major antioxidants, glutathione peroxidase. Glutathione peroxidase protects the body from free-radical damage. In this role as an antioxidant cofactor, selenium reduces the risk of degenerative diseases such as heart disease, arthritis, and certain cancers. In fact, the association between adequate selenium intake and reduced cancer risk has recently stimulated coverage by the media. Selenium's role as an antioxidant cofactor is extremely important, and new research has confirmed its role in strengthening the body to reduce the risk of cancer.

Benefits: Selenium promotes overall good health and well-being. It promotes both cardiovascular health and prostate health.

Ingredient Form: Selenomethionine, selenocysteine, selenate, selenium from yeast.

Effective Supplement Dosages: The adult RDI for selenium is 70 mcg. As a dietary supplement, 50 to 300 mcg per day is common.

Cofactors: Other antioxidants, antioxidant cofactors, and essential vitamins and minerals.

Concerns: Selenium is an essential nutrient. Low dietary intake causes adverse effects due to a weakening of the body's defenses against hydroperoxide free radicals. The symptoms of selenium deficiency include hair loss, growth disorders, pancreatic problems, and muscular discomfort and weakness. Selenium is also thought to be involved in thyroid gland function. Excessive selenium intake (which rarely, if ever, occurs) may result in fingernail and toenail changes, hair loss, fatigue, abdominal pain, nausea, increased dental caries, diarrhea, and irritability. Avoid taking excessive dosages of selenium because of these possible side effects. It is best used by adults in a daily dietary supplement formulation, and in children's formulas in lower dosages.

Use Guidelines: Take selenium-containing supplements as part of your daily nutrition program.

Shark cartilage

Supplement Type: Concentrate

Overview: Shark cartilage is a rich source of mucopolysaccharides, which are found in connective tissues. Because of this, shark cartilage traditionally has been ingested in the hopes of treating a wide range of disorders in which connective tissues may be abnormal, such as osteoarthritis, severe eczema, and psoriasis. Shark cartilage has also been touted as being effective in the treatment of certain cancers due to its presumed antiangiogenesis effects. Angiogenesis is the development of new blood vessels; tumors need to form new blood vessels to grow. If the generation of new blood vessels is inhibited, then it is thought that tumor cell growth will slow down. While this is an intriguing thought, clinical studies have not yet confirmed the tumor-inhibiting effects of shark cartilage, in humans. The use of shark cartilage supplements has grown partly because some people believe that taking shark cartilage supplements will prevent cancer from developing. (This use was promoted in popular books during the 1990s, which reported the fact that sharks don't get cancer. Unfortunately, this claim is not true. Sharks not only get cancer, they even get cancer of their cartilages!) There is a lack of scientific evidence to conclusively support this same claim in humans. However, high-quality shark cartilage is beneficial for promoting and maintaining healthy connective tissues.

Benefits: Supports connective tissue growth and maintenance.

Ingredient Form: Purified shark cartilage, 18% to 25% mucopolysaccharides.

Effective Supplement Dosages: 500 to 3,000 mg per day, used for several weeks at a time.

Cofactors: Glucosamine.

Concerns: Shark cartilage is not an essential nutrient, but its dietary intake is associated with connective tissue health. For adults only; not for children or pregnant or lactating women unless used under a doctor's supervision. Not for use by people with cardiovascular disorders. Use under medical supervision if you are suffering from a disease. Not for use by anyone concerned about the antiangiogenesis effects.

Use Guidelines: Use shark cartilage supplements on a periodic basis when needed.

Shiitake mushroom (also *Lentinula edodes*)

Supplement Type: Botanical

Overview: Shiitake mushroom contains phytonutrients that stimulate immune system function. While many popular books tout shiitake mushroom as a cure for cancer, studies to support this claim are lacking. It has been used to enhance the immune system and as supportive therapy in the treatment of diseases.

Benefits: Supports immune system function.

Ingredient Form: Standardized shiitake mushroom extract.

Effective Supplement Dosages: Use as directed on product labels.

Cofactors: Other immune system–stimulating botanicals.

Concerns: Shiitake mushroom is not an essential nutrient. It has been used in Asia to support immune system function. For adult use only; not for use by children or by pregnant or lactating women unless under a doctor's supervision. Use only periodically, when stimulation of immune system function is desired. Consult your doctor if you are using shiitake mushroom to stimulate your immune system as part of the treatment of a disease.

Use Guidelines: Use shiitake supplements periodically to boost immune system function.

Silicon

Supplement Type: Mineral

Overview: Silicon is a trace mineral, needed in small amounts. It is involved in the formation of bones and connective tissues. Silicon is also found in skin, hair, nails, and other body tissues. There is some evidence that older adults may require higher silicon intakes to compensate for the loss of silicon from aging tissues. Note that silica (silicon dioxide) may be listed on the labels of some supplements. Silica is found in plants and also in minerals such as quartz and flint. If your supplement lists silica, remember that it is not equivalent to an equal amount of silicon. If the supplement you are taking does not list the exact amount of silicon it contains, call the manufacturer to verify the source of the silicon and the daily dose of silicon contained in the product.

Benefits: Silicon is required in the diet for normal growth, development, and maintenance of health. It is especially important in bone and connective tissue formation and maintenance.

Ingredient Form: Silicon, derived from silicic acid and silicates (including silica) from the herb horsetail *(Equisetum arvense)*, is commonly found in dietary supplements.

Effective Supplement Dosages: Currently a reference daily intake (RDI) has not been established. Nutritionists estimate that the daily dietary intake of silicon is between 20 and 50 mg per day. Dietary supplements commonly contain 1 to 15 mg of silicon per daily dose.

Cofactors: Vitamins and minerals, or as part of a calcium-magnesium bone formulation.

Concerns: Silicon occurs naturally in low amounts in foods and is used in supplements. No major health concerns about silicon overdose or toxicity have been reported. Very high intakes of silicon over a long period may contribute to kidney stone (renal calculi) formation. While no clear deficiency symptoms due to poor intake of silicon have been clinically verified, it is generally regarded as an essential trace mineral required for proper bone and connective tissue growth, development, and maintenance. Silicon supplements are safe for all ages and both sexes when used as directed.

Use Guidelines: Take silicon-containing supplements daily as part of your nutrition program.

Silicon dioxide (Sipernat): *see* Excipients

Sodium

Supplement Type: Mineral

Overview: Sodium is the body's main extracellular cation, which helps regulate fluid balance, particularly in blood. It also helps regulate the pressure of fluids, assists with the absorption of nutrients in the intestines, functions in muscle contraction and nerve impulse transmission, and has a role in the active transport of nutrients across cell membranes. Maintain adequate but not excessive sodium intake for optimal health. Most people will get adequate amounts from food sources. Use salt sparingly, if at all. Consult your doctor if you think you may have high blood pressure due to salt intake.

Benefits: Daily adequate intake of sodium is required for maintenance of good health.

Ingredient Form: Sodium is found in the diet as sodium chloride.

Effective Supplement Dosages: Dietary supplements in tablet, capsule, and softgel form are usually free from sodium, because most people get too much sodium and are trying to reduce their dietary intake of sodium. The daily reference value for sodium is 2,400 mg per day for adults. Sodium is contained in most powdered beverage supplements, due to its natural occurrence in the food ingredients used in these products, or it is added to improve taste.

Cofactors: The other main electrolytes, chloride and potassium.

Concerns: Excessive intake of sodium, from salt and processed foods containing high amounts of sodium, may lead to the development of elevated blood pressure in some individuals. There is some evidence that frequent intake of salt-preserved or salt-pickled foods increases the risk of stomach cancer. Sodium depletion can occur under conditions of dehydration or malnutrition and in renal disease. Physically active people require higher-than-average sodium intakes to prevent sodium depletion. Sodium depletion can result in dizziness, fainting, and impaired physical performance.

Use Guidelines: Use of sodium-containing supplements is recommended only if you know you need to increase your dietary sodium intake.

Soy (also *Glycine max*)

Supplement Type: Botanical

Overview: Consumption of soybeans and soybean-derived products has been associated with many health benefits, including reduction of the risk of cancer and cardiovascular diseases. The research concerning these beneficial health effects is so impressive that a new health claim concerning the consumption of soy and reduction of cardiovascular disease risk is currently under review by the FDA. Soy is loaded with healthy essential nutrients, including protein, essential fatty acids, fiber, vitamins, and minerals. It also contains an interesting group of health-promoting and protective bioflavonoids called isoflavones. The specific type of isoflavones found in soy include chiefly genistein and daidzein. They exhibit antioxidant activity and also phyto-estrogenic activity. This phytoestrogenic effect is responsible for soy's reduction of the sever-ity of symptoms during menopause. Soy also has been shown to help normalize gastroin-testinal function. Finally, ingestion of soy prod-ucts is associated with lower cancer risk, probably because of the phytonutrients. How-ever, keep in mind that you must be following a healthy diet to experience these health bene-fits. The soy protein health craze is well founded, and increasing your consumption of soy-based products is beneficial, especially for women.

Benefits: Soy promotes cardiovascular health and digestive system wellness and maintains overall well-being. Soy can allevi-ate menopausal symptoms.

Ingredient Form: In soy protein drinks, look for a high-quality soy concentrate such as Supro. For tablet or capsules, look for products that have standardized isoflavone content.

Effective Supplement Dosages: Choose soy protein drink supplements with 15 to 30 g of high-quality soy protein per day. For isoflavone dietary supplements, look for 25 to 60 mg of isoflavones per day.

Cofactors: Other bioflavonoids, and essential vitamins and minerals.

Concerns: Soy contains essential nutri-ents and the semiessential isoflavone bioflavo-noids. Soy-based products are well tolerated by most people; however, some individuals may be sensitive to soy. Soy protein drinks are safe for individuals age two or older, and soy is a common ingredient in infant formulas as well. Regular consumption of soy products promotes health. However, it is uncertain what effects the long-term ingestion of soy may have on males, due to the phytoestrogen content.

Use Guidelines: Use on a regular basis if desired.

Spirulina: *see* Greens powders

Spleen extracts: *see* Glandulars

Stearic acid: *see* Excipients

Stevia (also *Stevia rebaudiana*)
Supplement Type: Botanical
Overview: Stevia has a history of use as a noncaloric, natural sweetener. The phyto-nutrients, called steviosides, are reported to be about a hundred times sweeter than sugar. Stevia is used in weight loss products and products for diabetics. It may also have hypo-glycemic effects, and is added to dietary sup-plement formulas designed for this reason. Technically, the use of stevia as a sweetener for food products is not approved by the FDA. However, you will often find it in dietary sup-plement products as a natural sweetener.

Benefits: Natural sweetener. May have a hypoglycemic effect (lowering blood sugar).

Ingredient Form: Standardized stevia extract (40% to 80% steviosides).

Common Supplement Dosages: Refer to specific product directions.

Cofactors: None.

Concerns: Stevia is not an essential nutrient. It is sometimes used in supplement products to add sweetness and produce a mild hypoglycemic effect. For adults only; not for children or for pregnant or lactating women unless taken under medical supervision.

Use Guidelines: Use of stevia-containing supplements is optional.

St. John's wort (also *Hypericum perforatum*)

Supplement Type: Botanical

Overview: More than twenty-five clinical studies have confirmed that standardized St. John's wort extract can have antidepressant action. It has been discovered to be an effective treatment for mild to moderate depression. St. John's wort extracts also reduce anxiety and nervous unrest in some people. While there is still scientific debate over exactly which phytochemicals in St. John's wort are responsible for these actions, studies reveal that the standardized extracts will normalize serotonin levels and also GABA activity, in addition to its effects on the norepinephrine and dopamine systems. Its immune-modulating effects may also contribute to its antidepressant action, making it the most broad-spectrum antidepressant medication known. St. John's wort is one of the fastest-growing herbal supplements in the United States. Stick to using brands, which guarantee potency.

Benefits: Promotes positive mood, positive mental outlook, and feelings of well-being. St. John's wort is a safe and effective treatment for mild or moderate depression.

Ingredient Form: Standardized St. John's wort flower extract (0.3% hypericin).

Effective Supplement Dosages: Daily dosages found to be effective in clinical studies range from 300 to 900 mg per day of standardized St. John's wort extract.

Cofactors: Some dietary supplement formulas use other calming herbs, such as kava kava, hops, valerian, and passionflower, in conjunction with St. John's wort.

Concerns: St. John's wort is not an essential nutrient, but promotes positive mood and is useful as an herbal antidepressant. St. John's wort has been shown to be well tolerated in clinical studies of two to three months' duration. It has been shown to be as effective as the antidepressant drugs maprotiline, imipramine, bromazepam, diazepam, amitriptyline, and desipramine. Side effects are rare and include stomach upset, fatigue, and allergic rash. Some people may develop reversible photosensitivity, especially fair-skinned individuals, but this side effect has been reported only once. Not for use by children or by pregnant or lactating women, unless under a doctor's supervision. Do not use with antidepressant drugs or indinavir, PIs, and NNRTIs. Use for only a few months at a time. Depression is a serious condition and should not be self-treated. See your doctor and use St. John's wort under his or her supervision.

Use Guidelines: If you are depressed, see your doctor. Use St. John's wort under medical supervision. Its effects take from two to eight weeks to become apparent.

Suma (also *Pfaffia paniculata*)

Supplement Type: Botanical

Overview: Suma is a plant native to South America, where it is used for general health-promoting benefits, similar to the ginsengs. In fact, suma is sometimes called Brazilian ginseng. Its phytonutrients are reported to improve energy and increase overall vitality. Suma is a highly regarded health-promoting herb in South America. You will find it added to adaptogenic herbal formulas, and also to immune-stimulating supplements. While more clinical research is needed to verify suma's effects, its use is supported by a long traditional history.

Benefits: Suma is traditionally used as an adaptogen to improve energy, endurance, and vitality, and stimulate the immune system.

Ingredient Form: Standardized suma root extract (3% to 5% beta-ecdysterone).

Effective Supplement Dosages: For use as dietary supplement, 50 to 300 mg per day of standardized suma root extract. Higher dosages are for periodic use only.

Cofactors: Other herbal adaptogens, such as the ginsengs.

Concerns: Suma is not an essential nutrient. It has a history of use in South America as an adaptogenic health tonic. For adults only; not for children or for pregnant or lactating women unless used under medical supervision. Lower dosages, under 100 mg per day, have been reported to be well tolerated for daily use. Higher daily dosages should be limited to a few months at a time, when needed during stressful periods.

Use Guidelines: Use suma-containing supplements on an optional basis.

Taurine (also L-taurine)

Supplement Type: Amino acid

Overview: Taurine is a nonessential amino acid, and is one of the sulfur-containing amino acids. Taurine plays a major role in brain tissues and in nervous system functioning. It is involved in blood pressure regulation and in the transportation of electrolytes across cell membranes. It is found in the heart muscle, central nervous system, and brain. It is also considered an inhibitory neurotransmitter, which is calming to the brain. Taurine is found in the eye, where it is important for maintaining good vision and eye function. Taurine is also linked to maintaining cell membrane stability, and it displays antioxidant activity. Taurine is made from the amino acid cysteine. New research indicates that the direct precursor of taurine, hypotaurine, may also be important as an antioxidant and have benefits similar to those of taurine.

Benefits: Supports good health. Supports cardiovascular wellness and good vision.

Ingredient Form: L-taurine.

Effective Supplement Dosages: Taurine is sometimes found in supplements in small amounts, 50 mg per day, and in larger amounts, up to 5,000 mg, in protein supplements.

Cofactors: Other amino acids, antioxidants.

Concerns: Taurine is not an essential nutrient. More research is needed to determine the exact benefits of taurine supplementation. For adults only; not for use by those with liver or kidney disease, by children, or by pregnant or lactating women unless under a doctor's supervision. Taurine is considered safe when ingested as directed.

Use Guidelines: Use of taurine as a supplement is optional. Take taurine-containing supplements if you are concerned about promoting and maintaining cardiovascular and vision wellness.

Thymus extract: *see* Glandulars

Thyroid extract: *see* Glandulars

Tomato concentrate: *see* Beta-carotene, carotenoids

Trace Elements

Trace elements are substances that have been found occurring in the human body in extremely small amounts. Some supplement companies will include them in their formulas. The principal trace elements you may encounter in supplement products include nickel and tin. However, the exact requirements have not been clearly established by the National Research Council. In small microgram amounts, these trace elements are used in many national supplement brands.

Trans-ferulic acid: *see* Gamma-oryzanol

Tribulus (also *Tribulus terrestris*)

Supplement Type: Botanical

Overview: Tribulus is a botanical with ancient origins as a medicinal herb. Products containing tribulus have slowly been appearing on the U.S. market since 1996. The purported benefits include increased sex drive and increased muscle mass. Traditionally, tribulus is regarded as stimulating sexual performance and libido. Clinical studies have confirmed these benefits and have also reported an increase in testosterone levels in men, as well as increasing estrogen levels in women. In both men and women libido and fertility can be increased by taking tribulus supplements. However, researchers caution that in men, the increase in testosterone is often accompanied by a rise in estrogen, which may lead to gynecomastia in susceptible individuals. Due to reports that tribulus stimulates a rise in testosterone levels, many strength athletes have started using (and abusing) tribulus-containing supplements. However, there are no clinical studies that report conclusively on any benefits for use by athletes. The research is impressive on the role of tribulus in improving sexual function. One of the major products sold in Europe and also found on the U.S. market is called Tribestan, which you may want to try if it is available in your area.

Benefits: Tribulus supplements increase libido and sexual performance in men and women.

Ingredient Form: Standardized tribulus root extract (20% to 40% furanosterols). Tribulin is a special standardized tribulus root extract used in dietary supplement products.

Effective Supplement Dosages: Dosages for short-term use range from 250 to 600 mg per day.

Cofactors: None.

Concerns: Tribulus is not an essential nutrient. It has a long history of use as a traditional herbal medicine, and as a commercial herbal drug product in Europe for restoring sexual performance, fertility, and libido. Tribulus supplements are intended for short-term use only, two to three months. It is considered safe when used as directed. For use by adults only; not for use by children or by pregnant or lactating women. Consult your doctor if you are using tribulus to treat a medical condition.

Tryptophan (also L-tryptophan)

Supplement Type: Amino acid

Overview: Tryptophan is an essential amino acid. It occurs naturally in foods. Tryptophan was used for its calming and sleep-promoting effects. It is a precursor of the calming neurotransmitter serotonin. Serotonin helps control the sleep cycle, causing a feeling of drowsiness. L-tryptophan has been used safely by millions of people for decades. However, because in 1989 it was implicated as a possible cause of a rare blood disease, its use in supplements was banned by the FDA.

The outbreak of the rare blood disorder was linked to a specific batch of L-tryptophan, from a supplier in Japan, and was found to contain a contaminant, which most experts think was the agent causing the health problem; however, this issue has yet to be resolved with the FDA. Recently, a metabolite of tryptophan, 5-hydroxytryptophan (5-HTP), is being used in dietary supplements as a tryptophan replacement. Clinical studies have shown that 5-HTP is effective in treating depression and in promoting sustained weight loss by improving appetite control and preventing overeating.

Benefits: Tryptophan promotes calming and restful sleep.

Ingredient Form: As mentioned above, L-tryptophan is technically banned from use in supplements, however, some manufacturers are using L-tryptophan as an ingredient in amino acid complexes.

Effective Supplement Dosages: Effective dosages of L-tryptophan are 500 to 2,000 mg a day, taken before bedtime. Dosages of 5-HTP range from 50 to 200 mg per day. Note that most supplements contain 5-HTP as provided from the plant *Griffonia simplicifolia*.

Cofactors: Other calming or sleep-promoting ingredients, GABA, tyrosine, valerian, and kava kava.

Concerns: L-tryptophan's use as a dietary supplement was banned in the United States in 1989 after an outbreak of a rare blood disorder was linked to a certain brand of L-tryptophan. For adult use only; not for use by children or by pregnant or lactating women unless under a doctor's supervision.

Use Guidelines: Use of tryptophan supplements is optional.

Turmeric: *see* Curcumin

Tyrosine (also L-tyrosine)
   Supplement Type: Amino acid
   Overview: Tyrosine is a nonessential amino acid that is made in the body from the essential amino acid phenylalanine. Tyrosine in turn is a precursor of dopamine and norepinephrine, regulates appetite, and aids in melanin production. Tyrosine is also reported to enhance mental function and concentration, but more clinical studies are needed to determine the exact benefits.
   Benefits: Tyrosine supplements promote appetite control. Tyrosine is a mental energizer and relieves feelings of stress.
   Ingredient Form: L-tyrosine is used in dietary supplement formulas.
   Effective Supplement Dosages: Dosages for tyrosine range from 100 to 3,000 mg per day, and vary according to the product being used. A daily dosage between 500 and 1,500 mg is considered to be effective for most people.
   Cofactors: Phenylalanine, copper, folic acid, and vitamin B_6.
   Concerns: L-tyrosine is not an essential nutrient. Its use as a supplement can be beneficial for some people. It is considered safe and effective when used as directed. For adult use only; not for use by children or by pregnant or lactating women or those with high blood pressure, liver or kidney disease, or those taking MAOI drugs or St. John's wort, unless under a doctor's supervision. Caution: Tyrosine may trigger migraine headaches in some people due to a breakdown product called tyramine.

Uva ursi (also *Arctostaphylos uva ursi*)
   Supplement Type: Botanical
   Overview: Uva ursi's most popular use in dietary supplements is for its diuretic effects. The primary active phytonutrient is arbutin. Uva ursi is also recognized in Europe for its antimicrobial action in the urinary tract. Use only for short periods of time, and do not overdose.
   Benefits: Uva ursi is a mild diuretic and promotes urinary tract health.
   Ingredient Form: Standardized uva ursi leaf extract (20% to 30% arbutin).
   Effective Supplement Dosages: 100 to 300 mg per day of standardized uva ursi leaf extract; for periodic use only, one to two weeks.
   Cofactors: Cranberry extract.
   Concerns: Uva ursi is not an essential nutrient. Its use as a dietary supplement should be limited to one to two weeks, or longer under a doctor's supervision. For use by adults only; not for use by children or by pregnant or lactating women unless under a doctor's supervision. Side effects include nausea, vomiting, and gastric distress. Overdosing uva ursi can result in serious illness or death.
   Use Guidelines: Use uva ursi supplements periodically as needed.

Valerian (also *Valeriana officinalis*)

Supplement Type: Botanical

Overview: Valerian has sedative and sleep-promoting actions. Valerian is reported to promote good-quality sleep, without the hangover side effect sometimes experienced with prescription and over-the-counter sleep aid drugs. Note that valerian is foul-smelling; some companies add vanilla or peppermint to mask this smell. However, the odor is an indication that you are getting a high-quality product.

Benefits: It is used as an effective sleep aid, to improve your ability to fall asleep and stay asleep. Valerian has also been shown to be effective in improving sleep in individuals with mild insomnia. The valerenic acid contained in valerian increases the activity of calming neurotransmitters.

Ingredient Form: Standardized valerian root extract (0.8% to 1% valerenic acid).

Effective Supplement Dosages: To promote sleep, use 200 to 400 mg of standardized valerian root extract before bedtime. Do not use for longer than two to three weeks at a time unless directed by your doctor, which may be required for severe insomnia. If sleep disturbance continues, consult your doctor.

Cofactors: Kava kava, passionflower, hops, and chamomile.

Concerns: Valerian root extract is not an essential nutrient. It is beneficial to promote duration and quality of sleep. Valerian is considered safe and effective when used as directed for short periods of time. For adult use only; not for use by children, by pregnant or lactating women, or by individuals on medication. Those with liver disease should avoid it.

Use Guidelines: Valerian is safe to use on a periodic basis.

Valine (also L-valine)

Supplement Type: Amino acid

Overview: Valine is an essential amino acid. It is one of the branched-chain amino acids (BCAAs) and is found in muscle tissue and other proteins. It is also an important source of energy during exercise, along with the other BCAAs, isoleucine and leucine. It is involved in tissue repair, tissue growth, and muscle metabolism. BCAA supplements can be very useful if you regularly engage in strenuous physical activity for more than one hour per day. New studies also report that taking BCAA supplements reduces feelings of fatigue and prolongs athletic performance.

Benefits: Valine is an essential amino acid required for growth and maintenance of good health.

Ingredient Form: L-valine is used in dietary supplements, and is found together with other amino acids in protein products.

Effective Supplement Dosages: For people involved in exercise or undergoing physical stress, the usual dosage is 800 to 3,000 mg per day of valine supplements. This is in addition to the valine supplied from your dietary proteins.

Cofactors: The other BCAAs, isoleucine and leucine.

Concerns: Valine is an essential nutrient. Its supplemental use was first established in hospitals to help stressed and injured patients heal more quickly and maintain nitrogen balance. For adults only; not for use by children or by pregnant or lactating women unless under a doctor's supervision.

Use Guidelines: Use valine supplements on a regular basis, along with the other BCAAs, when you need to increase your intake of BCAAs—for example, during periods of healing, stress, and increased physical activity.

Vanadium

Supplement Type: Mineral

Overview: Vanadium is a trace mineral present in the body in minute amounts. Vanadium is involved in metabolic pathways and is needed for cellular metabolism, for the formation of bones and teeth, and for growth and reproduction. Recent attention has been focused on vanadium's role in glucose metabolism and its insulin-mimetic effects, which may increase glucose utilization. Vanadium is known to inhibit cholesterol synthesis at pharmacological dosages. Clinical studies using vanadium supplements have not confirmed its beneficial use in diabetes, in promoting weight loss, or to enhance muscle building. Use in the management of non-insulin-dependent diabetes mellitus is experimental and should only be considered under medical supervision.

Benefits: Adequate dietary vanadium intake is required for maintenance of good health.

Ingredient Form: Forms used in supplements include vanadyl sulfate and vanadate.

Effective Supplement Dosages: No reference daily intake (RDI) has been established for vanadium. Dietary intake is estimated to range from 10 to 20 mcg per day. Dietary supplement intake is not warranted, except under medical supervision for therapeutic reasons.

Cofactors: None.

Concerns: There are no identified deficiency diseases linked to inadequate vanadium intake, though researchers believe that inadequate vanadium consumption may be related to cardiovascular disease, kidney disease, and reproductive disorders. Excessive intake of vanadium can be toxic. Symptoms include black discoloration of the tongue, slowed growth, diarrhea, hypoglycemia, and anorexia. If intake is excessive enough, it can lead to death. Vanadium toxicity is also linked with bipolar disorder (manic depression). A tolerable upper intake level for vanadium has not been established. Use only under a doctor's supervision.

Use Guidelines: Optional use on a regular basis in small amounts, under medical supervision.

Vinpocetine

Supplement Type: Metabolite

Overview: Vinpocetine is a new dietary supplement ingredient you will find appearing in some products designed to enhance mental function. In Europe, vinpocetine has a history of use as a cerebral vasodilator, which means it increases blood flow to the brain. It is used for treatment of ischemic cerebral diseases. Clinical studies have confirmed vinpocetine's safety and effectiveness for this purpose. It's too soon to determine how the FDA will ultimately respond to the appearance of vinpocetine in dietary supplement products. Vinpocetine is an interesting dietary supplement ingredient, because it has been sold in Europe as a drug. As with many of the new dietary supplement ingredients, some of them are or were used as drugs. It is also interesting to note that, like ginkgo, vinpocetine's main benefits are a result of improved blood flow.

Benefits: Improves blood flow in the brain, and can improve mental wellness and brain function.

Ingredient Form: Vinpocetine.

Effective Supplement Dosages: Vinpocetine has been used in clinical studies in dosages ranging from 10 to 20 mg, three times per day.

Cofactors: Ginkgo, phosphatidylserine, lecithin.

Concerns: Vinpocetine is not an essential nutrient. It should be used with caution due to its newness on the U.S. market. For adults only; not for use by children or by pregnant or lactating women, unless under a doctor's supervision. Use vinpocetine supplements for short-term use as determined by your doctor.

Use Guidelines: Use vinpocetine periodically when needed.

Vitamin A (also Retinol, 3,4-didehydroretinol)
Supplement Type: Vitamin

Overview: Vitamin A is an essential fat-soluble vitamin required for maintenance of normal mucous membranes and for normal vision. Vitamin A refers to a group of compounds that display vitamin A activity. Retinol is the principal vitamin A, and belongs to a class of chemicals known as the retinoids. Retinol and other retinoids occur in animal tissues. Beta-carotene and other carotenoids also display vitamin A activity, and are sometimes referred to as provitamin A, because they are converted to vitamin A in the body as needed. Carotenoids occur in plants and have the added benefit of providing antioxidant activity. Vitamin A is one of the most essential vitamins and should be part of your daily dietary supplement program. To avoid any potential side effects, choose supplements that provide Vitamin A as a combination of one of the retinoids and beta-carotene, or entirely from beta-carotene if your daily supplement dosage is over 3,500 IU per day.

Benefits: Dietary supplement intake of vitamin A is known to improve immune function, improve day and night vision, reduce eye fatigue, and improve skin function and structure. Vitamin A therapy is used in the treatment of skin disorders such as acne, eczema, and psoriasis. It is also used as supportive therapy in the treatment of respiratory illnesses such as allergies, asthma, bronchitis, and emphysema.

Ingredient Forms: Dietary supplements contain vitamin A acetate and vitamin A palmitate. However, because there is some concern about a possible buildup of toxic levels of this fat-soluble vitamin in these forms, beta-carotene (which does not pose the same risk) is commonly blended with these retinoids, or used as the sole source of vitamin A activity in dietary supplements.

Effective Supplement Dosages: The Reference daily intake (RDI) of vitamin A is 5,000 IU per day for adults. Dietary supplements commonly contain between 2,500 IU and 15,000 IU per daily dosage. Higher dosages of vitamin A are commonly used for therapeutic purposes, and should be taken under medical supervision.

Cofactors: Essential vitamins and minerals.

Concerns: Inadequate intake of vitamin A can lead to night blindness, glare blindness, loss of appetite, increased susceptibility to infection, impaired growth, and development of rough, dry skin. Vitamin A deficiency occurs commonly in children, the elderly, and individuals with chronic fat malabsorption. Excessive intake of vitamin A (the retinoid forms) can accumulate in the body and may cause toxic side effects. Symptoms of vitamin A overdosing include headaches, vomiting, dry mucous membranes, bone abnormalities, and liver damage. Toxicity can occur from prolonged intake of 50,000 IU per day in adults and as little as 20,000 IU per day in children. Acute vitamin A poisoning rarely occurs, but you should contact your doctor or poison control center immediately if accidental overdose occurs in adults or children. Pregnant women should not take more than 5,000 IU's of preformed vitamin A daily. Do not take vitamin A supplements if you have kidney failure. Use only B-carotene (not preformed vitamin A) if you are using an oral contraceptive pill. Otherwise vitamin A supplements are safe for all ages and sexes when taken as directed.

Use Guideline: Use vitamin A supplements daily as part of your nutritional health program.

Vitamin B$_1$ (also Thiamine, thiamine pyrophosphate)

Supplement Type: Vitamin

Overview: Vitamin B$_1$ is a water-soluble vitamin involved in many metabolic reactions. It is converted in the body into coenzymes that aid in carbohydrate metabolism. Vitamin B$_1$ also functions in the production of ribose, which is needed for the production of RNA and DNA. It is also involved in maintenance of nervous system functioning. Try taking higher amounts of B$_1$ during periods of mental and physical stress.

Benefits: Adequate intake of vitamin B$_1$ is essential for good health.

Ingredient Form: Vitamin B$_1$ is found in supplements as thiamine hydrochloride and thiamine mononitrate.

Effective Supplement Dosages: The Reference daily intake (RDI) of vitamin B$_1$ is 1.5 mg per day for adults. However, this and other B vitamins are commonly taken in amounts well above the RDI. Common dosages found to be safe and effective range from 1.5 to 90 mg per day. Higher dosages are used by athletes and for therapeutic purposes, as much as 300 to 500 mg per day for short periods of time, up to several months.

Cofactors: The other B vitamins.

Concerns: The classic vitamin B_1 deficiency disease is beriberi and is characterized by muscle weakness, muscle atrophy, depression, and heart failure. Other deficiency symptoms include abnormalities in carbohydrate metabolism, fatigue, loss of appetite, constipation, confusion, and poor muscle coordination. Toxicity from excessive vitamin B_1 intake is rarely reported in healthy adults, since it is water-soluble and readily cleared out of the body. One study using a dosage of 500 mg per day of vitamin B_1 for one month did not report any side effects. However, high dosages are not recommended for long periods of use (more than a few months) unless prescribed by your doctor. Vitamin B_1 supplements are safe for all ages and both sexes when taken as directed.

Use Guidelines: Take vitamin B_1 supplements daily as part of your nutritional health program.

Vitamin B_2 (also Riboflavin)

Supplement Type: Vitamin

Overview: Vitamin B_2 is an essential water-soluble vitamin. It is involved in the production of energy from carbohydrates, fatty acids, and amino acids. Vitamin B_2 is involved in the regeneration of one of the body's most important antioxidants, glutathione. Include vitamin B_2 in your daily supplement program. Dosages between 100 and 300 mg are sometimes used by athletes, and for clinical reasons in the management of migraine headaches, carpal tunnel syndrome, anxiety, depression, stress, and cataract treatment and prevention. However, it is best to use high dosages of vitamin B_2 for only short periods of time, up to a few months. If you plan on taking large dosages of vitamin B_2 for a medical condition, do so only under medical supervision.

Benefits: Essential for good health.

Ingredient Form: Dietary supplements contain vitamin B_2 as riboflavin.

Effective Supplement Dosages: The RDI for vitamin B_2 is 1.7 mg per day. Dietary supplements contain doses of this vitamin ranging from 1.7 to over 100 mg per day.

Cofactors: The other B vitamins.

Concerns: The symptoms of vitamin B_2 deficiency include cracked skin, inflamed lips, impaired growth, hair loss, cataract formation, seborrheic dermatitis, and behavioral changes characterized by depression, moodiness, nervousness, and irritability. Excessive intake of vitamin B_2 does not appear to readily produce notable side effects. However, taking megadoses of vitamin B_2 for long periods of time without doctor supervision is not recommended. Vitamin B_2 supplements are safe for all ages and both sexes when used as directed.

Use Guidelines: Take vitamin B_2 supplements daily as part of your nutritional health program.

Vitamin B_3 (also Niacin, nicotinic acid, nicotinamide)

Supplement Type: Vitamin

Overview: Vitamin B_3 is a water-soluble essential vitamin. It is functionally active as part of two important coenzymes—nicotinamide adenine dinucleotide (NAD) and nicotinamine adenine dinucleotide phosphate (NADP). NAD and NADP are present in every living cell and are involved in many vital metabolic processes, including energy production, fatty acid production, glycolysis, and the reduction of cholesterol and fatty acids in the bloodstream. Niacin supplementation was shown to reduce blood levels of the bad LDL cholesterol while increasing the good HDL cholesterol. Vitamin B_3 should be included in your daily dietary supplement program. Maintain moderate dietary supplement intake for good health. Increase daily dosages as required for management of healthy fatty acid and cholesterol blood levels. Take megadoses of vitamin B_3 only under medical supervision, and only for short periods of time.

Benefits: Vitamin B_3 is required for good health, and can be used to help reduce cholesterol and maintain healthy levels.

Ingredient Forms: High dosages of vitamin B_3 as nicotinic acid, greater than 50 mg, can cause the capillaries to dilate. This causes a condition known as "niacin flush." Because of this, individuals who desire to take vitamin B_3 in amounts over 50 mg per day should use a supplement containing the flush-free forms of vitamin B_3, such as inositol hexanicotinate, nicotinamide, and niacinimide.

Effective Supplement Dosages: The RDI for vitamin B_3 is 20 mg. Common dosages found in dietary supplements range from 20 to 100 mg per day. Megadoses of vitamin B_3 (as nicotinic acid) are used under medical super-

vision to reduce cholesterol and can range up to 1 to 3 g per day. Prolonged use of these high therapeutic dosages of vitamin B_3 can cause liver damage and nausea as well as bouts of the annoying niacin flush. See Chapter 6 for dietary supplements that are safe and effective for lowering cholesterol levels and maintaining healthy blood lipid levels.

Cofactors: The other B vitamins.

Concerns: The classic niacin deficiency disease is pellagra, characterized by dermatitis, inflamed mucous membranes, and dementia. Other symptoms of vitamin B_3 deficiency include elevated fatty acid blood levels, fatigue, depression, confusion, and headaches. Excessive dosages of vitamin B_3 as nicotinic acid can cause niacin flush, where the skin reddens, burns, and itches; this can last up to several hours. Prolonged use of high amounts of vitamin B_3 can cause liver dysfunction. Vitamin B_3 supplements are safe for all ages and both sexes when used as directed.

Use Guidelines: Take vitamin B_3 supplements daily as part of your nutritional health program.

Vitamin B_5 (also Pantothenic acid)

Supplement Type: Vitamin

Overview: Vitamin B_5 is an essential water-soluble vitamin. It has many important metabolic functions, primarily as a component of coenzyme A. Coenzyme A is important in the Krebs cycle (one of the body's energy-producing pathways) and in the metabolism of fatty acids. This makes vitamin B_5 important in the production of energy from carbohydrates and fatty acids. It is also involved in cholesterol and steroid synthesis. Include vitamin B_5 as part of your daily dietary supplement program. Intake of higher dosages may be indicated during times of physical or emotional stress.

Benefits: Vitamin B_5 is essential for good health, production of energy, and production of hormones.

Ingredient Form: Vitamin B_5 is supplied in dietary supplements as D-calcium pantothenate.

Effective Supplement Dosages: The adult RDI for vitamin B_5 is 10 mg. Dietary supplements commonly contain 5 to 30 mg per daily dosage. Dosages up to 100 mg per day are found in high potency "stress-fighting" vitamin B complex formulas.

Cofactors: The other B vitamins.

Concerns: A deficiency in vitamin B_5 can cause various symptoms, including insomnia, vomiting, burning feet, irritability, weakness, cramps, and reduced immune function. Excessive dosages of vitamin B_5 for short periods of time are reported to be nontoxic. Dosages as high as 10,000 to 20,000 mg per day can result in diarrhea and water retention. Intake at these high levels is not recommended. While taking megadoses of vitamin B_5 is common, do not exceed 200 mg per day without medical supervision and for specific medical reasons. Vitamin B_5 supplements are safe for all ages and both sexes when used as directed.

Use Guidelines: Take vitamin B_5 supplements daily as part of your nutritional health program.

Vitamin B_6 (also Pyridoxine hydrochloride)

Supplement Type: Vitamin

Overview: Vitamin B_6 is an essential water-soluble vitamin. It is important in enzyme function, cell division, production of red blood cells, immune system function, transamination, amino acid production, and energy production. Include vitamin B_6 as part of your dietary supplement program. If you want to take high dosages of this vitamin as part of nutritional therapy, do so under medical supervision. Individuals who consume large amounts of protein should increase their vitamin B_6 intake accordingly.

Benefits: B_6 maintains good health, boosts immunity, protects against the development of some nervous system disorders, and is used in the nutritional treatment of PMS and carpal tunnel syndrome.

Ingredient Form: Dietary supplements supply vitamin B_6 as pyridoxine hydrochloride (pyridoxine HCl).

Effective Supplement Dosages: The adult RDI for vitamin B_6 is 2 mg per day. A tolerable upper intake level of 100 mg per day has been established.

Cofactors: The other B vitamins.

Concerns: Deficiency symptoms due to inadequate vitamin B_6 intake include poor wound healing, fatigue, seizures, anemia, depression, and skin disorders. While vitamin B_6 is relatively nontoxic, high amounts (over 2 g per day) taken over several months have been reported to cause nervous system disorders, including tingling and numbness of the arms and legs. Vitamin B_6 supplements are safe for all ages and both sexes when used as directed. However, it is not recommended to take greater than 50 mg per day for extended periods of time without a doctor's supervision.

Use Guidelines: Take vitamin B_6 supplements daily as part of your nutritional health program.

Vitamin B_{12} (also Cyanocobalamin)

Supplement Type: Vitamin

Overview: Vitamin B_{12} is an essential water-soluble vitamin, required for healthy metabolism and proper nerve function. Vitamin B_{12} is important for new cell growth, nerve tissue development, folate metabolism (which is important to maintain healthy homocysteine levels), DNA synthesis, and energy production. It is also required for the production of red blood cells. In addition to vitamin B_{12}'s role in maintaining overall health, its use as an energy enhancer is of interest to athletes, the elderly, and anyone who is experiencing low energy levels. Vitamin B_{12}'s role in maintaining homocysteine levels is vital to maintaining cardiovascular health.

Benefits: Adequate intake of vitamin B_{12} is essential for good health.

Ingredient Form: Vitamin B_{12} is supplied in supplements as cyanocobalamin.

Effective Supplement Dosages: The RDI for vitamin B_{12} is 6 mcg. Vitamin B_{12} is available in dosages of 3 to 200 mcg. Some B_{12} supplements contain as much as 1,000 mcg per day dosages.

Cofactors: The other B vitamins.

Concerns: Vitamin B_{12} deficiency symptoms include loss of appetite, irritability, fatigue, constipation, headaches, tongue soreness, and pernicious anemia. Pernicious anemia results from the malabsorption of vitamin B_{12} due to a failure of the gastric mucosa to secrete intrinsic factor, a chemical needed for proper absorption of the vitamin. If you think you have pernicious anemia, taking extra vitamin B_{12} is not a valid treatment, because the disease is due to the lack of intrinsic factor, not a lack of dietary vitamin B_{12}. If you suspect your fatigue is due to pernicious anemia, consult your doctor for proper treatment, which usually includes vitamin B_{12} injections. Excessive intake of vitamin B_{12} does not appear to produce acute toxic side effects. However, megadoses of vitamin B_{12} are not recommended. Vitamin B_{12} supplements are safe for all ages and both sexes when used as directed.

Use Guidelines: Include vitamin B_{12} in your daily dietary supplement program.

Vitamin C (also Ascorbic acid)

Supplement Type: Vitamin

Overview: Vitamin C is a water-soluble essential vitamin that functions primarily in the production of collagen, the intercellular tissues that hold the body's cells together. It helps heal wounds, fights infection, maintains healthy capillaries, and promotes healthy gums and teeth. Vitamin C is a very important antioxidant and protects cells from damage; it also prevents the oxidation of folate. It assists in the metabolism of tyrosine and phenylalanine, and aids in the absorption of iron. Vitamin C should be part of your daily dietary supplement program. The most common reason for taking megadoses of vitamin C is for the prevention and treatment of colds and respiratory ailments. Research studies provide mixed results using vitamin C for the management of such diseases, with some studies reporting a significant benefit and others not. If you choose to take megadoses of vitamin C during illness, make sure to contact your doctor if symptoms persist more than a day, or if fever develops.

Benefits: Maintaining adequate intake is required for good health and protection from free-radical damage. Vitamin C is commonly used as supportive nutritional therapy in the treatment of several disorders, including bleeding gums, the common cold, allergies, asthma, and emotional stress. It is thought to promote cardiovascular wellness and protect against cancer.

Ingredient Form: Vitamin C is contained in dietary supplements as ascorbic acid. Buffered vitamin C is also available and is recommended if you have gastrointestinal problems or take high dosages of vitamin C on a regular basis. Ester-C is a special brand of vitamin C.

Effective Supplement Dosages: The adult RDI for vitamin C is 60 mg. Most health practitioners recognize that a daily dosage of between 250 and 500 mg is suitable for normal daily nutritional needs. Higher dosages of vitamin C are commonly taken, especially during cold season. Most adults experience no side effects from a daily intake as high as 1,000 mg per day. Dosages as high as 5,000 mg per day are not uncommon, taken for short periods. But there are some vitamin C fanatics who take very high dosages all the time. If you are taking large amounts of vitamin C for medical reasons, do so under medical supervision to make sure that your medical condition is properly treated.

Cofactors: Bioflavonoids and the essential vitamins and minerals.

Concerns: Scurvy is one of the best-known vitamin deficiencies, and results from prolonged inadequate vitamin C intake. Scurvy is a serious disease characterized by weakening of collagenous tissues and structures, such as the skin, gums, tendons, and cartilage. This results in widespread hemorrhaging of capillaries and tissues. Scurvy is rarely seen in adults in the United States but is sometimes observed in infants and the elderly. Excessive intake of vitamin C, over 3,000 mg per day, has been known to cause headaches, frequent urination, diarrhea, and nausea in some individuals. While vitamin C is considered nontoxic, consumption of the vitamin in excessive amounts for long periods of time is not recommended, as is true for all dietary supplement ingredients. Vitamin C supplements are safe for all ages and both sexes when taken as directed.

Use Guidelines: Take vitamin C supplements daily as part of your nutritional health program.

Vitamin D (also Ergocalciferol, cholecalciferol)

Supplement Type: Vitamin

Overview: Vitamin D is essential for growth, especially the normal growth and development of bones and teeth. Its major function is in assisting in calcium and phosphorus metabolism, including their intestinal absorption and utilization. Vitamin D should be part of your daily dietary supplement program. New guidelines for vitamin D intake have recently established an adequate intake level of 600 IU per day for the elderly. Do not take megadoses of vitamin D. If you have osteoporosis, there are prescription forms of vitamin D that may be indicated if your doctor finds that you have a problem with vitamin D metabolism and that it is contributing to your bone wellness problems. Do not take vitamin D if you have known hypercalcemia (high blood calcium levels).

Benefits: Vitamin D is essential for proper development and maintenance of bones and teeth.

Ingredient Form: Out of the four forms of vitamin D, vitamin D_2 (ergocalciferol, also called calciferol) and vitamin D_3 (cholecalciferol) are the most biologically active and are used in dietary supplements.

Effective Supplement Dosages: The adult RDI for vitamin D is 400 IU. The adult tolerable upper intake level has been established at 2,000 IU per day. Dietary supplements usually contain a dosage of 400 IU per day, up to 800 IU per day.

Cofactors: The essential vitamins and minerals. Also calcium, magnesium, boron, silicon, and other nutrients in bone maintenance formulas.

Concerns: Maintaining proper vitamin D status is vital for people of all ages. In fact, the widespread use of milk fortified with vitamin D was initiated to ensure development of strong bones in children, and is also useful for adults to maintain strong bones and healthy teeth. Vitamin D deficiency is characterized by inadequate bone mineralization. It causes abnormalities such as soft bones, bowlegs, poor teeth, and skeletal deformity. In children a vitamin D deficiency can result in rickets. In adults poor vitamin D status and defects in vitamin D metabolism are associated with osteoporosis, weak bones, and increased bone fractures. Infants and children not fed vitamin D–fortified milk and adults with poor vitamin D status who do not get adequate exposure to sunlight are at risk. The human body has the ability to make vitamin D_3 in the skin from a sterol called 7-dehydrocholesterol, which is stimulated by exposure to UV light. Excessive intake of vitamin D may lead to side effects, especially in children. These side effects include calcium buildup in soft tissues, kidney stone development, and irreversible kidney and cardiovascular damage. Vitamin D supplements are safe for all ages and both sexes when used as directed.

Use Guidelines: Take vitamin D supplements daily as part of your nutritional health program.

Vitamin E (also Alpha-tocopherol)

Supplement Type: Vitamin

Overview: Vitamin E is an essential fat-soluble nutrient. It is mainly known for its role as an antioxidant protecting the body from free-radical damage; it also protects tissue lipids and vitamin A from oxidation. Vitamin E assists in red blood cell formation and aids in the regulation of prostanoid synthesis. Prostanoids are compounds that are important in the reproductive process, blood platelet aggregation, energy production, and synthesis of DNA and RNA. Daily dietary supplement intake of vitamin E is necessary. It is estimated that the average intake of vitamin E from food sources is less than the RDI. Along with the other antioxidants, vitamin E plays a vital role in protecting the body from free-radical damage. Free radical damage leads to premature aging and contributes to development of degenerative diseases.

Benefits: Vitamin E is essential for promotion and maintenance of good health and prevention of premature aging due to free-radical damage. Its antioxidant function contributes to a reduced risk of developing certain degenerative diseases, such as coronary heart disease, cataracts, certain cancers, and arthritis. In major long-term clinical studies men and women who took a daily dosage of 100 IU of vitamin E per day for at least two years experienced a lowered risk of cardiovascular diseases. Vitamin E also enhances the action of the immune system. It lessens the severity of prostaglandin-mediated disorders, such as inflammation and premenstrual syndrome. Vitamin E helps improve circulatory irregularities such as nocturnal leg cramps

and blood platelet adhesion. Vitamin E also inhibits the conversion of dietary nitrites to harmful nitrosamines in the stomach. Nitrosamines are strong tumor promoters and are implicated in causing gastrointestinal cancers.

Ingredient Forms: The most biologically active form of vitamin E is naturally occurring d-alpha-tocopherol, which is an oil. Other natural forms of vitamin E include d-alpha-tocopheryl acetate (an oil) and d-alpha-tocopheryl acid succinate (a powder). There are also natural mixed tocopherols consisting of d-alpha-tocopherol, d-beta-tocopherol, d-gamma-tocopherol, and d-delta-tocopherol. Natural vitamin E is isolated from vegetable oils; soy oil is the most common. Synthetic forms of vitamin E are also biologically active, and are preceded with the letters *dl*. Synthetic forms found in dietary supplements include dl-alpha-tocopherol, dl-alpha-tocopheryl acetate, and dl-tocopheryl acid succinate. Note that because vitamin E is a powerful antioxidant, it can start losing its potency when exposed to air, heat, and light. When d-alpha-tocopherol is enclosed in soft gelatin capsules, this acts as an effective barrier and keeps the vitamin E oil stable. The vitamin E acetates, also oils, are more stable when exposed to air. For solid dosage types of dietary supplements, such as tablets and capsules, vitamin E succinate "powdered" forms were developed; these are also stable when exposed to air. Tablet, capsule, and powdered dietary supplements may also contain the oil forms of vitamin E in low amounts.

Effective Supplement Dosages: The adult RDI for vitamin E is 30 IU. Optimal daily intakes of vitamin E for nutritional purposes should be maintained at 100 to 400 IU from natural vitamin E sources, and 200 to 600 IU from synthetic vitamin E sources. Higher dosages may be indicated for larger or more active people, and for therapeutic reasons. Vitamin E is best taken with meals.

Cofactors: The other antioxidants.

Concerns: Inadequate vitamin E intake is associated with a higher risk of developing degenerative diseases. Symptoms of vitamin E deficiency are not clearly established but can include signs of muscle weakness, abnormal deposition of fat in the muscles, rupture of red blood cells, and increased destruction of cell membranes. Deficiency of vitamin E contributes to premature aging. Vitamin E is relatively nontoxic. Long-term use of dosages ranging from 100 IU to 800 IU per day have not had reported side effects. Several year-long studies using 100 IU per day have reported a decrease in the occurrence of cardiovascular disease, with no apparent side effects. Use only under medical supervision if you have a coagulation disorder or severe high blood pressure. Vitamin E supplements are safe for all ages and both sexes when used as directed.

Use Guidelines: Take vitamin E supplements daily as part of your nutritional health program.

Vitamin K (also Phylloquinone, menadione)
Supplement Type: Vitamin

Overview: Vitamin K is an essential lipid-soluble vitamin that functions in the synthesis of prothrombin, a substance vital for blood clotting. Without vitamin K, the blood clotting process cannot be initiated. Individuals who are physically active, involved in athletics, employed in physical jobs where bumps and bruises frequently occur, or who need it for medical reasons could benefit from supplemental intake of vitamin K.

Benefits: Required for proper blood clotting, healing of fractures, and possibly prevention of osteoporosis.

Ingredient Form: Vitamin K_1 (phylloquinone) and vitamin K_3 (menadione) are used in supplements.

Effective Supplement Dosages: The adult RDI for vitamin K is 80 mcg. Dietary supplements contain modest amounts of vitamin K, ranging from 20 to 200 mcg.

Cofactors: The other essential vitamins and minerals.

Concerns: Vitamin K deficiency is rare because vitamin K_2 (menaquinone) is formed by intestinal bacteria and is widely available in plant and animal foods. Inadequate vitamin K status can lead to an increased tendency to hemorrhage. Most instances of vitamin K deficiency are found in infants. However, individuals on antibiotic therapy for long periods of time, where the intestinal bacteria are killed off, can be at risk for developing a vitamin K deficiency. Also, chronic aspirin intake can interfere with the metabolic pathways in which vitamin K is involved, and can therefore impair normal blood clotting. Vitamin K is relatively nontoxic, and overdosing of vitamin K rarely occurs in adults. Taking megadoses of vitamin K is not advised, and may cause hemolytic anemia (separation of the hemoglobin from red blood cells) and liver problems. Do not take vitamin K supplements if you are taking coumadin (Warfarin) or other anticoagulant drugs. It reverses the effects of these drugs. Vitamin K supplements are safe for all ages and both sexes when used as directed.

Use Guidelines: Take vitamin K supplements daily as part of your nutritional health program.

Wheat germ oil: *see* Gamma-oryzanol

White willow bark (also *Salix alba, Salix purpurea,* and other *Salix* species)

Supplement Type: Botanical

Overview: White willow bark has a long history of use for reducing fever and relieving pain. In the early 1900s the active ingredient, salicin (salicylic acid or salicylate), was identified. Later on, salicin was used to make the world's first aspirin, acetylsalicylic acid. In Europe, white willow bark is used to treat fever, headaches, and rheumatic diseases. If you are taking aspirin and supplement products containing white willow bark, make sure you are not overdosing on total salicylates. Ask your doctor or pharmacist to check the total amount. Symptoms of excessive salicylate intake include ringing in the ears and gastrointestinal irritation.

Benefits: Natural pain reliever.

Ingredient Form: Standardized white willow bark (6% to 12% salicin).

Effective Supplement Dosages: The range of total salicin is 60 to 120 mg per day when used to relieve pain as a botanical drug. This would take about 1,000 to 2,000 mg of white willow bark supplement standardized to 6% salicin.

Cofactors: Other pain-relieving supplements, such as boswellia and DL-phenylalanine.

Concerns: White willow bark is not an essential nutrient. It is a botanical medicine for relieving pain and fever. It should not be used to replace drugs recommended by your doctor. For adult use only; not for use by children or by pregnant or lactating women unless under a doctor's supervision. Do not use if you have gastritis or ulcers. Always use under medical supervision when treating an illness.

Use Guidelines: Use white willow supplements periodically as needed.

Yam (also Wild yam root, colic root, rheumatism root, *Dioscorea villosa*)

Supplement Type: Botanical

Overview: Traditionally used as an anti-inflammatory, especially for gastrointestinal pain and rheumatoid arthritis. However, good clinical studies are lacking to confirm the exact benefits yam has to offer. Yam is a supplement ingredient that has not undergone rigorous scientific evaluation but has been shown to be safe and effective based on a long history of traditional use. Yam should not be used in place of drug therapy, but may be beneficial as supportive nutritional therapy for the conditions listed above.

Benefits: Nutritional support for inflammatory conditions of the gastrointestinal system and rheumatoid arthritis.

Ingredient Form: Standardized yam root (4% to 6% diosgenine).

Effective Supplement Dosages: As a dietary supplement, 150 to 600 mg per day.

Cofactors: None.

Concerns: Yam is not an essential nutrient. Its use for medical conditions should be under medical supervision. For adults only; not for use by children or by pregnant or lactating women. For short-term use only, as directed by your doctor.

Use Guidelines: The use of yam supplements is optional.

Yeast (also Brewer's yeast, *Saccharomyces cerevisiae*)

Supplement Type: Botanical

Overview: In Europe yeast products are available as herbal drugs for treating loss of appetite, chronic forms of acne, and acute diarrhea. They are sometimes taken before traveling to prevent traveler's diarrhea. In the United States, yeast supplements have been sold for similar health reasons and also as a "superfood." It contains vitamins and minerals, especially chromium and the B vitamins. Yeast supplements were very popular during the 1960s and 1970s,

but as more supplement products have entered the marketplace, their popularity has decreased.

Benefits: Promotes overall health. Maintains regular gastrointestinal function.

Ingredient Form: Concentrated, purified *Saccharomyces cerevisiae*. Hansen CBS 5926 is a standardized, high-quality brand of yeast from Europe, that can be found in some health food stores.

Effective Supplement Dosages: 250 to 750 mg per day. Higher dosages may be used as recommended by your health professional.

Cofactors: None.

Concerns: Yeast contains some essential nutrients, but it is not considered an essential nutrient. Its use in the United States as a dietary supplement has been primarily as a superfood health supplement. For adult use only; not for use by children or by pregnant or lactating women unless under a doctor's supervision. Not for people with yeast allergies. Some common side effects include flatulence and headaches. If using it for diarrhea, consult your doctor if symptoms persist more than forty-eight hours. Make sure to replace lost fluids and electrolytes when treating diarrhea.

Use Guidelines: Periodic use of yeast supplements is optional.

Yohimbe (also *Pausinystalia yohimbe*)

Supplement Type: Botanical

Overview: Traditionally yohimbe has been used as a male aphrodisiac. Chemically, yohimbe bark contains the chemical substance called yohimbine. In Western medicine, the drug yohimbine is considered an effective treatment for erectile impotence. It is a presynaptic alpha-2-adrenergic blocking agent, and results in increasing nervous system firing rates. It also has a blood vessel dilating effect. In the 1960s studies were conducted using a combination drug called nux vomica, which contained yohimbine and methyl testosterone. Nux vomica was found to be effective after two to three weeks of use in most cases, but various side effects were observed (see below). Keep in mind, however, that no conclusive studies using the botanical yohimbe have been published that show the same effects. Please note that this nux vomica was not the same as the more commonly available homeopathic preparation known by the same name. Homeopathic preparations of nux vomica contain no yohimbine or methyltestosterone. Why are so many men taking yohimbe supplements despite all the potential side effects and the fact that a doctor can prescribe an effective drug? Perhaps one reason is that purchasing a male sexual potency supplement is easier than going to the doctor to get a prescription and having to admit to erectile dysfunction. Also, most of the male sexual potency formulas contain other ingredients as well, to promote other biological effects, and are taken by men who have normal sexual function in an attempt to improve on it. Keep in mind that the use of yohimbe can result in the same side effects as taking the drug yohimbine. Also, it takes two to four weeks to see improvements, so avoid taking megadoses of yohimbe supplements with the mistaken expectation of immediate results.

Benefits: Improves male sexual function.

Ingredient Form: Standardized yohimbe bark extract (6% to 12% yohimbine).

Effective Supplement Dosages: The dosages of the drug yohimbine found to be effective in studies ranged from 5.4 to 10 mg of yohimbine, taken three times per day. This would be about 100 to 170 mg, three times per day, of a yohimbe bark extract standardized to 6% yohimbine. Restrict use to four to six weeks; use only under a doctor's supervision.

Cofactors: Arginine, carnitine, ginseng, zinc, vitamin E, and ginkgo.

Concerns: Yohimbe is not an essential nutrient. It is used in dietary supplements to supply its primary active phytochemical, yohimbine. Side effects reported when using yohimbine include nervousness, irritability, insomnia, headache, skin flushing, anorexia, nausea, gastric distress, diarrhea, vomiting, palpitations, tachycardia, dysuria, pain, increased blood pressure, dizziness, sweating, weight gain, constipation, and anxiety. To be used only by adult males suffering from erectile dysfunction. Use under medical supervision. Yohimbine is also a monoamine oxidase (MAO) inhibitor. Do not use if you are taking any medication or if you have any disease condition, especially a heart, liver, or kidney disease. Do not overdose on yohimbe; it can cause death.

Use Guidelines: Use of yohimbe supplements is optional.

Yucca (also *Yucca aloifolia, Yucca gluca, Yucca whipplei,* and other *Yucca* species)

Supplement Type: Botanical

Overview: Attention was drawn toward yucca during the 1970s, when a preliminary research study reported beneficial effects on arthritis. Scientists believe that the saponin content of yucca is responsible for the observed effects. However, additional research studies are needed to confirm the effectiveness of yucca, its long-term safety, and dosages. Yucca is also used in other products, such as soaps and shampoos. This is due to the foaming action of the saponins.

Benefits: May benefit people with arthritis as supportive therapy.

Ingredient Form: Standardized yucca extract (saponins).

Effective Supplement Dosages: Follow directions on product labels.

Cofactors: Other antiarthritic ingredients, such as glucosamine, boswellia, chondroitin sulfate, antioxidants, white willow, and so on.

Concerns: Yucca is not an essential nutrient. Yucca is an approved food ingredient, and its use in foods has not resulted in any reported side effects. However, the use of yucca in dietary supplements is relatively recent, and the long-term effects of standardized yucca extracts are unknown. Use with caution, and not for more than several months. Use under medical supervision, especially if treating a disease condition. For adults only; not for use by children or by pregnant or lactating women unless under a doctor's supervision. May cause gastrointestinal upset.

Use Guidelines: Use of yucca is optional.

Zinc

Supplement Type: Mineral

Overview: Zinc is a component of over two hundred enzymes that play important roles in cell replication, tissue repair, and growth. Zinc is also involved in the production, storage, and secretion of hormones, including testosterone and growth hormone. It is well known for its role in reproductive system health and prostate gland functioning. Consider trying higher zinc intake, up to 25 mg per day, for prostate health, improved vision, enhanced wound healing, and improved immune system function. Do not take megadoses of zinc. Periodic intake of up to 60 mg per day taken during the cold and flu season are well tolerated by most people.

Benefits: Maintaining adequate zinc status is vital for good health. Improved immune function, healing, fertility, skin health, and vision are just some of the benefits of zinc. Zinc supplementation also can restore or improve the sense of taste and smell in some individuals with zinc deficiency.

Ingredient Forms: Inorganic zinc molecules and organic chelates of zinc, including zinc carbonate, zinc oxide, zinc citrate, zinc arginate, zinc picolinate, zinc orotate, and zinc gluconate, are found in dietary supplements.

Dosages: The adult RDI for zinc is 15 mg. Dietary supplements intended for daily use typically contain 5 to 15 mg per day. Special use formulas for prostate health, wound healing, and enhanced immunity contain larger amounts of zinc, usually 15 to 25 mg per day.

Cofactors: The other essential vitamins and minerals, especially copper. Prolonged high zinc intake can interfere with the absorption and metabolism of copper and other minerals. Make sure your dietary supplement contains an adequate dosage of copper. If your doctor puts you on high dosages of zinc for medical reasons, make sure that your copper intake is increased as well.

Concerns: Inadequate dietary intake of zinc can cause growth disorders, loss of appetite, skin changes, immune system disorders, delayed sexual maturation in children, night blindness, and impaired hearing, taste, and smell. Excessive zinc intake can cause copper deficiency, lowering of beneficial HDL cholesterol, nausea, gastrointestinal disorders, depressed immune function, headaches, dizziness, and other metabolic disturbances. Zinc supplements are safe for all ages and both sexes when used as directed.

Use Guidelines: Use zinc-containing supplements as part of your daily nutritional health program.

LEARN THE NEW RULES OF WEIGHT LOSS AND
PERMANENT WEIGHT MAINTENANCE, USING
A PINCH OF SCIENCE
AND
A DASH OF COMMON SENSE

NATURAL-THIN
WEIGHT LOSS PROGRAM

THE ULTIMATE WEIGHT LOSS PLAN
THAT GETS YOU
FROM FAT TO FIRM

- *TRIM YOUR BELLY, BUTT, AND THIGHS*
- *LEARN HOW TO "EAT DOWN" THE POUNDS*
- *TURN ON YOUR WEIGHT LOSS POWER*
- *REACH YOUR "FAT LOSS POTENTIAL"*
- *SCIENTIFICALLY PROVEN TECHNIQUES*
- *UNDERSTAND WHY SO MANY DIETS?*

Know the new rules:

- *OF LOSING WEIGHT*
- *FAT LOSS NUTRITION*
- *FOR EATING DOWN THE POUNDS*
- *FOR EATING OUT*
- *FOR SWEATING DOWN THE POUNDS, THE BEST*
  EXERCISE FOR LOSING THE WEIGHT, AND KEEPING IT OFF
- *FOR THINKING OFF THE POUNDS, YES, THINKING OFF THE POUNDS*
- *OF PERMANENT WEIGHT MANAGEMENT—SCIENTIFICALLY PROVEN*
  TO BE THE BEST

INTRODUCTORY REMARKS ABOUT
WEIGHT LOSS AND WEIGHT MAINTENANCE
THE NATURAL-THIN WAY

Under section heading "NATURAL-THIN EATING PLAN," you will find "Daily Food Intake Goals" and the "Natural-Thin Meal and Snack Examples" subsections.

The Daily Food Intake Goals subsection contains BEST FOODS LISTS for the major food groups. It provides recommended servings per day for men and women, for during weight loss periods, and for weight maintenance.

Then, the Natural-Thin Meal and Snack Examples provides you with a quick menu-style reference of meals and snacks, mixing and matching the different foods from the Daily Food Intake Goals BEST FOODS LISTS. Remember these lists and menus are only examples. You can follow them exactly or use them as guidance for creating your own personal meal/snack eating plan.

The LEAN AND MEAN NUTRITION TIPS section offers tips and guidelines about foods to avoid and preferred types of foods. While it encourages low-fat foods, this does not mean that you cannot include moderate fat foods into your eating plan. But keep in mind that the scientific research shows when people are on a reduced calorie, low-fat diet, they lose body fat faster than on a moderate or high-fat diet. Also, most people have gained their weight from eating high-fat foods, which are more easily stored as body fat and easily overeaten. In any case, not overeating is the most important nutritional factor for weight maintenance and losing excess body fat.

Finally, remember that obesity is considered a disease, and while I always recommend that everyone, both overweight and obese individuals, seek medical supervision when undergoing a weight-loss program, individuals classified as obese have to make sure they are under doctor supervision. So, start out by using the NATURAL-THIN MEASUREMENT LOG to see how your body composition rates.

APPENDIX

Natural-Thin
Weight Loss Program

Are you already eating some of the right foods? Do you do some exercise? Have you already lost some weight? Losing weight is everybody's favorite side effect of being healthy. But maybe, in spite of your best efforts, you still have a few pounds to lose or are still overweight, and you're not quite sure why or what to do about it.

Well, the what-to-do-about-it part is easy: Just start following my Natural-Thin guidelines, and the pounds will start to disappear as you watch your slim, attractive body begin to emerge. I designed the Natural-Thin approach to be your guide to getting trim and staying that way. It offers you the medically proven tools you need to take control of your weight condition and reach your weight goals. The Natural-Thin plan is based on the most recent scientific studies and integrates nutrition, physical, and behavioral factors. Together, they stimulate your body into being a fat-burning machine instead of a fat-storing machine.

When most people think of weight loss and weight maintenance, they think diet, diet, diet. But I want you to think of this important area of your life differently for a moment. I want you to focus on the end result of following a program that will result in being trimmer. I want you to think about the numerous health benefits you will achieve. I want you to visualize the feelings of accomplishment, pride, and success you will experience when you attain your personal weight goal. I want you to think about the possibility of living a longer and healthier life.

You see, in these terms, losing weight and maintaining a healthy weight are not about diet—they're about attitude and lifestyle. They're about being honest with yourself and realizing that if you have a problem with weight management, you need to include in your life those supplements, foods, and behaviors that will make you trim and keep you thin.

Scientists have discovered a lot about weight management during the past fifty years. They have discovered that the majority of us will experience a weight management problem sometime during our lives. Your weight problem is unique to you. For some it may mean gaining just a few unwanted pounds or moving up one clothing size. For others it's dealing with obesity and life-threatening diseases.

What you must realize is that people with weight problems, whether it's a matter of 5 pounds or 100 pounds, share the same frustrations. When your best efforts to be thin are unsuccessful yet the desire to be thin remains, it makes the most sensible person try almost anything. Well, learn from your past. If you do, you will understand that you need a total weight management approach, the Natural-Thin way.

The Natural-Thin approach recognizes that as a person with a history of weight management problems, you have special metabolic needs. You need a daily regimen of food and supplements that will help your body burn fats and better control your appetite. You need to develop your fat-loss potential to make your body better at burning fat than at storing it. The Natural-Thin weight management system will give you the tools and skills you need to put you back in control of your body weight.

INTRODUCTION TO THE NATURAL-THIN PROGRAM

The science of getting trim and staying thin involves making your life work for you, not against you. This means setting goals and including in your life the foods, supplements, and behaviors that will result in losing the weight you want, then following a lifestyle that will allow you to keep it off. This *is* possible!

What most people with weight problems have in common is that their lifestyles, and the foods that have made them overweight, have ruined their metabolism, creating a fat-building metabolism instead of a fat-burning metabolism. Rebuilding your fat-loss potential starts with eating the right foods, engaging in the right physical activity, and adopting new mental strategies. For some of you, rebuilding your fat-loss potential may require taking special supplements to help with appetite control and stimulate your metabolism to burn more fat. The medical studies are very impressive and report that naturally occurring plant-based appetite control supplements and thermogenic nutrients and foods have been shown to assist in weight loss and weight maintenance in the following ways:

- Stimulate the metabolism to burn more calories
- Promote the metabolism of fatty acids in adipose tissue (body fat)
- Elevate the basal metabolic rate

- Promote lipid oxidation
- Exert an appetite suppressant effect
- Help preserve lean body mass, including muscle, while losing fat
- Promote weight loss in low-energy-adapted women
- Increase feelings of fullness and satisfaction
- Control appetite and cravings

The major factor for maximizing your fat-loss potential is to eat foods that will stimulate the burning of calories and discourage the storage of unwanted body fat. These Natural-Thin foods are included in the following section. The next important factor is to choose exercises that maximize fat burning and also build up the body. This is sensible exercise, not strenuous exercise that just wears you down and defeats your efforts. The Natural-Thin exercise suggestions are easy to follow and quickly become part of your daily life. Finally, the Natural-Thin behavioral strategies will help you reinforce your new fat-burning lifestyle and help you deal with food situations that have sabotaged you in the past.

While you are probably sitting at the edge of your seat and are eager to plunge into developing your fat-loss potential, it's important to think about why it is you still have a problem with weight. You have probably heard the statistic that most people who lose weight gain it back during the next five years. This statistic tells you an impor-

tant lesson that you should not forget: Gimmick diets don't work for most people. Why? It's simple. The one thing that most of these plans have in common is that they prescribe a low-calorie diet and a structured eating program. So when you make your pledge and stick to the diet, you will usually lose weight in the short term. But the majority of people can't stick to such a rigid program and return to their old ways of eating once they lose some weight. Also, a diet that is too low in calories is usually not properly balanced nutritionally, with the result that dieters lose a lot of muscle mass. This in turn slows their metabolism, that is, their calorie-burning rate. That's why so many people who have been on the diet roller coaster a few times find it hard to lose weight once they gain it back—the very essence of their fat-burning ability is reduced. So when you finish a gimmick diet, you're likely to be worse off than you were before you started.

Another factor that enters into the equation is aging. Studies show that when we age, our metabolism slows down. This means that the metabolism is not using up as many calories as it once did. People with weight problems need to consider their life in the present, not the past when their metabolism was burning more calories per day.

When designing the Natural-Thin weight management approach, I carefully considered many factors: the metabolic and behavioral aspects of why people have weight problems, what nutrients and foods are best to stimulate weight loss while maintaining health and empowering the metabolism, what the most common behaviors are among people with weight problems, how to phase in new behaviors to help with weight management, and what natural products and foods can help you control your appetite.

The Natural-Thin dietary supplement guidelines combine essential vitamins and minerals with premium standardized herbal extracts. They include thermogenic nutrients that help your body burn more energy and that promote a more efficient metabolism. (See Chapter 18.)

Appetite control nutrients support the brain's food intake control center. Energy-stimulating supplements help support your energy systems and also support the adrenal glands, which are important for maintaining your fat-loss potential.

The Natural-Thin eating plan includes appetite-satisfying foods that will enhance your metabolism, not work against it—foods that offer rich taste, fiber, and nutrition while offering the thermogenic edge to develop your fat-loss potential. These foods help burn more calories during the digestion process and are more likely to be used as energy instead of being stored as fat. These foods include low-fat proteins, leafy vegetables, and whole grains.

The Natural-Thin exercise section lists the best fat-burning, metabolism-stimulating exercises for accelerating the fat-loss process. I also include the results of a recent research project that determined the best training program for women to maintain and even build up bone mass.

The Natural-Thin behavioral strategies section covers this important and often neglected part of your weight management program. Making "thin" an attitude will empower you and increase the chances of success.

The Natural-Thin planning and goal setting section provides some simple charts to keep track of your weekly success and meal planning. One characteristic observed among the masters of weight control is that they always write down their accomplishments—and their menus. This is part of making weight management a lifelong skill.

FOLLOWING THE NATURAL-THIN APPROACH

Here are a few things to do before you start your Natural-Thin program.

First, fat-proof your house by getting rid of processed and packaged foods you overeat. Start writing down and keeping track of the foods you catch yourself overeating. Be creative and come up with some healthy alternatives that are less likely to make you lose control.

Second, read through the food guidelines and plan out your meals and snacks for the next week.

Third, approach your Natural-Thin eating as a skill—yes, a skill. This means eating with the purpose of getting trim and staying trim. Always think before you put any food in your mouth: "Is this food going to help me attain my Natural-Thin goals, or will it sabotage them?"

Fourth, consult your doctor before starting this or any weight loss program, to monitor your health as you lose weight. For safest results, continue to be monitored.

NATURAL-THIN EATING PLAN

When planning menus and selecting foods, remember that you choose what goes into your mouth. So why not choose foods that keep you trim and healthy, foods that maximize your fat-loss potential and energize you? Choose foods that are natural, wholesome, high in fiber, and low in fat. Here are some rules to remember:

- Minimize salt intake.
- Avoid high-fat snacks such as chips, cake, and ice cream.
- Choose fresh foods and whole-grain foods when possible.
- Drink at least eight 8-ounce glasses of water per day, or more if active.
- Take your recommended dietary supplements daily.
- Split food intake over three or four small meals and one or two snacks per day.
- Don't overeat!

How many calories are required to promote healthy weight loss and weight maintenance? Most people realize that even with the best fat-burning metabolism, you need to reduce calories when trying to lose weight. This means reducing total daily caloric intake to around 1,000 to 1,200 calories a day for women, and 1,200 to 1,400 calories a day for men. You will find that you may need to make adjustments to this depending on your personal activity level, age, size, and how your metabolism increases while on the Natural-Thin program. You can expect that during the first week or two you may lose as much as 10 to 15 pounds. However, experts agree that after this initial weight loss period, fine-tuning your rate of weight loss to between 1 and 2 pounds per week is best. Studies have shown that if you lose weight too fast, even under the best circumstances, you will end up losing muscle mass as well as body fat. Part of your Natural-Thin goal is to encourage beneficial weight loss, which means preserving muscle mass while losing body fat. So be patient and settle into the 1- to 2-pound-a-week weight loss rule for best results.

How many calories should you be eating a day once you have lost the weight you want to lose? This is a question most people with a weight maintenance problem have a hard time coming to terms with. But the results of a recent survey published in the April 1998 issue of the *Journal of the American Dietetic Association* will shed some light on the issue of calories. The study took a look at over four hundred men and women who had lost on average 60 pounds and maintained the weight loss for five years. The study reported that these winners at weight control continued consumption of a lower-calorie, low-fat diet. Women reported eating an average of 1,306 calories per day, while men reported consuming 1,685 calories per day. Both men and women kept fat intake to about 24 percent of their total daily calories.

Weight loss specialists have found that the body burns calories better during the day than at night. This means paying close attention to your food intake at dinner and if you have an after-dinner snack. For many people, this also means cutting back on the amount of complex carbohydrates (from pasta, bread, and rice) that they eat in the evening. Many people who are overweight develop a condition that the medical community refers to as insulin resistance. Insulin is the hormone in your body that is needed to stimulate the passage of nutrients from the bloodstream into your cells. When you are insulin-resistant, your body does not do this job efficiently, and many of the nutrients you eat, especially the ones from carbohydrates, end up back at the liver, where they are converted to fat. That's why some of the low-carbohydrate diets you may have tried in the past had only a short-term effect. So if you find that your rate of weight loss is slow, instead of reducing the calories

even further, try cutting back on your daily servings of carbohydrate foods for a week or two by substituting a vegetable serving for a serving from the grain/bread/cereal/rice group of foods; especially in the evenings. Along with a regular exercise program, studies have revealed that you can start seeing improvements in your insulin resistance condition in a few weeks, assuming you are otherwise healthy and do not have any serious medical conditions such as diabetes.

What if you're eating at a restaurant? Remember that eating out does not mean pigging out; the calories are not free. Too many people with weight problems simply blow it when they eat out. They've stuck to their eating plan and lost weight—then choose to reward themselves with a fat-laden, calorie-rich feast. This makes no sense at all. If you have a problem with weight maintenance, then you need to stick to your eating plan all the time. Yes, you can eat at fancy restaurants. But you can't eat all the rolls, salad with dressing, an appetizer, the entree, and dessert and expect to stay trim. Create a new strategy when eating out.

Planning means success in weight loss. Plan your meals and snacks each day. If you plan your eating, then you increase your chances of sticking to your plan and not throwing meals together in a last-minute frenzy to satisfy your hunger. It is no surprise that you will need to eat three meals and two or three snacks each day. Write out your menus for the day and week ahead. Have a healthy snack with you in your car, for the times when you are on the run. This will be a much better alternative than pulling into a fast food restaurant, where you will end up eating over a thousand calories. Be prepared.

Daily Food Intake Goals

The following daily food choice guide summarizes your daily food intake goals for weight loss and weight maintenance. Adults of all ages should aim for eating the lower number of servings recommended each day, keeping fat and sugar intake to a minimum. This will provide about 1,200 to 1,400 calories, which meets the needs of most inactive women and the elderly. However, many adults need more than this, depending on body size and physical activity. So men and all active individuals should aim for the middle to upper number of servings per day. This will result in approximately 2,800 to 3,000 calories per day. Adjust the number of servings to achieve fat loss or weight maintenance to suit your personal metabolism.

The Best Foods Lists provide general daily food intake goals for men and women who are losing weight or maintaining weight. These lists are then followed by meal and snack examples. All you have to do is turn to the meal you want—lunch, for example—and you will find several meal examples to guide you in selecting the foods you should eat. For best results, select the healthy foods you like to eat.

BEST FOODS LIST 1:

FRUITS

*2 servings a day for men during
   weight loss*
*2–4 servings a day for men during
   weight maintenance*

*2 servings a day for women during
   weight loss*
*2–4 servings a day for women during
   weight maintenance*

SERVING EXAMPLES
1 apple
1 banana
1 orange
1 grapefruit
1 pear
1 tangerine
1 nectarine
1 peach
1 slice of watermelon
2 kiwis
2 plums
3 small apricots
½ cup cantaloupe
½ cup honeydew melon
½ cup chopped fresh fruit

½ cup unsweetened applesauce

½ cup berries

¼ cup dried fruit, like raisins

Occasional Fruit Choices
   (once or twice a week):

Avocado

Papaya

Olives

Canned fruit

BEST FOODS LIST 2:

VEGETABLES

3–5 servings a day for men during weight
   loss and during weight maintenance

3–5 servings a day for women during
   weight loss and during weight
   maintenance

SERVING EXAMPLES

Servings sizes: 1 cup raw, leafy vegetables,
   ½ cup all other vegetables (cooked or
   chopped raw), or 6 oz. vegetable juice

Alfalfa sprouts

Asparagus

Bamboo shoots

Bean sprouts

Broccoli

Cabbage

Cauliflower

Collard greens

Celery

Cucumbers

Eggplant

Endive

Green Beans

Kale

Lettuce

Mushrooms

Okra

Onions

Parsley

Peppers

Potato, sweet potato, or yam
   (limit to one a day)

Radishes

Snow peas

Spaghetti squash

Spinach

Squash

String beans

Swiss chard

Tomatoes

Tomato juice

Turnip greens

Vegetable juice

Water chestnuts

Yellow wax beans

Zucchini

Occasional vegetable choices
   (once or twice a week):

Artichokes

Beets

Brussels sprouts

Carrots

Corn

BEST FOODS LIST 3:

BREAD, CEREAL, RICE, PASTA
AND OTHER GRAIN PRODUCTS

4–6 servings a day for men during
weight loss
6–11 servings a day for men during
weight maintenance

3–4 servings a day for women during
weight loss
5–6 servings a day for women during
weight maintenance

SERVING EXAMPLES

Serving sizes include: 1 slice of bread,
1 oz. ready-to-eat cereal, ½ cup cooked
cereal, rice, or pasta

Whole-grain bread
Whole-grain pasta
Whole-grain bagels (½ bagel per
serving)
Whole-grain pita
English muffin
Muffins, biscuits, or rolls with 2 or fewer
grams of fat
Unbuttered popped corn
Pretzels
Rice cakes
Melba toast
Breakfast cereal
Oatmeal
Grits
Couscous

Kasha
Quinoa

Occasional bread/grain choices include
unpackaged breads and rolls that do
not have Nutrition Facts information
(and which can be easily overeaten),
highly processed products, low-fat
snack foods like chips and crackers,
no-fat baked goods

BEST FOODS LIST 4:

HIGH PROTEIN FOODS: MEAT, POULTRY,
FISH, AND ALTERNATIVES

3 servings a day for men during weight
loss
3 servings a day for men during weight
maintenance

SERVING EXAMPLES

2 servings a day for women during
weight loss
2–3 servings a day for women during
weight maintenance

Serving sizes will vary depending on
the type of food eaten: Meats: 3–5
ounces
Poultry, fish, and seafood: 4–6 ounces
Beans: 1–1½ cups cooked beans
Eggs: 2–3 eggs or ½ cup egg substitute
or 4–5 egg whites
Organic peanut butter: 3–5 tablespoons

FISH AND SEAFOOD

Abalone, anchovy, bass, carp, catfish, clams, cod, crab, flounder, grouper, haddock, halibut, lobster, perch, pike, pollack, monkfish, mussels, ocean perch, oysters, red snapper, salmon, sardines, shark, shrimp, sole, squid, swordfish, tuna, whitefish.

Avoid bluefish, mackerel, and trout while losing weight.

MEAT AND POULTRY

Beef: eye round, top round

Pork: reduced fat brands, low-fat ham

Poultry: skinless chicken breasts, low-fat tenders, white meat turkey, sliced turkey breast, 93% fat free ground turkey, canned turkey chunks

Eggs: hard boiled, poached, scrambled, microwaved

Dried Beans: all types, e.g., kidney, black, navy, soy beans, etc.

Tofu

Occasional protein choices: less lean beef, like pot roast, porterhouse steak, brisket, ribs, and lamb, smoked fish, frankfurters (eat only no-fat brands), oil-packed canned fish and seafood, bacon (only use lean Canadian bacon); nuts

BEST FOODS LIST 5:

DAIRY/DAIRY SUBSTITUTES

2 servings a day for men during weight loss

2–3 servings a day for men during weight maintenance

2 servings a day for women during weight loss

2–3 servings a day for women during weight maintenance

8 ounces nonfat milk

8 ounces nonfat yogurt

2 ounces nonfat or reduced-fat cheeses

BEST FOODS LIST 6:

CONDIMENTS

3 servings per day

Herbs and spices

Relish

Mustard

BEST FOODS LIST 7:

BEVERAGES

6–10 8-ounce glasses of filtered water, or more if you are very active or on hot days

Naturally decaffeinated coffee

Herbal teas

No-calorie diet beverages, limit to 1–2 servings a day

Diet hot chocolate, under 30 calories per serving, limit to 1 serving a day

NATURAL-THIN BREAKFAST EXAMPLES

Breakfast is the most important meal of the day. These meal options are quick and convenient, so there's no excuse for skipping. For those of you rushing out the door, you can take a meal bar with you. Remember, skipping breakfast is associated with overeating later in the day. Pay attention to what type of breakfast works best for you; one that is high in protein, or high in carbohydrates, or balanced. But always maintain a low-fat intake at breakfast.

½ cup orange or grapefruit juice
8 ounces skim milk or nonfat soy milk
½ bagel
1 tablespoon low-cal jelly
Herbal tea or naturally decaffeinated coffee

1 serving of oat bran cereal
1 cup skim milk or nonfat soy milk
1 banana
Herbal tea or naturally decaffeinated coffee

½ cup orange or grapefruit juice
8 ounces skim milk or nonfat soy milk
2 small pancakes (nonfat)
2 tablespoons low-cal jelly or syrup
Herbal tea or naturally decaffeinated coffee

2 eggs
1 slice of lean ham (or vegetarian equivalent)
1 cup skim milk or nonfat soy milk
1 slice wheat toast
1 tablespoon low-cal jelly
½ grapefruit
Herbal tea or naturally decaffeinated coffee

⅔ cup bran cereal
1 cup skim milk or nonfat soy milk
1 orange
Herbal tea or naturally decaffeinated coffee

2 eggs
1 slice of Canadian bacon (1 oz) (or vegetarian equivalent)
1 slice wheat toast
1 tablespoon low-cal jelly
1 cup skim milk or nonfat soy milk
1 orange
Herbal tea or naturally decaffeinated coffee

½ cup grapefruit or orange juice
2 small waffles (nonfat)
2 tablespoons low-cal jelly
1 cup skim milk or nonfat soy milk
Herbal tea or naturally decaffeinated coffee

NATURAL-THIN LUNCH EXAMPLES

Like breakfast, lunch is a very essential meal that many people neglect. Skipping lunch is associated with overeating at dinner and late into the evening. Lunch should be a balanced meal with a plentiful amount of carbohydrates, a moderate amount of protein, and little fat. Most people have a tendency to overeat at lunch, thinking that they will burn off the excess calories. However, be cautioned that researchers have determined that when you eat too many calories and too much fat for lunch, you will feel bogged down an hour later. So keep lunches lean and under 400 to 500 calories for a midday lift. Again, pay attention to how you respond to different meals in terms of feeling energetic and having appetite control until your midday snack.

Chicken Sandwich, 3 ounces skinless chicken breast, 2 slices whole-grain bread, 1 sliced tomato, lettuce, onion
1 serving of fruit
Beverage

1½ cups cooked whole-grain pasta
4 ounces low-cal tomato sauce
2 tablespoons nonfat Parmesan cheese
1 serving fruit
Beverage

3 ounces canned tuna (in water)
1 slice wheat toast
1 sliced tomato
1 serving of fruit

1 cup tossed salad w/ 1 tablespoon low-cal dressing
Beverage

1 cup cooked whole-grain rice
1 serving of vegetables
1 cup tossed salad w/ 1 tablespoon low-cal dressing
Beverage

3 ounces chicken breast (skinless) sliced over lettuce
Sliced tomato and onion
1 serving fruit
Beverage

Turkey sandwich, 3 ounces white meat turkey, 2 slices wheat bread, 1 sliced tomato, lettuce, onion
1 serving of fruit
Beverage

9 ounces tofu
1 slice wheat toast
1 fruit serving
3 ounces raw carrot
1 cup tossed salad, w/ 1 tablespoon low-cal dressing
Beverage

NATURAL-THIN DINNER CHOICES

This is the meal at which most people overdo it—for many reasons. Many people with weight problems think that not eating during the day and eating a lot of food at night is the answer. But you know that that is not true. Dinner should be a balanced meal that is not too high in carbohydrates and is low in fat, because this is the time of day when your metabolism is slowing down—which means that your body is more likely to store any excess calories as body fat.

3 ounces chicken breast, skinless
1 slice lowfat melted natural cheese
1 biscuit with 1 tablespoon low-cal jelly
2 cups tossed salad, w/ 1 tablespoon
   low-cal dressing and 1 sliced tomato
1 sliced green pepper
Beverage

3 ounces lean beef
½ cup cooked noodles with ½ cup cooked
   broccoli
½ cup cooked asparagus
1 cup skim milk or nonfat soy milk
Beverage

3 ounces baked fish
½ cup corn
½ cup carrots
1 baked potato w/ 1 slice lowfat natural
   cheese, melted
Beverage

Lean 3–5 ounce turkey burger on bun
2 cups tossed salad w/ 1 tablespoon
   low-cal dressing
½ cup cooked mushrooms
½ cup cooked green beans
Beverage

3–4 ounces chicken breast
Baked potato with 1 slice melted lowfat
   natural cheese
1 cup cooked broccoli
½ cup cooked asparagus
2 cups tossed salad w/ 1 tablespoon
   low-cal dressing
Beverage

1–1½ cups cooked kidney beans
½ cup cooked brown rice
½ cup cooked cauliflower
2 cups tossed salad w/ 1 tablespoon
   low-cal dressing
Beverage

3 ounces lean lamb
Baked potato with 1 slice melted lowfat
   natural cheese
1 cup cooked carrots
½ cup cooked beets
½ cup unsweetened applesauce
2 cups tossed salad w/ 1 tablespoon
   low-cal dressing
Beverage

NATURAL-THIN SNACK CHOICES

When it comes to weight loss and maintenance, snacks can be your salvation. They will help you control your blood sugar levels and appetite so that you will not overeat at your main meals. But be aware that people with weight problems frequently gain most of their weight from overeating snacks. A few crackers leads to half the box; one piece of fruit leads to two, three, and so on. Maintain control when eating snacks so that they work for you, not against you. Eating trim is a habit of eating the right foods in the right amounts at the right times of the day. You know when you will crave foods. Most people experience cravings due to a drop in blood sugar in the late afternoon and late evening. So plan to have a healthy, appetite satisfying snack for these crucial times of the day.

1 serving fruit

1 health food bar

8 ounces nonfat yogurt

Piece of whole-grain toast

Rice cake

Low-fat frozen waffle with a tablespoon of no-fat cottage cheese or jam

Any of the vegetables from the food list

4 ounces low-sodium tomato juice

1 piece of low-fat natural cheese

60- to 90-calorie frozen fruit bar

60- to 90-calorie chocolate sorbet bar

1 tablespoon no-fat fudge topping

Diet hot chocolate (fewer than 60 calories)

No-fat soup (fewer than 120 calories)

Diet beverage

Egg-white omelet, made with two egg whites, vegetables, and mushrooms

LEAN AND MEAN NUTRITION TIPS

This section has been designed to help you embrace your Natural-Thin program. It provides useful tips for home or on the road. It also provides a broad range of information ranging from when to go food shopping to how to eat out at restaurants.

Foods to Avoid

Bagged snack food (face it, you can't eat just one)

Cakes, doughnuts, and pies

Canned foods

Salt and salty foods

Alcohol

Butter, margarine, oils, and cooking fats

Fatty meats

Candy

Fast foods

Ice cream

Eat More Fat-Free and Fat-Reduced Foods

As a result of the realization that too much fat makes *you* fat and is unhealthy, many companies have designed a diversity of fat-free foods. However, this does not mean that these foods are calorie-free. In fact, they are usually high in sugar, so make sure to read the labels. Eating a bag of fat-free snacks can still add up to hundreds of calories. So when eating these foods, keep track of the calories.

Fat-free or low-fat butter sprinkles

Fat-free or low-fat cake

Fat-free or low-fat cheeses

Fat-free or low-fat chips

Fat-free or low-fat cookies

Fat-free or low-fat cream cheese

Fat-free or low-fat crackers

Fat-free or low-fat frozen entrees
Fat-free or low-fat ice cream
Fat-free or low-fat sour cream

Shopping Tips

Weight loss starts by shopping right in the supermarket. Most people gain weight from overeating foods that they bring into their own homes.

Never go shopping when you're hungry. Eat something before you go so you won't be tempted by hunger to buy junk foods.

Prepare a shopping list before you go, to avoid impulse buying.

Be a smart shopper when choosing dressings as flavorings. Some are much higher in calories than others. Select no-fat salad dressings and condiments.

Buy foods that are low in sodium.

Read all labels on canned and packaged foods. Try to avoid foods that don't give nutritional information. This will protect you from eating foods with hidden amounts of calories, fats, and sodium.

Select lean and white meats and other high-protein foods that are lower in the "bad" fats. This includes lean poultry, egg whites, fish, seafood, and beans (which also contain fiber and complex carbohydrates).

Select fresh or frozen vegetables rather than canned, because of their higher nutritional value.

When purchasing canned tuna, chicken, and turkey, always make sure that it is processed in water. (Remember, every tablespoon of oil contains about 14 grams of fat.)

Always choose nonfat and low-fat dairy products: milk, cheese, and yogurt.

Food Flavoring Tips

Use sprinkle-on spices or powders to flavor vegetables, meats, poultry, seafood, fish, etc. Be creative in how you season food; look for suggestions in magazines and books.

Use herb seasoning mixtures made without salt or MSG, fresh herbs, or low-sodium soy sauce to enhance food flavor.

Use nonfat plain yogurt and low-fat cottage cheese in place of mayonnaise and sour cream.

Add nonfat dressings to baked potatoes and other foods for flavor.

Use all-fruit jellies to add flavor to bread, waffles, and pancakes.

Natural-Thin Cooking Tips

Avoid the use of MSG (monosodium glutamate).

Always trim any excess fats and skins from meats, poultry, etc.

Broil, bake, steam, microwave and grill foods; this will reduce the added fat from cooking oils used in frying.

Use spray cooking oils such as Pam rather than regular oils (one tbs. of oil equals 126 calories and 14 grams of fat).

Use low-fat cheese made from low-fat milk instead of regular processed cheese. Swiss cheese has the least amount of sodium with about 100 milligrams per ounce.

Use nonstick frying pans, pressure cooker, steamer baskets, roast racks to cook foods. These tools aid in separating unnecessary fats from foods.

Natural-Thin Restaurant Tips

Choose restaurants that offer a variety of foods that fall under your meal plan.

Before going out, eat a snack to avoid overeating at the restaurant.

Don't eat from the bread basket or load up your salad with salad dressing.

Order an entree with a vegetable; avoid the selections that are made with cream sauces.

Ask the server how food is being prepared, to ensure there is no hidden fat through additives such as butter, sour cream, oils, etc. For example, when ordering a baked potato, ask for it to be served plain. Double-check how the vegetables are prepared; steamed is the best.

Ask to have sauces and dressings served on the side.

Study your menu and look for broiled meats and fish. These tend to be the best choices at most restaurants.

Seafood restaurants offer low-fat meals such as broiled sole, swordfish, etc.

At steakhouses, order a lean cut of meat such as filet, ground steak, or grilled skinless chicken breast, preferably broiled.

Remember restaurant servings tend to vary in size. Be aware of portion size; if it's on your plate, you will probably eat it all up. Choose restaurants that serve modest servings of high-quality gourmet foods, not large quantities of low-quality foods.

Don't always feel that you have to clean your plate. Have the waiter remove your plate immediately so it won't tempt you into finishing it all up.

Natural-Thin Tips for Eating on the Run

Pack fruit, cereal, air-popped popcorn, and other healthy foods from the snack list. You know you are going to get hungry and need to eat, so bring along something healthy instead of being tempted into the loads of high-fat foods you will encounter along your journey.

Prepare lunch if you know you'll be on the road or on an airplane.

Don't put yourself in a position where there is no healthy food available.

Order special meals when making plane reservations. Kosher food plates, fruit plates, and other meals are available when preordered through a travel agent or the airline.

Bring bottled water with you to ensure you meet your daily requirement.

Natural-Thin General Eating Tips

Plan to eat meals at approximately the same time every day. This will increase the efficiency of the body's digestive process.

Eat fresh foods whenever possible.

Reduce salt intake as much as possible. (Use a salt shaker with fewer holes or a wooden salt mill filled with coarse sea salt.)

Keep a food diary to keep track of what you are eating. Your food intake will dictate how the scale moves; up or down.

Try not to eat in front of the TV, when reading the paper, etc. This will allow you to focus on enjoying the meal. There is a tendency to overeat when you are distracted.

Try not to go into the kitchen at any other time but mealtime. This will keep you from being tempted.

Don't skip meals.

Avoid eating late at night. This is the time when the metabolism will be most unlikely to burn calories. It's one of the habits you most need to break.

Keep track in your food diary of the times you are most likely to snack. Have some type of low-calorie alternatives, such as fruit or celery and carrot sticks, readily available.

Drink eight or more glasses of filtered water every day. Squeeze fresh lemon and/or lime in your water for added flavor. For some, this makes it easier to drink the daily quota.

Use calorie-free beverages, such as low-sodium club soda or flavored sugar-free seltzer. Avoid artificially sweetened beverages.

NATURAL-THIN FAT BURNING EXERCISE GUIDELINES

Experts agree that exercise can play an important part in your weight management program. Incorporating some type of exercise in your trim lifestyle can help increase your rate of fat loss and provide you with lots of other health benefits. Some of these benefits include:

- Increased metabolic rate
- Reduced body fat
- Increased energy
- Improved muscle tone
- Stronger bones
- Improved cardiovascular fitness
- Better posture
- Longevity benefits
- Increased strength
- Better sleep

The list of exercise benefits continues to grow as more research is performed on people of all ages. However, be advised that if you have never exercised, have not exercised in the past few months, are over thirty-five, or are very overweight, be sure to consult a doctor before starting an exercise program, and review the precautions listed in the beginning of this section. It is important to start slowly, at a pace that will not exhaust you or cause you to become dizzy or out of breath. Your body will respond quickly to exercise, but just how quickly depends on your personal constitution. As you get accustomed to a particular level of exercise, you will be able to increase your exercise intensity to derive more benefits. Here is what some of the recent research has reported on how the body responds to exercise.

Exercise Versus Physical Activity

Many people who move around a lot and are active will indeed burn up more calories per day than a person who is less active. But there is a difference between exercise and physical activity. Physical activity is a general term used to describe the act of expending energy by moving your body around. Physical activity can be light, like sitting down and watching television, or heavy, like working in the garden all day. Exercise, on the other hand, is a specific type of physical activity designed and undertaken to meet specific goals. Gener-

ally, exercise programs are structured for improved aerobic fitness, body building, and improved flexibility.

Increasing your activity level is a good start toward improving your health and burning extra calories. Keep the body moving around as much as possible. One of the simplest types of exercise to promote fat loss is walking. When you walk for exercise, you will need to keep up a steady pace for 45 minutes or longer to achieve fat-burning results. One recent study conducted on women walking four nights per week found that they all lost weight and improved their fitness.

Some guidelines for starting a walking program, after you have received your physician's approval: Walk three to four times per week. Begin at a walking rate that is comfortable for your level of fitness. Include a five- to ten-minute warm-up and cool-down period. Each week increase the pace of walking; add 5 to 10 minutes every two weeks, until your program lasts 45 to 60 minutes. Before you know it, you will be walking off pounds of fat per month. By adding a pair of hand weights to your walking routine, you will burn more calories and firm and strengthen your shoulders and arms.

How Hard Should You Exercise?

Your individual fitness level will determine the intensity and duration at which you exercise. You do not have to exercise strenuously and work up a sweat to derive benefits from exercise. As indicated above, even a regular walking exercise program is great. Consistency is the key to success, so make your exercise program an enjoyable part of your life, something to look forward to.

Beginners should start by walking or by following along with one of the many TV exercise shows. Once you are in shape and your physician gives you the okay, you should target your exercise sessions to maintain a steady heart rate of about 65 percent of your maximum heart rate for your age. One way to determine this is with the following formula.

$$\text{Exercise heart rate} = (220 - \text{age}) \times 0.65$$

For a forty-two-year-old women this would be:

$$178 \times 0.65 = 115 \text{ beats per minute}$$

As you get more fit, you may increase your exercise heart rate to 70 percent of maximum. However, only do so under the advice of your doctor.

There are three phases to a typical aerobic exercise session, whether you're a beginner or an advanced exerciser: warm-up, aerobic exercise, and cool-down. Each phase has a specific purpose.

Warm-up phase. This phase prepares the body for the aerobic phase, and helps reduce the chance of injury. You should warm up for between 5 and 10 minutes, combining stretching with limbering exercises. Examples of warm-up exercises include arm circles, leg circles, small kicks, knee lifts, and stretching. These exercises should be performed in a very smooth and controlled fashion at a moderate pace.

Aerobic phase. There are a variety of exercises that qualify as aerobic, which basically means working the large muscle groups to increase breathing rate and heart rate, which increases your demand for oxygen and promotes fat-burning. Start slowly and increase the intensity of your exercise activity to a pace you can endure without getting out of breath or dizzy.

Cool-down phase. The purpose of the cool-down phase is to provide a transition between vigorous aerobic work and less aerobically taxing exercise. This period should last between 5 and 10 minutes. Cool-downs should consist of light activity, such as slow walking and stretching. This will allow your heart rate to decrease gradually, while your body movements help the blood flow through your body.

Muscle Building Exercises

Along with aerobic-type exercises such as walking, running, or cycling, adding muscle-building exercises to your fitness program will help to tone your body, sculpt muscle, and in some cases build up bone mass.

There are many types of exercise programs you can follow, from using the most sophisticated weight training machines to doing calisthenics using your body weight.

Muscle-building exercises are generally short in duration and high in intensity—for example, lifting heavy weights for only a minute or so. They involve working various muscle groups of your body through using weights or calisthenics. Many of you can start by lifting your own body weight as you follow along with one of the fitness shows on television, or working with weights at home or at the gym. It's a good idea to consult with a certified fitness trainer who can help you design a weight training program that is compatible with your physical condition and time requirements.

How much weight training is needed to see results? Well, contrary to what most people believe, a recent study measured increased muscle mass in women who exercised only 45 minutes twice a week. They started by performing two sets of ten repetitions for each of six different exercises. Then after a few weeks, they performed three sets of ten repetitions for each exercise. Here is the program they followed, which consisted of two supervised sessions per week, with six types of weight-lifting exercises performed each session. The first session consisted of: dumbbell bench presses, seated dumbbell press, lat pull-down, dumbbell curl, leg extension, and leg curl. The second session consisted of fly, upright row, lat pull-down, easy biceps curl, leg extension, and leg curl. The study reported that the exercises rested for about 30 to 60 seconds between sets of a particular exercise, and 2 to 3 minutes between each type of exercise.

An added benefit of weight-lifting exercise is increase in bone mass. In a recent study published in the December 1997 issue of the *Journal of Sports Medicine and Physical Fitness,* premenopausal women followed a weight-lifting program for six months, and at the end of the study there was an increase in bone mass observed, as well as increased strength and muscle mass. The women in this study exercised for 1 hour three times a week. They also varied their training intensity, with light, moderate, and heavy days.

Natural-Thin Exercise Guidelines
Before beginning any exercise program, consult with your physician, who will help determine your fitness level and the level of exercise you are capable of safely performing.

Schedule a fixed time to exercise and stick to it. Treat your exercise time as you would any other appointment.

Drink plenty of fluids before and after exercising to prevent dehydration.

Wear appropriate athletic footwear and clothing that is comfortable and suitable for the indoor or outdoor temperature.

Use quality exercise equipment that is well made and has smooth action.

Never exercise to the point of heavy breathing or dizziness. If exercise becomes fatiguing, stop immediately and rest.

Exercise with a partner when possible. This makes your exercise a social event and increases your chances of keeping up with it. Never exercise alone when lifting weights; always have a partner or spotter assist you.

Summary of Common Exercises

COMMON AEROBIC EXERCISES

Cycling, outdoors

Cycling, stationary

Running, outdoors

Treadmill

Aerobic dancing

Rowing machine

Walking and fast walking

Basketball

Tennis and racquetball

Hiking

Swimming

Cross-country skiing, outdoors

Cross-country skiing machine

Stair-climber machines

COMMON STRENGTH/
BODY BUILDING EXERCISES

Upper Body Exercises

Shoulders (barbell presses or lateral raises)

Chest (bench presses or lying dumb-bell fly)

Back (lat pull-downs or seated cable rowing)

Trapezius (barbell shrugs or upright rowing)

Biceps (barbell curls or dumbbell curls)

Triceps (press-downs or lying barbell extensions)

Stomach (sit-ups or leg raises)

Lower Body Exercises

Thighs (seated leg extensions)

Hamstrings (lying leg curl)

Calves (calf raises)

NATURAL-THIN BEHAVIORAL STRATEGIES

An important part of the Natural-Thin weight management lifestyle to maximize your fat-loss potential is to take into consideration your eating behavior. Scientists have determined that people who have a problem with weight management generally have a problem with controlling their amount of eating. It is important for you to realize that you need to pay close attention to your eating patterns and learn from your history with food and dieting. Your history with food will give you the answers you need to become successful at being trim.

Think about the times of the day and the types of foods that are associated with your compulsion to overeat. Is it in the mid-afternoon, the late evening, or when you go out to eat? Once you identify which foods you tend to overeat and the times of day you overeat them, then getting back your control is simply a matter of planning. Plan to have healthy, appetite-satisfying foods around to keep you from bingeing. A simple rule of thumb is not to skip meals or let yourself get hungry, even if this means having a small snack an hour before your dinner. In fact, studies have demonstrated that people who have a predinner snack are more likely to eat fewer calories for dinner.

The next time you are tempted to binge or overeat at a restaurant, remember this: Behavior predicts your weight. Yes, when you start returning to your old ways of eating, you may be able to get away with it for a few days or weeks, but eventually you will see the pounds of fat returning to your body.

The mind is unbelievably powerful—put it to work for you. Researcher William P. Morgan researched the role psychological factors play in influencing metabolic rate. He found that both posthypnotic suggestion and suggestion in the nonhypnotic state can increase the resting and exercising metabolic rate. This means that your thoughts, feelings, and sensations can influence your metabolism. So keep a positive attitude, and maximize the role your "mental edge" can play in your weight-management program.

Natural-Thin Behavior Tips

Take control of food in your life, and do not let food control you.

Learn from your history with food; recognize your eating patterns and the foods you tend to overeat.

Set realistic weight-management goals and stick to them. Most experts agree that losing fat at the rate of 1 to 2 pounds a week is healthy for most people.

Increase your physical activity and stick to your exercise program.

Schedule a time in your daily routine to exercise. Following a consistent pattern will ensure success.

Approach being trim as a skill and lifelong commitment.

Realize that gimmicky diets don't work for long-term weight management for the majority of people, because they often demand too many changes too fast. Give yourself daily, weekly, and monthly goals that will allow you to slowly phase into a trimmer lifestyle.

Protect your weight loss accomplishments, even when they fall short of your ultimate goal. Make it a point to maintain what you lose.

Don't eat out of boredom, depression, stress, or other negative emotions. Become aware of these times and become involved in activities that are more constructive and positive. Go for a walk instead, or get engrossed in something that diverts your attention from eating.

Watch out for the weekends. In a study that examined weekly rhythms of eating, the researcher determined that more total calories and bigger meals were consumed on weekends. This was associated with longer weekend mealtimes and a greater number of people present.

Always lose weight for yourself first, not your spouse, family, or friends. Hold yourself personally accountable for all aspects of your weight management plan. Take charge of your attitude. Don't let someone else decide it for you.

Commit yourself to consistent self-improvement.

When you are craving food, go to the gym, take a walk, or become involved in a rewarding activity. The craving will pass in a few minutes, but losing the weight takes much, much longer.

Become the most positive and enthusiastic person you know. Think like a champion. Being a champion means having the spirit and dedication to develop skills that will pay off in the end, allowing you to reap all the rewards that go along with being Natural-Thin.

NATURAL-THIN PLANNING AND GOAL-SETTING LOG SHEETS

Regular use of the Food Eating Log and Body Measurement Log sheets will help you keep your weight loss plan on track.

First, use the Body Measurement Log to determine your starting body measurements. Note that you will have to perform some simple math calculations to determine your BMI. Once you determine your BMI, this number will indicate your level of overweightness. Along with your waist circumference measurement, you will also be able to determine your risk level for developing type 2 diabetes, hypertension, and cardiovascular disease.

Second, start using the Food Eating Log to track your eating patterns and to determine which foods you tend to overeat, and the times of day you overeat. You can also use the Food Eating Log sheets to plan your meals.

One of the habits of the slim and trim is that they keep track of their body measurements and foods they eat. When they start overeating, or start gaining weight, they take immediate action to maintain their healthy body weight.

FOOD EATING LOG

	BREAKFAST	MORNING SNACK	LUNCH
SUNDAY			
MONDAY			
TUESDAY			
WEDNESDAY			
THURSDAY			
FRIDAY			
SATURDAY			

FOOD EATING LOG

AFTERNOON SNACK	DINNER	EVENING SNACK

NATURAL-THIN BODY MEASUREMENT LOG

MEASUREMENT	START	ULTIMATE GOAL	DATE	DATE	DATE	DATE	DATE	DATE	DATE	DATE	DATE
Weight (pounds)											
Height (inches)											
Waist circumference*											
Upper right arm											
Chest											
Hips											
Right thigh											
Body mass index (BMI) (refer to calculation below chart)											
Percentage body fat (optional)											

*Take your waist circumference by lining up the tape measure at the top of your right hip bone (iliac crest).

A safe rate of weight loss is considered to be 1 to 2 pounds of body fat per week.

Body mass index (BMI) is a measurement calculated using your weight and height measurements. BMI is calculated as follows: $[\text{pounds}/\text{inches}^2] \times 704.5$. For example, for an individual who weighs 195 pounds and is 70 inches tall, the BMI is calculated as follows: $[195/70^2] \times 704.5$. First square your height, $70 \times 70 = 4,900$, then use this number to divide your weight by $[195/4,900] = 0.0397959$, then times this number by $704.5 = 28$ BMI.

How to use the BMI number and waist circumference to determine if your body weight is healthy or not: You are considered underweight if your BMI is less than 18.5. You are considered to be a normal weight if your BMI is 18.5 to 24.9 You are considered overweight if your BMI is between 25 and 29.9. You are considered to be in Obesity Class I if your BMI is 30 to 34.9. You are considered to be in Obesity Class II if your BMI is 35 to 39.9. You are considered to be in the Extreme Obesity Class III if your BMI is 40 or greater. Concerning your waist measurement, men who have a waist measurement equal to or under 40 inches and are classified as overweight have an increased risk for developing type 2 diabetes, hypertension, and cardiovascular disease. Men who have a waist measurement over 40 inches and are classified as Obese have an increased risk of developing these diseases as their level of obesity increases. Women who have a waist measurement equal to or under 35 inches and are classified as overweight have an increased risk for developing type 2 diabetes, hypertension, and cardiovascular disease. Women who have a waist measurement over 35 inches and are classified as Obese have an increased risk of developing these diseases as their level of obesity increases.

There are several ways you can determine your percentage body fat, which include the use of skinfold calipers, water-weighing methods, bioelectrical impedance machines, and infra-red interactance method using the Futrex Analyzer. Note that all of these methods will display variations, and for most people using the BMI and waist determinations will be adequate. Individuals who are athletic, or want a better understanding of where their weight changes are coming from, body fat or muscle mass, should seek a qualified individual to determine the percentage of body fat.

SELECTED REFERENCES

The following are some key scientific references consulted during the writing of this book. This list should serve as a valuable resource for readers interested in reading the primary literature on dietary supplements and learning firsthand about their scientific validation.

Abbey, M., P. J. Nestel, and P. A. Baghurst. "Antioxidant Vitamins and Low-Density-Lipoprotein Oxidation." *American Journal of Clinical Nutrition* 58 (1993): 525–32.

Acheson, K. J., et al. "Caffeine and Coffee: Their Influence on Metabolic Rate and Substrate Utilization in Normal Weight and Obese Individuals." *American Journal of Clinical Nutrition* 33 (1980): 989–97.

Adami, S., et al. "Ipriflavone Prevents Radical Bone Loss in Postmenopausal Women with Low Bone Mass over Two Years." *Osteoporosis International* 7 (1997): 119–25.

Adelekan, D. A., and D. I. Thurnham. "Plasma Ferritin Concentrations in Anemic Children: Relative Importance of Malaria, Riboflavin Deficiency, and Other Infections." *American Journal of Clinical Nutrition* 50 (1990): 453–6.

Adler, A. J., and B. J. Holub. "Effect of Garlic and Fish-Oil Supplementation on Serum Lipid and Lipoprotein Concentrations in Hypercholesterolemic Men." *American Journal of Clinical Nutrition* 65 (1997): 445–50.

Adlercreutz, H., et al. "Excretion of the Lignans Enterolactone and Enterodiol and of Equol in Omnivorous and Vegetarian Postmenopausal Women and in Women with Breast Cancer." *Lancet* 2 (1982): 1295–8.

Adon, M. B., T. Lloyd, and V. Matkovic. "Supplementation Trials with Calcium Citrate Malate: Evidence in Favor of Increasing the Calcium RDA During Childhood and Adolescence." *Journal of Nutrition* 124 (1994): 1412–7.

Afanas'ev, B. G., V. A. Zhestovskii, K. V. Mazunov, and K. L. Maevskii. "Comparison of the Effects of Siberian Ginseng and Oxygen/Salt Beverage on Development of

Adaptation to the Heat" (in Russian). *Voprosy Pitania* 1 (1973): 3–9.

Agnusdei, D., et al. "Effects of Ipriflavone on Bone Mass and Calcium Metabolism in Postmenopausal Osteoporosis." *Bone and Mineral* 19 (1992): S43–8.

Agnusdei, D., et al. "Short-Term Treatment of Paget's Disease of Bone with Ipriflavone." *Bone and Mineral* 19 (1992): S35–42.

Ai, C., and L. Li. "Stereostructure of Salvianolic Acid B and Isolation of Salvianolic Acid C from Salvia Miltiorrhiza." *Journal of Natural Products* 51, no. 1 (1988): 145–9.

Alam, N., B. Wojtyniak, and M. M. Rahaman. "Anthropometric Indicators and Risk of Death." *American Journal of Clinical Nutrition* 49 (1989): 884–8.

Alfieri, M. A. H., J. Pomerleau, D. M. Grace, and L. Anderson. "Fiber Intake of Normal Weight, Moderately Obese, and Severely Obese Subjects." *Obesity Research* 3, no. 6 (1995): 541–7.

Alfthan, G., et al. "Selenium Metabolism and Platelet Glutathione Peroxidase Activity in Healthy Finnish Men: Effects of Selenium Yeast, Selenite, and Selenate." *American Journal of Clinical Nutrition* 53 (1991): 120–5.

Alhomida, A. S., et al. "Age, Sex, and Diabetes-Related Changes in Total, Free, and Acyl Carnitine in Human Plasma." *Medical Science Research* 23 (1995): 167–9.

Allain, H., et al. "Effect of Two Doses of Ginkgo Biloba Extract on the Dual-Coding Test in Elderly Subjects." *Clinical Therapeutics* 15, no. 3 (1993): 549–58.

Aloia, J. F., A. Vaswani, R. Ma, and E. Flaster. "To What Extent Is Bone Mass Determined by Fat-Free or Fat Mass?" *American Journal of Clinical Nutrition* 61 (1995): 1110–4.

Amaducci, L., et al. "Use of Phosphatidylserine in Alzheimer's Disease." *Annals of New York Academy of Sciences* 40 (1991): 245–9.

Amatruda, J. M., T. L. Biddle, M. L. Patton, and D. H. Lockwood. "Vigorous Supplementation of a Hypocaloric Diet Prevents Cardiac Arrhythmias and Mineral Depletion." *American Journal of Medicine* 74 (1983): 1016–22.

Ambrus, J. L., H. B. Lassman, and J. J. De Marchi. "Absorption of Exogenous and Endogenous Proteolytic Enzymes." *Clinical Pharmacology and Therapeutics* 8, no. 3 (1968).

Anderson, J. W., L. Story, B. Sieling, and W.-J. L. Chen. "Hypocholesterolemic Effects of Oat-Bran or Bean Intake for Hypercholesterolemic Men." *American Journal of Clinical Nutrition* 40 (1984): 1146–55.

Anderson, R. A., et al. "Elevated Intakes of Supplemental Chromium Improve Glucose and Insulin Variables in Individuals with Type 2 Diabetes." *Diabetes* 46 (1997): 1786–91.

Andersson, B., K. Terning, and P. Bjorntorp. "Dietary Treatment of Obesity Localized in Different Regions: The Effect of Dietary Fibre on Relapse." *International Journal of Obesity* 11, supplement 1 (1987): 79–85.

Andon, M. B., M. Peacock, R. L. Kanerva, and J. A. S. De Castro. "Calcium Absorption from Apple and Orange Juice Fortified with Calcium Citrate Malate." *Journal of the American College of Nutrition* 15, no. 3 (1996): 313–6.

Antila, H., et al. "Serum Iron, Zinc, Copper, Selenium, and Bromide Concentrations After Coronary Bypass Operation." *Journal of Parenteral and Enteral Nutrition* 14, no. 1 (1990): 85–9.

Araghiniknam, M., et al. "Antioxdant Activity of Dioscorea and Dehydroepiandrosterone (DHEA) in Older Humans." *Life Sciences* 59, no. 11 (1996): 147–57.

Arase, Y., et al. "The Long-Term Efficacy of Glycyrrhizin in Chronic Hepatitis C Patients." *Cancer* 79, no. 8 (1997): 1494–1500.

Arenas, J., et al. "Carnitine in Muscle, Serum, and Urine of Nonprofessional Athletes: Effects of Physical Exercise, Training, and L-carnitine Administration." *Muscle and Nerve* 14 (1991): 598–604.

Arenas, J., et al. "Effects of L-carnitine on the Pyruvate Dehydrogenase Complex and Carnitine Palmitoyl Transferase Activities in Muscle of Endurance Athletes." *FEBS Letters* 341 (1994): 91–3.

Aronstam, A., and D. L. Aston. "A Comparative Trial of a Controlled-Release Iron Tablet Preparation ('Ferrocontin' Continus) and Ferrous Fumarate Tablets." *Pharmatherapeutica* 3, no. 4 (1982): 263–7.

Arrigo, A., R. Casale, M. Buonocore, and C. Ciano. "Effects of Acetyl-l-carnitine on Reaction Times in Patients with Cerebro-vascular Insufficiency." *International Journal of Clinical Pharmacological Research* 10, nos. 1–2 (1990): 133–7.

Asano, K., et al. "Effect of Eleutheroccocus Senticosus Extract on Human Physical Working Capacity." *Planta Medica* 3 (1986): 175–7.

Astin, J. A. "Why Patients Use Alternative Medicine: Results of a National Study." *JAMA* 279, no. 19 (1998): 1548–53.

Astrup, A., J. Madsen, J. J. Holst, and N. J. Christensen. "The Effect of Chronic Ephedrine Treatment on Substrate Utilization, the Sympathoadrenal Activity, and Energy Expenditure During Glucose-Induced Thermogenesis in Man." *Metabolism* 35, no. 3 (1986): 260–5.

Astrup, A., E. Vrist, and F. Quaade. "Dietary Fibre Added to Very Low Calorie Diet Reduces Hunger and Alleviates Constipation." *International Journal of Obesity* 14 (1990): 105–12.

Auer, W., et al. "Hypertension and Hyperlipidaemia: Garlic Helps in Mild Cases." *British Journal of Clinical Practice* 69 (1990): 3–6.

August, D., et al. "Determination of Zinc and Copper Absorption at Three Dietary Zn-Cu Ratios by Using Stable Isotope Methods in Young Adult and Elderly Subjects." *American Journal of Clinical Nutrition* 50 (1989): 1457–63.

Augusti, K. T. "Hypocholesterolaemic Effect of Garlic Allium Sativum Linn." *Indian Journal of Experimental Biology* 15 (1977): 489–90.

Avenell, A., P. R. Richmond, M. E. J. Lean, and D. M. Reid. "Bone Loss Associated with High Fibre Weight Reduction Diet in Postmenopausal Women." *European Journal of Clinical Nutrition* 48 (1994): 561–6.

Avorn, J., et al. "Reduction of Bacteriruria and Pyuria After Ingestion of Cranberry Juice." *JAMA* 271 (1994): 751–54.

Aybak, M., A. Sermet, M. O. Ayyildiz, and A. Z. Karakilcik. "Effect of Oral Pyridoxine Hydrochloride Supplementation on Arterial Blood Pressure in Patients with Essential Hypertension." *Arzneimittel-Forschung* 45, no. 12 (1995): 1271–3.

Babin, F., et al. "Nervonic Acid in Red Blood Cell Sphingomyelin in Premature Infants: An Index of Myelin Maturation?" *Lipids* 28, no. 7 (1993): 627–30.

Baburin, E. F., P. V. Porkalov, and V. V. Polonskij. "Effects of Siberian Ginseng Whole Plant and Ginseng (Korean) on Physical Conditions of Scuba Divers" (in Russian). *Lek. Sredstva Dall'nego Vostoka* 10 (1970): 67–71.

Bach, D., and L. Ebeling. "Long-Term Drug Treatment of Benign Prostatic Hyperplasia: Results of a Prospective Three-Year Multicenter Study Using Sabal Extract IDS 89." *Phytomedicine* 3, no. 2 (1996): 105–11.

Baetgen, D. "Erfolge in der Keuchhusten-Behandlung mit Echinacin." *Therapiewoche* 34 (1984): 5115–9.

Bak, J. F., N. Moller, and O. Schmitz. "Effects of Growth Hormone on Fuel Utilization and Muscle Glycogen Snythase Activity in Normal Humans." *American Journal of Physiology* 260 (1991): 736–42.

Ballot, D. E., et al. "Fortification of Curry Powder with NaFe(111)EDTA in an Iron-Deficient Population: Report of a Controlled Iron-Fortification Trial." *American Journal of Clinical Nutrition* 49 (1989): 162–9.

Banderet, L. E., and H. R. Lieberman. "Treatment with Tyrosine, a Neurotransmitter Precursor, Reduces Environmental Stress in Humans." *Brain Research Bulletin* 22 (1989): 759–62.

Banerjee, U., and J. Izquierdo. "Antistress and Antifatigue Properties of Panax Ginseng: Comparison with Piracetam." *Acta Physiologica Latino Americana* 32 (1982): 277–85.

Barbul, A., S. A. Lazarou, H. L. Wasserkrug, and G. Efron. "Arginine Enhances Wound Healing and Lymphocyte Immune Responses in Humans." *Surgery* 108 (1990): 331–7.

Barlet, A., et al. "Wirksamkeit eines Extraktes aus Pygeum africanum in der medikamentosen Therapie von Miktionsstorungen infolge einer benignen Prostatahyperplasie: Bewertung objektiver und subjektiver Parameter; Eine placebokontrollierte doppelbline Multizenterstudie." *Wiener Klinische Wochenschrift* 102 (1990): 667–73.

Baron, J. A., et al. "A Randomized Controlled Trial of Low Carbohydrate and Low Fat/High Fiber Diets for Weight Loss." *American Journal of Public Health* 76, no. 11 (1986): 1293–6.

Barrie, S. A., J. V. Wright, and J. E. Pizzorno. "Effects of Garlic Oil on Platelet Aggregation, Serum Lipids, and Blood Pressure in Humans." *Journal of Orthomolecular Medicine* 2, no. 1 (1987): 15–21.

Barrie, S. A., J. V. Wright, J. E. Pizzorno, E. Kutter, and P. C. Barron. "Comparative Absorption of Zinc Picolinate, Zinc Citrate, and Zinc Gluconate in Humans." *Agents and Actions* 21 (1987): 223–8.

Barsacchi, R., et al. "Myocardial Vitamin E Is Consumed During Cardiopulmonary Bypass: Indirect Evidence of Free Radical Generation in Human Ischemic Heart." *International Journal of Cardiology* 37 (1992): 339–43.

Barth, S., et al. "Influences of Ginkgo Biloba on Cyclosporin A Induced Lipid Peroxidation in Human Liver Microsomes in Comparison to Vitamin E, Glutathoine, and N-acetylcysteine." *Biochemical Pharmacology* 41, no. 10 (1991): 1521–6.

Bascom, R., A. Kagey-Sobotka, and D. Proud. "Effect of Intranasal Capsaicin on Symptoms and Mediator Release." *Journal of Pharmacology and Experimental Therapeutics* 259 (1991): 1323–7.

Baskaran, K., et al. "Antidiabetic Effect of a Leaf Extract from Gymnema Sylvestre in Non-insulin-dependent Diabetes Mellitus Patients." *Journal of Ethnopharmacology* 30 (1990): 295–305.

Bassi, P., et al. "Estratto standardizzato di Pygeum Africanum nel trattamento dell'ipertrofia prostatica benigna: Studio clinico controllato versus placebo." *Minerva Urologica e Nefrologica* 39 (1987): 45–50.

Bates, C. J., et al. "Riboflavin Status in Gambian Pregnant and Lactating Women and Its Implications for Recommended Dietary Allowances." *American Journal of Clinical Nutrition* 34 (1981): 928–35.

Bauer, R., and H. Wagner. "Echinacea Species as Potential Immunostimulatory Drugs." *Economic and Medical Plant Research* 1 (1991): 253–321.

Baumann, G., S. Felix, U. Sattelberger, and G. Klein. "Cardiovascular Effects of Forskolin (HL 362) in Patients with Idiopathic Congestive Cardiomyopathy—A Comparative Study with Dobutamine and Sodium Nitroprusside." *Journal of Cardiovascular Pharmacology* 16, no. 1 (1990): 93–100.

Bazzarre, T. L., et al. "Plasma Amino Acid Responses of Trained Athletes to Two Successive Exhaustion Trials with and without Interim Carbohydrate Feeding." *Journal of the American College of Nutrition* 11, no. 5 (1992): 501–10.

Beattie, V. A., C. A. Edwards, J. P. Hosker, D. R. Cullen, J. D. Ward, and N. W. Read. "Does Adding Fibre to a Low Energy, High Carbohydrate, Low Fat Diet Confer Any Benefit to the Management of Newly Diagnosed Overweight Type II Diabetics?" *BMJ* 296 (1988): 1147–9.

Beckman, K. B., and B. N. Ames. "The Free Radical Theory of Aging Matures." *Physiological Reviews* 78, no. 2 (1998): 547–81.

Belfiore, F., V. Borzi, E. Napoli, and G. M. Rabuazzo. "Enzymes Related to Lipogenesis in the Adipose Tissue of Obese Subjects." *Metabolism* 25, no. 5 (1976): 483–93.

Belizan, J. M., et al. "Reduction of Blood Pressure with Calcium Supplementation in Young Adults." *JAMA* 249, no. 9 (1983): 1161–5.

Belko, A. Z., et al. "Effects of Exercise on Riboflavin Requirements of Young Women." *American Journal of Clinical Nutrition* 37 (1983): 509–17.

Bell, K. M., L. Plon, W. E. Bunney, and S. G. Potkin. "S-adenosylmethionine Treatment of Depression: A Controlled Clinical Trial." *American Journal of Psychiatry* 145, no. 9 (1988): 1110–4.

Bell, L. P., K. J. Hectorn, H. Reynolds, and D. B. Hunninghake. "Cholesterol-Lowering Effects of Soluble-Fiber Cereals as Part of a Prudent Diet for Patients with Mild to Moderate Hypercholesterolemia." *American Journal of Clinical Nutrition* 52 (1990): 1020–6.

Bellizzi, M. C., et al. "Vitamin E and Coronary Heart Disease: The European Paradox." *European Journal of Clinical Nutrition* 48 (1994): 822–31.

Bellone, J., et al. "Effects of Phenylalanine, Histidine, and Leucine on Basal and GHRH-Stimulated GH Secretion and on PRL, Insulin, and Glucose Levels in Short Children: Comparison with the Effects of Arginine." *Journal of Pediatric Endocrinology and Metabolism* 3, no. 9 (1996): 523–31.

Bellone, J., et al. "Methionine Potentiates Both Basal and GHRH-Induced GH Secretion in Children." *Clinical Endocrinology* 47 (1997): 61–4.

Ben-Amotz, A., and Y. Levy. "Bioavailability of a Natural Isomer Mixture Compared with Synthetic All-Trans B-carotene in Human Serum." *American Journal of Clinical Nutrition* 63 (1996): 729–734.

Berdyshev, V. V. "Effects of Siberian Ginseng and Physical Training on Marines in Tropical Climates." *Lek. Sredstv. Dal'nego Vostoka* 10 (1970): 64–6.

Berges, R., J. Windeler, H. Trampisch, T. Senge, and the B-sitosterol Study Group "Randomised, Placebo-Controlled, Double-Blind Clinical Trial of B-sitosterol in Patients with Benign Prostatic Hyperplasia." *Lancet* 345 (June 1995): 1529–32.

Berglund, B., and P. Hemmingson. "Effects of Caffeine Ingestion on Exercise Performance at Low and High Altitudes in Cross-Country Skiers." *International Journal of Sports Medicine* 3 (1982): 234–6.

Berliner, J. A., and J. W. Heinecke. "The Role of Oxidized Lipoproteins in Atherogenesis." *Free Radical Biology and Medicine* 20, no. 5 (1996): 707–27.

Bersudsky, Y., M. Kotler, M. Shifrin, and R. H. Belmaker. "A Preliminary Study of Possible Psychoactive Effects of Intravenous Forskolin in Depressed and Schizophrenic Patients." *Journal of Neural Transmission* 103 (1996): 1463–7.

Berthold, H. K., T. Sudhop, and K. von Bergmann. "Effect of a Garlic Oil Preparation on Serum Lipoproteins and Cholesterol Metabolism: A Randomized Controlled Trial." *JAMA* 279, no. 23 (1998): 1900–4.

Besset, A., et al. "Increase in Sleep-Related GH and PRl Secretion After Chronic Arginine Asparate Administration in Man." *Acta Endocrinologica* 99 (1982): 18–23.

Best, M. M., C. H. Duncan, V. Loon, and J. D. Wathen. "The Effect of Sitosterol on Serum Lipids." *American Journal of Medicine* (1955): 61–70.

Beveridge, J.M.R., H. L. Haust, and W. F. Connell. "Magnitude of the Hypocholesterolemic Effect of Dietary Sitosterol in Man." *Journal of Nutrition* 83 (1964): 119–22.

Bhate, H., G. Gerster, and E. Gracza. "Orale Pramedikation mit Zubereitungen aus Piper methysticum bei operativen Eingriffen in Epiduralanathesie." *Erfahrungsheilkunde* 6 (1989): 339–45.

Bhathema, S. J., et al. "Decreased Plasma Enkephalins in Copper Deficiency in Man." *American Journal of Clinical Nutrition* 43 (1986): 42–6.

Bierenbaum, M. L., R. P. Reichstein, H. N. Bhagavan, T. R. Watkins, and K. L. Jordan. "Relationship Between Serum Lipid Peroxidation Products in Hypercholesterolemic Subjects and Vitamin E Status." *Biochemistry International* 28, no. 1 (1992): 57–66.

Bingol, F., and B. Sener. "A Review of Terrestrial Plants and Marine Organisms Having Anti-inflammatory Activity." *International Journal of Pharmacognosy* 33, no. 2 (1995): 81–97.

Birdsall, T. C., and G. S. Kelly. "Berberine: Therapeutic Potential of an Alkaloid Found in Several Medicinal Plants." *Alternative Medicine Review* 2, no. 2 (1997): 94–103.

Bisler, H., R. Pfeifer, N. Kluken, and P. Pauschinger. "Wirkung von Robkastaniensamenextrakt auf die transkapillare Filtration bei chronisch venoser Insuffizienz." *Deutsche Medizische Wochenschrift* 111 (1986): 1321–9.

Bjerve, K. S., S. Fischer, F. Wammer, and T. Egeland. "Alpha-linolenic Acid and Long-Chain W-3 Fatty Acid Supplementation in Three Patients with 2–3 Fatty Acid Deficiency: Effect on Lymphocyte Function, Plasma and Red Cell Lipids, and Prostanoid Formation." *American Journal of Clinical Nutrition* 49 (1989): 290–300.

Blair, S., et al. "Physical Activity, Nutrition, and Chronic Disease." *Medical Science in Sports and Exercise* 28, no. 3 (1996): 335–349.

Bliznakov, E. G., and D. J. Wilkins. "Biochemical and Clinical Consequences of Inhibiting Coenzyme Q10 Biosynthesis by Lipid-Lowering HMG-CoA Reductase Inhibitors (Statins): A Critical Overview." *Advances in Therapy* 15, no. 4 (1998): 218–28.

Block, G., and E. Lanza. "Dietary Fiber Sources in the United States by Demographic Group." *Journal of the National Cancer Institute* 79 (1987): 83–91.

Blokhin, B. N. "Effect of Siberian Ginseng Root Extract and Leaf on Endurance in Physical Labor" (in Russian). *Lek. Sredstva Dall'nego Vostoka* 7 (1966): 191–4.

Blomstrand, E., P. Hassmen, S. Ek, B. Ekblom, and E. A. Newsholme. "Influence of Ingesting a Solution of Branched-Chain Amino Acids on Perceived Exertion During Exercise." *Acta Physiologica Scandinavica* 159 (1997): 41–9.

Blount, B. Mack, M. Wehr, C. MacGregor, J. Hiatt, R. Wang, G. Wickramasinghe, S. Everson, R. Ames, and B. Ames. "Folate Deficiency Causes Uracil Misincorporation into Human DNA and Chromosome Breakage: Implications for Cancer and Neuronal Damage." *Proceedings of the National Academy of Science of the United States of America* 94 (April 1997): 3290–5.

Blum, B., M. H. Stern, and K. I. Melville. "A Comparative Evaluation of the Action of Depressant and Stimulant Drugs on Human Performance." *Psychopharmacologia* 6 (1964): 173–7.

Blumberg, J. "Considerations of the Scientific Substantiation for Antioxidant Vitamins and B-carotene in Disease Prevention." *American Journal of Clinical Nutrition* 62 (1995): 52–6.

Blundell, J. E., and A. J. Hill. "On the Mechanism of Action of Dexfenfluramine: Effect on Alliesthesia and Appetite Motivation in Lean and Obese Subjects." *Clinical Neuropharmacology* 11, supplement 1 (1988): S121–34.

Boccafoschi, C., and S. Annoscia. "Confronto fra estratto di Serenoa repens e placebo mediate prova clinica controllata in pazienti con adenomatosi prostatica." *Urologia* 50 (1983): 1257–68.

Boden, G., X. Chen, J. Ruiz, G. D. V. van Rossum, and S. Turco. "Effects of Vanadyl Sulfate on Carbohydrate and Lipid Metabolism in Patients with Non-insulin-dependent Diabetes Mellitus." *Metabolism* 45, no. 9 (1996): 1130–5.

Bodigheimer, K., and D. Chase. "Wirksamkeit von Weißdorn-Extrakt in der Dosierung 3mal 100 mg taglich: Multizentrische Doppelblindstudie mit 85 herzinsuffizienten Patienten im Stadium NYHA II." *Munch. med. Wschr.* 136 (1994): S7–11.

Bodinet, C., and N. Beuscher. "Antiviral and Immunological Activity of Glycoproteins from Echinacea Purpurea Radix." *Planta Medica* 57, supplement 2 (1991): A33–4.

Bogden, J. D., et al. "Zinc and Immunocompetence in Elderly People: Effects of Zinc Supplementation for Three Months." *American Journal of Clinical Nutrition* 48 (1988): 655–63.

Bohnert, K.-J. "The Use of Vitex Agnus Castus for Hyperprolactinemia." *Quarterly Review of Natural Medicine* (1997): 19–21.

Bone, K. "Kava—A Safe Herbal Treatment for Anxiety." *British Journal of Phytotherapy* 3 (1993): 147–153.

Bongi, G. "Tadennan nella terapia dell'adenoma prostatico: Studio anatomo-clinico." *Minerva Urologica* 24 (1972): 129–39.

Bonithon-Kopp, C., C. Coudray, C. Berr, P-J. Touboul, J. M. Feve, A. Favier, and P. Ducimetiere. "Combined Effects of Lipid Peroxidation and Antioxidant Status on Carotid Atherosclerosis in a Population Aged 59–71 Years: The EVA Study." *American Journal of Clinical Nutrition* 65 (1997): 121–7.

Bordia, A. "Effect of Garlic on Human Platelet Aggregation In Vitro." *Atherosclerosis* 30 (1978): 355–60.

Bordia, A., H. C. Bansal, S. K. Arora, and S. V. Singh. "Effect of the Essential Oils of Garlic and Onion on Alimentary Hyperlipemia." *Atherosclerosis* 21 (1975): 15–19.

Bordia, A., H. K. Joshi, Y. K. Sanadhya, and N. Bhu. "Effect of Essential Oil of Garlic on Serum Fibrinolytic Activity in Patients with Coronary Artery Disease." *Atherosclerosis* 28 (1977): 155–9.

Bracher, F. "Phytotherapie der benigen Prostahyperplasie" (Phytotherapy in the Treatment of Benign Prostatic Hyperplasia). *Urologe Ausgabe A* 36 (1997): 10–7.

Braeckman, J. "The Extract of Serenoa Repens in the Treatment of Benign Prostratic Hyperplasia: A Multicenter Open Study." *Current Therapeutic Research* 55, no. 7 (1994): 776–85.

Brala, P. M., and R. L. Hagen. "Effects of Sweetness Perception and Caloric Value of a Preload on Short Term Intake." *Physiology and Behavior* 30 (1983): 1–9.

Brandis, S. A., and V. N. Pilovitskaya. "Effectiveness of Extracts of Siberian Ginseng Root and Ginseng Root (Korean) on Prolonged Physical Labor While Inhaling Gas Mixtures Enhanced with Oxygen" (in Russian) *Lek. Sredstva Dal'nego Vostoka* 7 (1966): 141–53.

Brandis, S. A., and V. N. Pilovitskaya. "Effectiveness of Siberian Ginseng Root Extract on Labor at High Temperature Conditions" (in Russian). *Lek. Sredstva Dall'nego Vostoka* 7 (1966): 155–6.

Brattstrom, L., B. L. Hultberg, and J. E. Hardebo. "Folic Acid–Responsive Postmenopausal Homocysteinemia." *Metabolism* 34, no. 1 (1985): 1073–7.

Brattstrom, L., B. Israelsson, J. O. Jeppsson, and B. L. Hultberg. "Folic Acid—An Innocuous Means to Reduce Plasma Homocysteine." *Scandinavian Journal of Clinical and Laboratory Investigation* 48 (1988): 215–21.

Brattstrom, L., B. Israelsson, B. Norrving, D. Bergqvist, J. Thorne, B. Hultberg, and A. Hamfelt. "Impaired Homocysteine Metabolism in Early-Onset Cerebral and Peripheral Occlusive Arterial Disease: Effects of Pyridoxine and Folic Acid Treatment." *Atherosclerosis* 81 (1990): 51–60.

Brattstrom, L., et al. "Pyridoxine Reduces Cholesterol and Low-Density Lipoprotein and Increases Antithrombin III Activity in Eighty-Year-Old Men with Low Plasma Pyridoxam 5-Phosphate." *Scandinavian Journal of Clinical and Laboratory Investigation* 50 (1990): 873–7.

Braunig, B., et al. "Echinaceae purpureae Radix: Zur Starkung der korpereigenen

Abwehr bei grippalen Infekten." *Zeitschrift fur Phytotherapie* 13 (1992): 7–13.

Bray, G. A. "Use and Abuse of Appetite-Suppressant Drugs in the Treatment of Obesity." *Annals of Internal Medicine* 199 (1993): 703–13.

Brekhman, I. I., and I. V. Dardymov. "Pharmacological Investigation of Glycosides from Ginseng and Eleutherococcus." *Lloydia* 32, no. 1 (1969): 46–51.

Bressa, G. M. "S-adenoysyl-1-methionine (SAMe) as Antidepressant: Meta-analysis of Clinical Studies." *Acta Neurologica Scandinavica* 154 (1994): 7–14.

Brevetti, G., et al. "Increases in Walking Distance in Patients with Peripheral Vascular Disease Treated with L-carnitine: A Double-Blind, Cross-over Study." *Circulation* 77, no. 4 (1988): 767–73.

Brighenti, F., G. Testolin, A. Giacca, F. Caviezel, and G. Pozza. "Dietary Selenium and Zinc Intake and the Medium-Term Se and Zn Status in Obese Persons on Low-Calorie Diets." *International Journal of Vitamin and Nutritional Research* 57 (1987): 185–92.

Brilla, L. R., and T. F. Haley. "Effect of Magnesium Supplementation on Strength Training in Humans." *Journal of the American College of Nutrition* 11, no. 3 (1992): 326–9.

Brittenden, J., S. D. Heys, and O. Eremin. "L-arginine and Malignant Disease: A Potential Therapeutic Role?" *European Journal of Surgical Oncology* 20 (1994): 189–92.

Broberg, S., and K. Sahlin. "Adenine Nucleotide Degradation in Human Skeletal Muscle During Prolonged Exercise." *Journal of Applied Physiology* 67, no. 1 (1989): 116–22.

Brock, C., and H. Curry. "Comparative Incidence of Side Effects of a Wax-Matrix and a Sustained-Release Iron Preparation." *Clinical Therapeutics* 7, no. 4 (1985).

Brosche, T., D. Platt, and H. Dorner. "The Effect of a Garlic Preparation on the Composition of Plasma Lipoproteins and Erythrocyte Membranes in Geriatric Subjects." *British Journal of Clinical Practice* 69 (1990): 12–9.

Brown E. D., et al. "Plasma Carotenoids in Normal Men after a Single Ingestion of Vegetables or Purified B-carotene." *American Journal of Clinical Nutrition* 49 (1989): 1258–65.

Brown, G., et al. "Regression of Coronary Artery Disease as a Result of Intensive Lipid-Lowering Therapy in Men with High Levels of Apolipoprotein B." *New England Journal of Medicine* 323 (1990): 1289–98.

Brown K., P. Morrice, and G. Duthie. "Vitamin E Supplementation Suppresses Indexes of Lipid Peroxidation and Platelet Counts in Blood of Smokers and Nonsmokers but Plasma Lipoprotein Concentrations Remain Unchanged." *American Journal of Clinical Nutrition* 60 (1994): 383–7.

Brown, M. R., et al. "A High Protein, Low Calorie Liquid Diet in the Treatment of Very Obese Adolescents: Long-Term Effect on Lean Body Mass." *American Journal of Clinical Nutrition* 38 (1983): 20–31.

Brune, M., L. Rossander, and L. Hallberg. "Iron Absorption: No Intestinal Adaptation to a High-Phytate Diet." *American Journal of Clinical Nutrition* 49 (1989): 542–5.

Bucci, L., and J. F. Hickson. "Ornithine Supplementation and Insulin Release in Bodybuilders." *International Journal of Sport Nutrition* 2 (1992): 287–91.

Bucci, L., et al. "Ornithine Ingestion and Growth Hormone Release in Bodybuilders." *Nutr Res* 10 (1990): 239–45.

Buck, C., A. P. Donner, and H. Simpson. "Garlic Oil and Ischemic Heart Disease." *International Journal of Epidemiology* 11 (1982): 294–5.

Budd, K. "Use of D-phenylalanine, an Enkephalinase Inhibitor, in the Treatment of Intractable Pain." *Advances in Pain Research and Therapy* 5 (1983): 305–8.

Burack, J. H., M. R. Cohen, J. A. Han, and D. I. Abrams. "Pilot Randomized Controlled Trial of Chinese Herbal Treatment for HIV-Associated Symptoms." *Journal of Acquired Immune Deficiency Syndromes and Human Retrovirology* 12 (1996): 386–93.

Burke, L. M., D. B. Pyne, and R. D. Telford. "Effect of Oral Creatine Supplementation on Single-Effort Sprint Performance in Elite Swimmers." *International Journal of Sport Nutrition* 6 (1996): 222–33.

Burney, P.G.J., G. W. Comstock, and J. S. Morris. "Serologic Precursors of Cancer: Serum Micronutrients and the Subsequent Risk of Pancreatic Cancer." *American Journal of Clinical Nutrition* 49 (1989): 895–900.

Burri, B. J., R. M. Dougherty, D. S. Kelley, and J. M. Iacono. "Platelet Aggregation in Humans Is Affected by Replacement of Dietary Linoeic Acid with Oleic Acid." *American Journal of Clinical Nutrition* 54 (1991): 359–62.

Butler, J., C. D. Thomson, P. D. Whanger, and M. F. Robinson. "Selenium Distribution in Blood Fractions of New Zealand Women Taking Organic or Inorganic Selenium." *American Journal of Clinical Nutrition* 53 (1991): 748–54.

Byerley, L. O., and A. Kirksey. "Effects of Different Levels of Vitamin C Intake on the Vitamin C Concentration in Human Milk and the Vitamin C Intake of Breast-Fed Infants." *American Journal of Clinical Nutrition* 41 (1985): 665–71.

Caballero, B., R. E. Gleason, and R. J. Wurtman. "Plasma Amino Acid Concentrations in Healthy Elderly Men and Women." *American Journal of Clinical Nutrition* 53 (1991): 1249–52.

Caceres, D. D., J. L. Hancke, R. A. Burgos, and G. K. Wikman. "Prevention of Common Colds with Andrographic Paniculata Dried Extract: A Pilot Double-Blind Trial." *Phytomedicine* 4, no. 2 (1997): 101–4.

Caffarra, P., and V. Santamaria. "The Effects of Phosphatidylserine in Patients with Mild

Cognitive Decline." *Clinical Trials Journal* 24, no. 1 (1987): 109–14.

Caldwell, M. D., H. T. Jonsson, and H. B. Othersen. "Essential Fatty Acid Deficiency in an Infant Receiving Prolonged Parenteral Alimentation." *Journal of Pediatrics* 81, no. 5 (1972): 894–8.

Campbell, W. W., and R. A. Anderson. "Effects of Aerobic Exercise and Training on the Trace Minerals Chromium, Zinc, and Copper." *Sports Medicine* 4 (1987): 9–18.

Cappiello, A., et al. "Augmentation of Fluvoxamine in Refractory Depression: A Single-Blind Study." *Biological Psychiatry* 38 (1995): 765–7.

Cappuccio, F. P., et al. "Lack of Effect of Oral Magnesium on High Blood Pressure: A Double-Blind Study." *BMJ* 291 (1985): 235–7.

Carbin, B.-E., B. Larsson, and O. Lindahl. "Treatment of Benign Prostatic Hyperplasia with Phytosterols." *British Journal of Urology* 66 (1990): 639–41.

Carey, M. C., J. J. Fennelly, and O. Fitzgerald. "Homocystinuria. II. Subnormal Serum Folate Levels, Increased Folate Clearance, and Effects of Folic Acid Therapy." *American Journal of Medicine* 45 (1968): 26–31.

Carlson, H. E., and J. H. Shah. "Aspartame and Its Constituent Amino Acids: Effects on Prolactin, Cortisol, Growth Hormone, Insulin, and Glucose in Normal Humans." *American Journal of Clinical Nutrition* 59 (1989): 427–32.

Carraro, J.-C., et al. "Comparison of Phytotherapy (Permixon) with Finasteride in the Treatment of Benign Prostate Hyperplasia." *Prostate* 29 (1996): 231–40.

Caruso, I., and V. Pietrogrande. "Italian Double-Blind Multicenter Study Comparing S-adenosylmethionine, Naproxen, and Placebo in the Treatment of Degenerative Joint Disease." *American Journal of Medicine* 83, supplement 5A (1987): 66–71.

Casarosa, C., et al. "Lack of Effect of a Lyposterolic Extract of Serenoa Repens on Plasma Levels of Testosterone, Follicle-Stimulating Hormone, and Luteinizing Hormone." *Clinical Therapeutics* 10, no. 5 (1988): 585–8.

Cassidy, A., S. Bingham, and K. D. R. Setchell. "Biological Effects of a Diet of Soy Protein Rich in Isoflavones on the Menstrual Cycle of Premenopausal Women." *American Journal of Clinical Nutrition* 60 (1994): 333–40.

Casson, P., et al. "Oral Dehydroepiandrosterone in Physiologic Doses Modulates Immune Function in Postmenopausal Women." *American Journal of Obstetrics and Gynecology* 169 (1993): 1536–9.

Casson, P., et al. "Replacement of DHEA Enhances T-lymphocyte Insulin Binding in Postmenopausal Women." *Fertility and Sterility* 63, no. 5 (1995): 1027–31.

Castaneda-Acosta, J., and N. H. Fisher. "Biomimetic Transformations of Parthenolide." *Journal of Natural Products* 56, no. 1 (1993): 90–8.

Castillo-Duran, C., et al. "Oral Copper Supplementation: Effect on Copper and Zinc Balance During Acute Gastroenteritis in Infants." *American Journal of Clinical Nutrition* 51 (1990): 1088–92.

Catanzanaro, J. A., and L. Green. "Microbial Ecology and Dysbiosis in Human Medicine." *Alternative Medicine Review* 2, no. 3 (1997): 202–9.

Cavagnini, F., C. Invitti, M. Pinto, C. Maraschini, A. Di Landro, A. Dubini, and A. Marelli. "Effect of Acute and Repeated Administration of Gamma Aminobutyric Acid (GABA) on Growth Horomone and Prolactin Secretion in Man." *Acta Endocrinologica* 93 (1980): 149–54.

Cenacchi, T., T. Bertoldin, C. Farina, M. Fiori, G. Crepaldi, and Participating Investigators. "Cognitive Decline in the Elderly: A Double-Blind, Placebo-Controlled Multicenter Study on Efficacy of Phosphatidylserine Administration." *Aging: Clinical Experimental Research* 5 (1993): 123–33.

Champault, G., J. C. Patel, and A. M. Bonnard. "A Double-Blind Trial of an Extract of the Plant Serenoa Repens in Benign Prostatic Hyperplasia." *British Journal of Clinical Pharmacology* 18 (1984): 461–2.

Chan, G., M. McMurry, K. Westover, K. Engelbert-Fenton, and M. Thomas. "Effects of Increased Dietary Calcium Intake upon the Calcium and Bone Mineral Status of Lactating Adolescent and Adult Women." *American Journal of Clinical Nutrition* 46 (1987): 319–23.

Chan, J. K., V. M. Bruce, and B. E. McDonald. "Dietary Alpha-linolenic Acid Is as Effective as Oleic Acid and Linoleic Acid in Lowering Blood Cholesterol in Normolipidemic Men." *American Journal of Clinical Nutrition* 53 (1991): 1230–4.

Chan, Y., M. Suzuki, and S. Yamamoto. "Dietary, Anthropometric, Hematological and Biochemical Assessment of the Nutritional Status of Centenarians and Ederly People in Okinawa, Japan." *Journal of the American College of Nutrition* 16, no. 3 (1997): 229–35.

Chapuy, M.-C., P. Chapuy, and P. J. Meunier. "Calcium and Vitamin D Supplements: Effects on Calcium Metabolism and Elderly People." *American Journal of Clinical Nutrition* 46 (1987): 324–8.

Charles, P., E. Eriksen, C. Hasling, K. Sondergard, and L. Mosekilde. "Dermal, Intestinal, and Renal Obligatory Losses of Calcium: Relation to Skeletal Calcium Loss." *American Journal of Clinical Nutrition* 54 (1991): 266–73.

Chasiotis, D., M. Bergstrom, and E. Hultman. "ATP Utilization and Force During Intermittent and Continuous Muscle Contractions." *Journal of Applied Physiology* 63, no. 1 (1987): 167–74.

Chawla, R. K., H. L. Bonkovsky, and J. T. Galambos. "Biochemistry and Pharmacology of S-adenosyl-l-methionine and Rationale for Its Use in Liver Diseases." *Drugs* 40, no. 3 (1990): 98–110.

Chawla, Y. K., P. Dubey, R. Singh, S. Nundy, and B. N. Tandon. "Treatment of Dyspepsia with Amalaki—An Ayurvedic Drug." *Indian Journal of Medical Research* 76 (1982): 95–98.

Chen, M. F., et al. "Effect of Ascorbic Acid on Plasma Alcohol Clearance." *Journal of the American College of Nutrition* 9, no. 3 (1990): 185–9.

Chen, M.-D., et al. "Zinc in Hair and Serum of Obese Individuals in Taiwan." *American Journal of Clinical Nutrition* 48 (1988): 1307–9.

Childs, S. J. "Dimethyl Sulfone (DMSO2) in the Treatment of Interstitial Cystitis." *Interstitial Cystitis* 21, no. 1 (1994): 85–8.

Chlebowski, R. T., et al. "Nutritional Status, Gastrointestinal Dysfunction, and Survival in Patients with AIDS." *American Journal of Gastroenterology* 84, no. 10 (1989): 1288–93.

Chochola, M., M. Zeman, P. Hrabak, S. Stary, A. Zak, and J. Skorepa. "Effect of Diet Enriched with Sea and Freshwater Fish on the Plasma Lipid Level After Three Months of Administration." *Sbornik Lekarsky* 87 (1985): 23–8.

Chrubasik, S., C. H. Ximpfer, U. Schutt, and R. Ziegler. "Effectiveness of Harpagophytum Procumbens in Treatment of Acute Low Back Pain." *Phytomedicine* 3, no. 1 (1996): 1–10.

Chwang, L.-C., et al. "Iron Supplementation and Physical Growth of Rural Indonesian Children." *American Journal of Clinical Nutrition* 47 (1988): 496–501.

Cirelli, M. G. "Five Years of Clinical Experience with Bromelains in Therapy of Edema and Inflammation in Postoperative Tissue Reaction, Skin Infections, and Trauma." *Clinical Medicine* (June 1967): 55–9.

Cirillo-Marucco, E., A. Pagliarulo, G. Tritto, A. Piccinno, and U. D. Rienzo. "L'Estratto di Serenoa repens (Permixon) nel trattamento precoce dell'ipertrofia prostatica" (Extract of Serenoa Repens [Permixon] in the Early Treatment of Prostatic Hypertrophy)." *Urologia* 50 (1983): 1269–77.

Clark, L. C., G. F. Combs, B. W. Turnbull, E. H. Slate, D. K. Chalker, J. Chow, L. S. Davis, R. A. Glover, A. Glover, G. F. Graham, E. G. Gross, A. Krongrad, J. L. Lesher, H. K. Park, B. B. Sanders, C. L. Smith, and J. R. Taylor. "Effects of Selenium Supplementation for Cancer Prevention in Patients with Carcinoma of the Skin." *JAMA* 276, no. 24 (1996): 1957–63.

Clark, L. C., et al. "Decreased Incidence of Prostate Cancer with Selenium Supplementation: Results of a Double-Blind Cancer Prevention Trial." *British Journal of Urology* 81 (1998): 730–4.

Clausen, J., S. A. Nielsen, and M. Kristensen. "Biochemical and Clinical Effects of an Antioxidative Supplementation of Geriatric Patients." *Biological Trace Element Research* 20 (1989): 135–51.

Clifton, P., and P. J. Nestel. "Effects of Dietary Cholesterol on Postprandial Lipoproteins in

Three Phenotypic Groups." *American Journal of Clinical Nutrition* 64 (1996): 361–7.

Clubley, M., C. E. Bye, T. A. Henson, A. W. Peck, and C. J. Riddington. "Effects of Caffeine and Cyclizine Alone and in Combination on Human Performance, Subjective Effects, and EEG Activity." *British Journal of Clinical Pharmacology* 7 (1979): 157–63.

Coburn, S., et al. "Response of Vitamin B-6 Content of Muscle to Changes in Vitamin B-6 Intake in Man." *American Journal of Clinical Nutrition* 53 (1991): 1436–42.

Coeugniet, E., and R. Kuhnast. "Rezidivierende Candidiasis: Adjuvante Immuntherapie mit verschiedenen Echinacin-Darreichungsformen." *Therapiewoche* 36 (1986): 3352–8.

Cohen, H. J., M. R. Brown, D. Hamilton, J. Lyons-Patterson, N. Avissar, and P. Liegey. "Glutathione Peroxidase and Selenium Deficiency in Patients Receiving Home Parenteral Nutrition: Time Course for Development of Deficiency and Repletion of Enzyme Activity in Plasma and Blood Cells." *American Journal of Clinical Nutrition* 49 (1989): 132–9.

Cohen, L., and R. Kitzes. "Infrared Spectroscopy and Magnesium Content of Bone Mineral in Osteoporotic Women." *Israel Journal of Medical Sciences* 17 (1981): 1123–5.

Cohen, L., and R. Kitzes. "Magnesium Sulfate in the Treatment of Variant Angina." *Magnesium* 3 (1984): 46–9.

Cohen, L., A. Laor, and R. Kitzes. "Lymphocyte and Bone Magnesium in Alcohol-Associated Osteoporosis." *Magnesium* 4 (1985): 148–152.

Cohen. M., and H. Bhagvan. "Ascorbic Acid and Gastrointestinal Cancer." *Journal of the American College of Nutrition* 14, no. 6 (1995): 565–78.

Cohen, N., et al. "Oral Vanadyl Sulfate Improves Hepatic and Peripheral Insulin Sensitivity in Patients with Non-insulin-dependent Diabetes Mellitus." *Journal of Clinical Investigation* 95 (1995): 2501–9.

Colditz, G. A., et al. "Patterns of Weight Change and Their Relation to Diet in a Cohort of Healthy Women." *American Journal of Clinical Nutrition* 51 (1990): 1100–5.

Collipp, P., et al. "Zinc Deficiency: Improvement in Growth and Growth Hormone Levels with Oral Zinc Therapy." *Annals of Nutrition and Metabolism* 26 (1982): 287–90.

Conforti, A., et al. "Serum Copper and Ceruloplasmin Levels in Rheumatoid Arthritis and Degenerative Joint Disease and their Pharmacological Implications." *Pharmacological Research Communications* 15, no. 9 (1983): 859–67.

Connor, W. E. "Effects of Omega-3 Fatty Acids in Hypertriglyceridemic States. *Seminars in Thrombosis and Hemostatis* 14, no. 3 (1988): 271–84.

Constantin-Teodosiu, D., S. Howell, and P. L. Greenhaff. "Carnitine Metabolism in Human Muscle Fiber Types During Submaximal Dyanic Exercise." *Journal of Applied Physiology* 80 (1996): 1061–4.

Contaldo, F., L. Scalfi, A. Coltorti, M. Mancini. "Postprandial Thermogenesis in Different Pathophysiological Conditions." *International Journal for Vitamin and Nutrition Research* 56 (1986): 211–6.

Cook, J. D., S. A. Dassenko, and S. R. Lynch. "Assessment of the Role of Nonheme-Iron Availability in Iron Balance." *American Journal of Clinical Nutrition* 54 (1991): 717–22.

Cook, J. D., S. A. Dassenko, and P. Whittaker. "Calcium Supplementation: Effect on Iron Absorption." *American Journal of Clinical Nutrition* 53 (1991): 106–11.

Cook, J. D., and D. A. Lipschitz. "Absorption of Controlled-Release Iron." *Clinical Pharmacology and Therapeutics* 32, no. 4 (1982): 531–9.

Cook, J. D., T. A. Morck, and S. R. Lynch. "The Inhibitory Effect of Soy Products on Nonheme-Iron Absorption in Man." *American Journal of Clinical Nutrition* 34 (1981): 2622–9.

Cook, J. D., B. S. Skikne, S. R. Lynch, and M. E. Reusser. "Estimates of Iron Sufficiency in the U.S. Population." *Blood* 68, no. 3 (1986): 726–31.

Cook, J. D., et al. "The Effect of High Ascorbic Acid Supplementation on Body Iron Stores." *Blood* 64, no. 3 (1984): 721–6.

Cook, J. D., et al. "Food Iron Absorption Measured by an Extrinsic Tag." *Journal of Clinical Investigation* 51 (1972): 805–15.

Cook, J. D., et al. "Gastric Delivery System for Iron Supplementation." *Lancet* 335 (1990): 1136–9.

Cooke, J. P., and P. S. Tsao. "Arginine: A New Therapy for Atherosclerosis?" *Circulation* 95 (1997): 311–12.

Corpas, E., M. R. Blackman, R. Roberson, D. Schofield, and S. M. Harman. "Oral Arginine-Lysine Does Not Increase Growth Hormone or Insulin-like Growth Factor I in Old Men." *Journal of Gerontology* 48, no. 4 (1993): M128–33.

Cossins, E., R. Lee, and L. Packer. "ESR Studies of Vitamin C Regeneration, Order of Reactivity of Natural Source Phytochemical Preparations." *Biochemistry and Molecular Biology International* 45, no. 3 (1998): 583–97.

Couzy, F., P. Kastenmayer, M. Vigo, J. Clough, R. Munoz-Box, and D. Barclay. "Calcium Bioavailability from a Calcium- and Sulfate-Rich Mineral Water, Compared with Milk, in Young Adult Women." *American Journal of Clinical Nutrition* 62 (1995): 1239–44.

Cox, I. M., M. J. Campbell, and D. Dowson. "Red Blood Cell Magnesium and Chronic Fatigue Syndrome." *Lancet* 337 (1991): 757–60.

Craig, A., and E. Richardson. "Effects of Experimental and Habitual Lunch-Size on Performance, Arousal, Hunger, and Mood." *International Archives of Occupational and Environmental Health* 61 (1989): 313–9.

Cravo, M. L., et al. "Hyperhomocysteinemia in Chronic Alcoholism: Correlation with Folate, Vitamin B12, and Vitamin B6 Status." *American Journal of Clinical Nutrition* 63, no. 2 (1996): 220–4.

Crofton, R. W., et al. "Inorganic Zinc and the Intestinal Absorption of Ferrous Iron." *American Journal of Clinical Nutrition* 50 (1989): 141–4.

Crolle, G., and E. D'Este. "Glucosamine Sulphate in the Management of Arthrosis: A Controlled Clinical Investigation." *Current Medical Research and Opinion* 7, no. 2 (1980): 104–9.

Cubasch, H., and D. Stocksmeier. "Deutliche Zunahme der T-Helferzellen" (Significant Increase of T-helper Lymphocytes)." *Therapiewoche* 42 (1992): 990–1000.

Cunliffe, W. J., and K. T. Holland. "Clinical and Laboratory Studies on Treatment with 20% Azelaic Acid Cream for Acne." *Acta Dermato-Venereologica* supplement 143 (1989): 31–4.

Cunnane, S. C. "The Profile of Long-Chain Fatty Acids in Serum Phospholipids: A Possible Indicator of Copper Status in Humans." *American Journal of Clinical Nutrition* 48 (1988): 1475–8.

Cunningham, J. J. "Micronutrients as Nutriceutical Interventions in Diabetes Mellitus." *Journal of the American College of Nutrition* 17, no. 1 (1998): 7–10.

Cunningham, J. J., et al. "Zinc and Copper Status of Severely Burned Children During TPN." *Journal of the American College of Nutrition* 10 (1991): 57–62.

Curatolo, P. W., and D. Robertson. "The Health Consequences of Caffeine." *Annals of Internal Medicine* 98, no. 5 (1983): 641–53.

Curhan, G. C., W. C. Willett, E. B. Rimm, and M. J. Stampfer. "Prospective Study of the Intake of Vitamins C and B6, and the Risk of Kidney Stones in Men." *Journal of Urology* 155 (1996): 1847–51.

Cynober, L., et al. "Action of Ornithine Alpha-ketoglutarate, Ornithine Hydrochloride, and Calcium Alpha-ketoglutarate on Plasma Amino Acid and Hormonal Patterns in Healthy Subjects." *Journal of the American College of Nutrition* 9, no. 1 (1990): 2–12.

D'Ambrosio, E., B. Casa, R. Bompani, G. Scali, and M. Scali. "Glucosamine Sulphate: A Controlled Clinical Investigation in Arthrosis." *Pharmatherapeutica* 2 (1981): 504–8.

D'Angelo, L., R. Grimaldi, M. Caravaggi., et al. "A Double-Blind Placebo Controlled Clinical Study on the Effect of Standardized Ginseng Extract on Psychomotor Performance in Healthy Individuals." *Journal of Ethnopharmacology* 16 (1986): 15–22.

Dahanukar, S. A., and U. M. Thatte. "Current Status of Ayurveda in Phytomedicine." *Phytomedicine* 4, no. 4 (1997): 359–68.

Dal Negro, R., G. Pomari, O. Zoccatelli, and P. Turco. "Changes in Physical Performance of Untrained Volunteers: Effects of L-carnitine." *Clinical Trials Journal* 23, no. 4 (1986): 242–8.

Dalery, K., et al. "Homocysteine and Coronary Artery Disease in French Canadian Subjects: Relation with Vitamins B12, B6, Pyridoxal Phosphate, and Folate." *Journal of Cardiology* 75, no. 16 (1995): 1107–11.

Das, B. S., et al. "Increased Plasma Lipid Peroxidation in Riboflavin-Deficient, Malaria-

Infected Children." *American Journal of Clinical Nutrition* 51 (1990): 859–63.

Daum, K., W. W. Tuttle, C. Martin, and L. Myers. "Effect of Various Types of Breakfasts on Physiologic Response." *Journal of the American Dietetic Association* 26 (1950): 503–9.

Davidson, G. P., et al. "Passive Immunisation of Children with Bovine Cartilage Containing Antibodies to Human Rotavirus." *Lancet* 23 (1989): 709–12.

Davis, A. T., P. G. Davis, and S. D. Phinney. "Plasma and Urinary Carnitine of Obese Subjects on Very-Low-Calorie Diets." *Journal of the American College of Nutrition* 9, no. 3 (1990): 261–4.

Davis, J., et al. "Fluid Availability of Sports Drinks Differing in Carbohydrate Type and Concentration." *American Journal of Clinical Nutrition* 51 (1990): 1054–7.

Davis, R., J. Kabbani, and N. Maro. "Aloe Vera and Wound Healing." *Journal of the American Podiatic Medical Association* 77, no. 4 (1987): 165–9.

Dawson-Hughes, B., S. S. Harris, and G. E. Dallal. "Plasma Calcidiol, Season, and Serum Parathyroid Hormone Concentrations in Healthy Elderly Men and Women." *American Journal of Clinical Nutrition* 65 (1997): 67–71.

Dawson-Hughes, B., et al. "A Controlled Trial of the Effect of Calcium Supplementation on Bone Density in Postmenopausal Women." *New England Journal of Medicine* 323, no. 13 (1990): 878–83.

De A Santos, O. S., and J. Grunwald. "Effect of Garlic Powder Tablets on Blood Lipids and Blood Pressure—A Six-Month Placebo Controlled, Double Blind Study." *British Journal of Clinical Research* 4 (1993): 37–44.

Decourt, P. "Experimentation de la gelee royale d'abeilles en pratique geriatrique." *Rev. Pathol. Gener. Physiol. Clin.* (1956): 1641–63.

Deehr, M. S., G. E. Dallal, K. T. Smith, J. D. Taulbee, and B. Dawson-Hughes. "Effects of Different Calcium Sources on Iron Absorption in Postmenopausal Women." *American Journal of Clinical Nutrition* 51 (1990): 95–9.

DeFronzo, R. A. "Obesity Is Associated with Impaired Insulin-Mediated Potassium Uptake." *Metabolism* 37, no. 2 (1988): 105–8.

Deitrick, R. E. "Oral Proteolytic Enzymes in the Treatment of Athletic Injuries: A Double-Blind Study." *Pennsylvania Medical Journal* (1965): 35–37.

de Lorgeril, M., S. Renaud, N. Marnelle, P. Salen, J. Martin, I. Monjaud, J. Guidollet, P. Touboul, and J. Delaye. "Mediterranean Alpha-linolenic Acid–rich Diet in Secondary Prevention of Coronary Heart Disease." *Lancet* 343 (1994): 1454–9.

Demke, D. M., G. R. Peters, O. I. Linet, C. M. Metzler, and K. A. Klott. "Effects of a Fish Oil Concentrate in Patients with Hypercholesterolemia." *Atherosclerosis* 70 (1988): 73–80.

Dengel, J. L., L. I. Karzel, and A. P. Goldberg. "Effect of an American Heart Association

Diet, with or without Weight Loss, on Lipids in Obese Middle-Aged and Older Men." *American Journal of Clinical Nutrition* 62 (1995): 715–21.

Denis, C., D. Dormois, M. T. Linossier, J. L. Eychenne, P. Hauseux, and J. R. Lacour. "Effect of Arginine Asparate on the Exercise-Induced Hyperammoniemia in Humans: A Two-Periods Crossover Trial." *Archives Internationales de Physiologie et de Biochimie* 99 (1991): 123–7.

Devaraj, S., D. Li, and I. Jialal. "The Effects of Alpha Tocopherol Supplementation on Monocyte Function: Decreased Lipid Oxidation, Interleukin 1B Secretion, and Monocyte Adhesion to Endothelium." *Journal of Clinical Investigation* 98, no. 3 (1996): 756–63.

Devine, A., R. Prince, and R. Bell. "Nutritional Effect of Calcium Supplementation by Skim Milk Powder or Calcium Tablets on Total Nutrient Intake in Postmenopausal Women." *American Journal of Clinical Nutrition* 64 (1996): 731–7.

Dhariwal, K. R., W. O. Hartzell, and M. Levine. "Ascorbic Acid and Dehydroascorbic Acid Measurements in Human Plasma and Serum." *American Journal of Clinical Nutrition* 54 (1991): 712–6.

Diaz, E., G. R. Goldberg, M. Taylor, J. M. Savage, D. Sellen, W. A. Coward, and A. M. Prentice. "Effects of Dietary Supplementation on Work Performance in Gambian Laborers." *American Journal of Clinical Nutrition* 53 (1991): 803–11.

Diehm, C., D. Vollbrecht, K. Amendt, and H. U. Comberg. "Medical Edema Protection—Clinical Benefit in Patients with Chronic Deep Vein Incompetence." *Vasa* 21 (1992): 188–91.

Diehm, C., H. J. Trampisch, S. Lange, and C. Schmidt. "Comparison of Leg Compression Stocking and Oral Horse-Chestnut Seed Extract Therapy in Patients with Chronic Venous Insufficiency." *Lancet* 147 (1996): 292–4.

Di Padova, C. "S-adenosylmethinoine in the Treatment of Osteoarthritis." *American Journal of Medicine* 83, no. 5A (1987): 60–4.

Diplock, A. T. "Antioxidant Nutrients and Disease Prevention: An Overview." *American Journal of Clinical Nutrition* 53 (1991): 189–93S.

Diplock, A. T. "Safety of Antioxidant Vitamins and B-carotene." *American Journal of Clinical Nutrition* 62 (1995): 1510–6S

Ditkoff, E. C., W. G. Crary, M. Cristo, and R. A. Lobo. "Estrogen Improves Psychological Function in Asymptomatic Postmenopausal Women." *Obstetrics and Gynecology* 78, no. 6 (1991): 991–95.

Ditzler, K., B. Gessner, W. F. H. Schatton, and M. Willems. "Clinical Trial on Neurapas versus Placebo in Patients with Mild to Moderate Depressive Symptoms: A Placebo-Controlled, Randomised Double-Blind Study." *Complementary Therapies in Medicine* 2 (1994): 5–13.

Dixon, Z. R., S. Feng-Shiun, B. A. Warden, B. J. Burri, and T. R. Neidlinger. "The Effect of a

Low Carotenoid Diet on Malondialdahyde-Thiobarbituric Acid (MDA-TBA) Concentrations in Women: A Placebo-Controlled Double-Blind Study." *Journal of the American College of Nutrition* 17, no. 1 (1998): 54–8.

Dodson, W. L., D. S. Sachan, S. Krauss, and W. Hanna. "Alterations of Serum and Urinary Carnitine Profiles in Cancer Patients: Hypothesis of Possible Significance." *Journal of the American College of Nutrition* 8, no. 2 (1989): 133–42.

Dollins, A., et al. "Effect of Inducing Nocturnal Serum Melatonin Concentrations in Daytime on Sleep, Mood, Body Temperature, and Performance." *Proceedings of the National Academy of Science of the United States of America* 91, no. 5 (1994): 1824–8.

Donkervoort, T., A. Sterling, J. van Ness, and P. J. Donker. "A Clinical and Urodynamic Study of Tadenan in the Treatment of Benign Prostatic Hypertrophy." *European Urology* 3 (1977): 218–25.

Donnan, P. T., M. Thomson, F. G. R. Fowkes, R. J. Prescott, and E. Housley. "Diet as a Risk Factor for Peripheral Arterial Disease in the General Population: The Edinburgh Artery Study." *American Journal of Clinical Nutrition* 57 (1993): 917–21.

Donnelly, J. E., D. J. Jacobsen, J. E. Whatley, J. O. Hill, L. L. Swift, A. Cherrington, B. Polk, Z. V. Tran, and G. Reed. "Nutrition and Physical Activity Program to Attenuate Obesity and Promote Physical and Metabolic Fitness in Elementary School Children." *Obesity Research* 4, no. 3 (1996): 229–43.

Dragan, I., V. Stroescu, I. Stoian, E. Georgescu, and R. Baloescu. "Studies Regarding the Efficiency of Supro Isolated Soy Protein in Olympic Athletes." *Olympic Scientific Congress,* July 14–18, 1992.

Dreikorn, K., and P. S. Schonhofer. "Stellenwert von Phytotherpeutika bei der Behandlung der benignen Prostathyperplasie." *Urolge A* 34, no. 2 (1995): 119–29.

Drexel, H., C. Breier, H.-J. Lisch, and S. Sailer. "Lowering Plasma Cholesterol with Beta-sitosterol and Diet." *Lancet* 1 (1981): 1157.

Dudman, N., X. Guo, R. Gordon, P. Dawson, and D. Wilcken. "Human Homocysteine Catabolism: Three Major Pathways and Their Relevance to Development of Arterial Occlusive Disease." *Journal of Nutrition* 126 (1996): 1295–1300.

Dudman, N., D. E. L. Wilcken, J. Wang, J. F. Lynch, D. Macey, and P. Lundberg. "Disordered Methionine/Homocysteine Metabolism in Premature Vascular Disease: Its Occurrence, Cofactor Therapy, and Enzymology." *Arteriosclerosis and Thrombosis* 13 (1993): 1253–60.

Duester, P. A., et al. "Magnesium Homeostasis During High-Intensity Anaerobic Exercise in Men." *Journal of Applied Physiology* 62, no. 2 (1987): 545–50.

Dufour, B., C. Choquenent, M. Revol, G. Faure, and R. Jorest. "Etude controlee des effets de l'extrait de Pygeum Africanum sur les symptomes fonctionnels de l'adenome prostatique." *Annales D'Urologie* 18 (1984): 193–5.

Duker, Eva-Maria. "Effects of Extracts from

Cimicifuga Racemosa on Gonadotropin Release in Menopausal Women and Ovariectomized Rats." *Planta Medica* 57, no. 5 (1991): 420–4.

Dustmann, H. O., G. Godolias, and K. Seibel. "Verminderung des Fubvolumens bei der chronischen venosen Insuffizienz im Stehversuch durch eine neue Wirkstoffkombination." *Therapiewoche* 34 (1984): 5077–86.

Duthie, G. G., et al. "Blood Antioxidants and Indices of Lipid Peroxidation in Subjects with Angina Pectoris." *Applied Nutritional Investigation* 10, no. 4 (1994): 313–6.

Dyckner, T., and P. O. Weste. "Effect of Magnesium on Blood Pressure." *BMJ* 286 (1983): 1847–9.

Eby, G. A., D. R. Davis, and W. W. Halcomb. "Reduction in Duration of Common Colds by Zinc Gluconate Lozenges in a Double-Blind Study." *Antimicrobial Agents and Chemotherapy* 25, no. 1 (1984): 20–4.

Edidin, D. V., et al. "Resurgence of Nutritional Rickets Associated with Breast-Feeding and Special Dietary Practices." *Pediatrics* 65, no. 2 (1980): 232–5.

Egorov, Y. N., and E. F. Baburin. "Effects of Siberian Ginseng on Nervous System of Humans" (in Russian). *Lek. Sredstva Dal' nego Vostoka* 7 (1966): 167–72.

Egsmose, C., et al. "Low Serum Levels of 25-hydroxyvitamin D and 1,25-dihydroxyvitamin D in Institutionalized Old People: Influence of Solar Exposure and Vitamin D Supplementation." *Age and Ageing* 16 (1987): 35–40.

Eichstadt, H., et al. "Crataegus-Extrakt hilft dem Patienten mit NYHA II-Herzinsuffizienz: Untersuchung der myokardialen und hamodyanmischen Wirkung eines standardsierten Crataegus-Praparates mit Hilfe computergestutzter Radionuklidventrikulographie." *Therapiewoche* 39 (1989): 3288–96.

Eisenberg, D. M., et al. "Trends in Alternative Medicine Use in the United States, 1990–1997." *JAMA* 280, no. 18 (1998): 1569–75.

Eisenberg, D. M., et al. "Unconventional Medicine in the United States: Prevalence, Costs, and Patterns of Use." *New England Journal of Medicine* 328, no. 4 (1993): 246–52.

Ek, J. "Plasma, Red Cell, and Breast Milk Folacin Concentrations in Lactating Women." *American Journal of Clinical Nutrition* 38 (1983): 929–35.

Elam, R. P., D. H. Hardin, R. A. L. Sutton, and L. Hagen. "Effects of Arginine and Ornithine on Strength, Lean Body Mass, and Urinary Hydroxyproline in Adult Males." *Journal of Sports Medicine and Physical Fitness* 29, no. 1 (1989): 52–6.

Elkins, R. N., et al. "Acute Effects of Caffeine in Normal Prepubertal Boys." *American Journal of Psychiatry* 138, no. 2 (1981): 178–83.

Ellis, J. M., and K. S. McCully. "Prevention of Myocardial Infarction by Vitamin B6." *Research Communications in Molecular Pathology and Pharmacology* 89, no. 2 (1995): 208–20.

Elmer, G. W., C. M. Surawicz, and L. V. McFarland. "Biotherapeutic Agents: A

Neglected Modality for the Treatment and Prevention of Selected Intestinal and Vaginal Infections." *JAMA* 275, no. 11 (1996): 870–6.

Elsair, J., J. Poey, P. Rochiccioli, R. Denine, R. Merad, and N. Benouniche. "Effets de l'administration per os a doses variables, d'aspartate d'arginine et de chlorhydrate d'arginine sur les taux d'hormone de croissance et d'acides gras libres du plasma chez l'enfant normal." *A Jeun Pathologie Biologie* (1980): 638–44.

Emili, E., M. Lo Cigno, and U. Petrone. "Risultati clinici su un nuovo farmaco nella terapia dell' impertrofia della prostata (Permixon)." *Urologia* 50 (1983): 1042–8.

Eng, R. H. K., R. Drehmel, S. M. Smith, and E. J. C. Goldstein. "Saccharomyces Cerevisiae Infections in Man." *Journal of Medical and Veterinary Mycology* 22 (1984): 403–7.

Enghofer, E., R. Eisenburger, and K. Seibel. "Venentonisierende Wirkung und therapeutische Wirksamkeit von Roßkastaniensamenextrakt bei der orthostatischen Fehlregulation." *Therapiewoche* 29 (1984): 4360–72.

Enoksson, S., E. Blaak, and P. Arner. "Forskolin Potentiates Isoprenaline-Induced Glycerol Output and Local Blood Flow in Human Adipose Tissue in Vivo." *Pharmacology and Toxicity* 81 (1997): 214–18.

Epstein, O., Y. Kato, and S. Sherlock. "Vitamin D, Hydroxyapatite, and Calcium Gluconate in Treatment of Cortical Bone Thinning in Postmenopausal Women with Primary Biliary Cirrhosis." *American Journal of Clinical Nutrition* 36 (1982): 426–30.

Erdlen, F. "Klinische Wirksamkeit von Venostasin Retard im Doppelblindversuch." *Medwelt* 40 (1989): 994–6.

Erler, M. "Robkastaniensamenextrakt bei der Therapie peripherer venoser Odeme: Ein klinischer Therapievergleich." *Medwelt* 42 (1991): 593–6.

Ernst, E. "St. John's Wort, an Anti-Depressant? A Systematic, Criteria-Based Review." *Phytomedicine* 2, no. 1 (1995): 67–71.

Eskelinen, A., and J. Santalahti. "Natural Cartilage Polysaccharides for the Treatment of Sun-Damaged Skin in Females: A Double-Blind Comparison of Vivda and Imedeen." *Journal of International Medical Research* 20 (1992): 227–33.

Essig, D., D. L. Costill, and P. J. Van Handel. "Effects of Caffeine Ingestion on Utilization of Muscle Glycogen and Lipid During Leg Ergometer Cycling." *International Journal of Sports Medicine* 1 (1980): 86–90.

Ettinger, B., G. D. Friedman, T. Bush, and C. P. Quesenberry. "Reduced Mortality Associated with Long-Term Postmenopausal Estrogen Therapy." *Obstetrics and Gyencology* 87, no. 1 (1996): 6–12.

Facchinetti, F., et al. "Oral Magnesium Successfully Relieves Premenstrual Mood Changes." *Obstetrics and Gynecology* 78, no. 2 (1991): 177–81.

Facchini, F., A. M. Coulston, and G. M. Reaven. "Relation Between Dietary Vitamin Intake and Resistance to Insulin-Mediated

Glucose Disposal in Healthy Volunteers." *American Journal of Clinical Nutrition* 63 (1996): 946–9.

Fairweather-Tait, S. J., et al. "Lactoferrin and Iron Absorption in Newborn Infants." *Pediatric Research* 22, no. 6 (1987): 651–4.

Farnsworth, N. R., A. D. Kinghorn, D. D. Soejarto, and D. P. Waller. "Siberian Ginseng (Eleutherococcus senticosus): Current Status as an Adaptogen." *Economic and Medicinal Plant Research* 1 (1985): 155–215.

Farquhar, J. W., R. E. Smith, and M. E. Dempsey. "The Effect of Beta-sitosterol on the Serum Lipids of Young Men with Arteriosclerotic Heart Disease." *Circulation* 14 (1956): 77–82.

Farquhar, J. W., and M. Sokolow. "Response of Serum Lipids and Lipoproteins of Man to Beta-sitosterol and Safflower Oil: A Long-Term Study." *Circulation* 17 (1958): 890–99.

Fava, M., et al. "Neuroendocrine Effects of S-adenosyl-l-methionine, a Novel Putative Antidepressant." *Journal of Psychiatric Research* 24, no. 2 (1990): 177–84.

Fawaz, F. "Zinc Deficiency in Surgical Patients: A Clinical Study." *Journal of Parenteral and Enteral Nutrition* 9, no. 3 (1985): 364–9.

Figge, H. L., J. Figge, P. F. Souney, A. H. Mutnick, and F. Sacks. "Nicotinic Acid: A Review of Its Clinical Use in the Treatment of Lipid Disorders." *Pharmacotherapy* 8, no. 5 (1988): 287–94.

Fine, K. D., C. A. Santa, and J. S. Fordtran. "Diagnosis of Magnesium-Induced Diarrhea." *New England Journal of Medicine* 324, no. 15 (1991): 1012–7.

Finley, E. B., and F. L. Cerklewski. "Influence of Ascorbic Acid Supplementation on Copper Status in Young Adult Men." *American Journal of Clinical Nutrition* 37 (1983): 553–6.

Fleming, C. R., L. M. Smith, and R. E. Hodges. "Essential Fatty Acid Deficiency in Adults Receiving Total Parenteral Nutrition." *American Journal of Clinical Nutrition* 29 (1976): 976–83.

Foldi, M., A.G.B. Kovach, L. Varga, and O. T. Zoltan. "Die Wirkung des Melilotus-Praparates esberiven auf die Lymphstromung." *Arzneimittel-Forschung* 16 (1962): 99–102.

Forgo, I., L. Kayaseeh, and J. J. Staubb. "Einfluss eines standardisierten Ginseng-Extrakes auf das Allgemeinbefinden. Die Reaktionsfahigkeit. Lungenfunktion und die Gonadalen." *Hormone Med. Welt* 32, no. 19 (1981): 751–6.

Foster, S. "Black Cohosh Cimicifuga Racemosa: A Literature Review." *HerbalGram* 45 (1999): 35–50.

Fotouchi, N., et al. "Carotenoid and Tocopherol Concentrations in Plasma, Peripheral Blood Mononuclear Cells, and Red Blood Cells after Long-Term B-carotene Supplementation in Men." *American Journal of Clinical Nutrition* 63 (1996): 55–58.

Franceschi, C., et al. "Oral Zinc Supplementation in Down's Syndrome: Restoration of Thymic Endocrine Activity and of Some

Immune Defects." *Journal of Mental Deficiency Research* 32 (1988): 169–81.

Franceschi, S., E. Bidoli, C. La Vecchia, R. Talamini, B. D'Avanzo, and E. Negri. "Tomatoes and Risk of Digestive-Tract Cancers." *International Journal of Cancer* 59 (1994): 181–4.

Franconi, F., et al. "Plasma and Platelet Taurine Are Reduced in Subjects with Insulin-Dependent Diabetes Mellitus: Effects of Taurine Supplementation." *American Journal of Clinical Nutrition* 61 (1995): 1115–9.

Franken, D. G., G. H. J. Boers, H. J. Blom, F.J.M. Trijbels, and P.W.C. Kloppenborg. "Treatment of Mild Hyperhomocysteinemia in Vascular Disease Patients." *Arteriosclerosis and Thrombosis* 14, no. 3 (1994): 465–70.

Freire, W. B. "Hemoglobin as a Predictor of Response to Iron Therapy and Its Use in Screening and Prevalence Estimates." *American Journal of Clinical Nutrition* 50 (1989): 1442–9.

Friederich, H. C., H. Vogelsberg, and A. Neiss. "Ein Beitrag zur Bewertung von intern wirksamen Venenpharkaka." *Zeitschrift Fur Hautkrankheiter* 53, no. 11 (1977): 369–74.

Fries, M. E., B. M. Chrisley, and J. A. Driskell. "Vitamin B6 Status of a Group of Preschool Children." *American Journal of Clinical Nutrition* 34 (1981): 2706–10.

Frolova, I. A., V. A. Oleneva, I. I. Sirota, and G. D. Nikiforova. "Effect of Pyridoxine on Patterns of Lipid Metabolism in Patients with Alimentary Obesity" (in Russian). *Voprosy Meditsinskoi Khimii* 21 (1975): 299–306.

Fuhrman, B., et al. "Consumption of Red Wine with Meals Reduces the Susceptibility of Human Plasma and Low Density Lipoprotein to Lipid Peroxidation." *American Journal of Clinical Nutrition* 61 (1996): 549–54.

Gabric, V., and H. Miskic. "Behandlung des Benignen Prostata-Adenoms und der chronischen Prostatatitis." *Therapiewoche* 37 (1987): 1775–88.

Galduroz, J. C. F., and E. A. Carlini. "The Effects of Long-Term Administration of Guarana on the Cognition of Normal, Elderly Volunteers." *Sao Paulo Medical Journal* 114, no. 1 (1996): 1073–8.

Garland, C. F., F. C. Garland, and E. D. Gorham. "Can Colon Cancer Incidence and Death Rates Be Reduced with Calcium and Vitamin D?" *American Journal of Clinical Nutrition* 54 (1991): 193–201S

Garry, P. J., G. M. Owen, E. M. Hooper, and B. A. Gilbert. "Iron Absorption from Human Milk and Formula with and without Iron Supplementation." *Pediatric Research* 15 (1981): 822–8.

Garry, P. J., et al. "Nutritional Status in a Healthy Elderly Population: Vitamin C." *American Journal of Clinical Nutrition* 36 (1982): 332–9.

Gastelu, Daniel. *All About Bioflavonoids.* Garden City Park, N.Y.: Avery Publishing Group, in press.

Gastelu, Daniel. *All About Carnitine.* Garden City Park, N.Y.: Avery Publishing Group, in press.

Gastelu, Daniel. *All About Sports Nutrition.* Garden City Park, N.Y.: Avery Publishing Group, in press.

Gastelu, Daniel, and Edmund R. Burke. *Avery's Sports Nutrition Almanac.* Garden City Park, N.Y.: Avery Publishing Group, 1999.

Gastelu, Daniel, and Fred Hatfield. *Dynamic Nutrition for Maximum Performance.* Garden City Park, N.Y.: Avery Publishing Group, 1997.

Gastelu, Daniel and Fred Hatfield. *Performance Nutrition: The Complete Guide.* Santa Barbara, Calif.: International Sports Sciences Association, 1995.

Gaull, G. E., D. K. Rassin, and J. A. Sturman. "Enzymatic and Metabolic Studies of Homocystinuria: Effects of Pyridoxine." *Neuropadiatrie* 1, no. 2 (1969): 199–226.

Gaziano, J. M., et al. "Discrimination in Absorption or Transport of B-carotene Isomers after Oral Supplementation with Either All-trans- or 9-cis-b-carotene." *American Journal of Clinical Nutrition* 61 (1995): 1248–52.

Geßner, B., and P. Cnota. "Untersuchung der Vigilanz nach Applikation von Kava-Kava-Extrakt, Diazepam oder Placebo." *Z. Phytother.* 15 (1994): 30–7.

Gey, K. F., P. Puska, P. Jordan, and U. K. Moser. "Inverse Correlation Between Plasma Vitamin E and Mortality from Ischemic Heart Disease in Cross-Cultural Epidemiology." *American Journal of Clinical Nutrition* 53 (1991): 326–4S

Ghigo, E., et al. "Arginine Abolishes the Inhibitory Effect of Glucose on the Growth Hormone Response to Growth Hormone-Releasing Hormone in Man." *Metabolism* 41, no. 9 (1992): 1000–3.

Ghigo, E., et al. "Arginine Potentiates the GHRH- but Not the Pyridostigmine-Induced GH Secretion in Normal Short Children: Further Evidence for a Somatostatin Suppressing Effect of Arginine." *Clinical Endocrinology* 32 (1990): 763–7.

Gibson, R. S., et al. "A Growth-Limiting, Mild Zinc-Deficiency Syndrome in Some Southern Ontario Boys with Low Height Percentiles." *American Journal of Clinical Nutrition* 49 (1989): 1266–73.

Gibson, S. A. "Are High-Fat, High-Sugar Food and Diets Conducive to Obesity?" *International Journal of Food Sciences and Nutrition* 47 (1996): 405–15.

Gillilan, R. E., B. Mondell, and J. R. Warbasse. "Quantitative Evaluation of Vitamin E in the Treatment of Angina Pectoris." *American Heart Journal* 93, no. 4 (1977): 444–9.

Giomberardino, M. A., et al. "Effects of Prolonged L-carnitine Administration on Delayed Muscle Pain and CK Release After Eccentric Effort." *International Journal of Sports Medicine* 17 (1996): 320–4.

Giovannucci, E., et al. "Intake of Carotenoids and Retinol in Relation to Risk of Prostate Cancer." *Journal of the National Cancer Institute* 87, no. 23 (1995): 1767–76.

Gogos, C. A., F. E. Kalfarentzos, and N. C. Zoumobs. "Effect of Different Types of Total Parental Nutrition on T-lymphocyte Subpopulations and NK Cells." *American Journal of Clinical Nutrition* 51 (1990): 119–22.

Golay, A. "Blunted Glucose-Induced Thermogenesis: A Factor Contributing to Relapse of Obesity." *International Journal of Obesity* 17 (1993): S23–7.

Goldenbeg, R. L., et al. "The Effect of Zinc Supplementation on Pregnancy Outcome." *JAMA* 274, no. 6 (1995): 463–75.

Goldin, B. R., H. Adlercreutz, S. L. Gorbach, M. N. Woods, J. T. Dwyer, T. Conlon, E. Bohn, and S. N. Gershoff. "The Relationship Between Estrogen Levels and Diets of Caucasian American and Oriental Immigrant Women." *American Journal of Clinical Nutrition* 44 (1986): 945–53.

Goldman, J. A., R. H. Lerman, J. H. Contois, and J. N. Udall. "Behavioral Effects of Sucrose on Preschool Children." *Journal of Abnormal Child Psychology* 14, no. 4 (1986): 565–77.

Goldstein, A., S. Kaizer, and R. Warren. "Psychotropic Effects of Caffeine in Man: II. Alertness, Psychomotor Coordination, and Mood." *Journal of Pharmacology and Experimental Therapeutics* 150, no. 1 (1965): 146–53.

Golikov, P. P. "Effects of Liquid Extracts of Siberian Ginseng and Ginseng (Korean) on Mental Work of Humans" (in Russian). *Lek. Sredstva Dal'nego Vostoka* 5 (1963): 233–40.

Golledge, C. and Thomas V. Riley. "'Natural' Therapy for Infectious Diseases." *Medical Journal of Australia* 164 (January 1996): 94–5.

Gomes, J.A.C., D. Venkatachalapathy, and J. I. Haft. "The Effect of Vitamin E on Platelet Aggregation." *American Heart Journal* 91, no. 4 (1976): 425–9.

Gonder-Frederick, L., D. J. Cox, S. A. Bobbitt, and J. W. Pennebaker. "Mood Changes Associated with Blood Glucose Fluctuations in Insulin-Dependent Diabetes Mellitus." *Health Psychology* 8, no. 1 (1989): 45–59.

Gonder-Frederick, L., J. L. Hall, J. Vogt, D. J. Cox, J. Green, and P. E. Gold. "Memory Enhancement in Elderly Humans: Effects of Glucose Ingestion." *Physiology and Behavior* 41 (1987): 503–4.

Gonella, M., G. Calabrese, G. Vagelli, G. Pratesi, S. Lamon, and S. Talarico. "Effects of High CaCO3 Supplements on Serum Calcium and Phosphorus in Patients on Regular Hemodialysis Treatment." *Clinical Nephrology* 24, no. 3 (1985): 147–50.

Goodwin, J. S., W. C. Hunt, P. Hooper, and P. J. Garry. "Relationship Between Zinc Intake, Physical Activity, and Blood Levels in High-Density Lipoprotein Cholesterol in a Healthy Elderly Population." *Metabolism* 34, no. 6 (1985): 519–23.

Gordeuk, V. R., G. M. Brittenham, M. A. Hughes, and L. J. Keating. "Carbonyl Iron for Short-Term Supplementation in Female Blood Donors." *Transfusion* 27 (1987): 80–5.

Gordeuk, V. R., G. M. Brittenham, C. E. McLaren, M. A. Hughes, and L. J. Keating.

"Carbonyl Iron Therapy for Iron Deficiency Anemia." *Blood* 67, no. 3 (1986): 745–52.

Grandhi, A., A. M. Mujumdar, and B. Patwardhan. "A Comparative Pharmacological Investigation of Ashwagandha and Ginseng." *Journal of Ethnopharmacology* 44 (1994): 131–5.

Grasso, M., et al. "Comparative Effects of Alfuzosin Versus Serenoa Repens in the Treatment of Symptomatic Benign Prostatic Hyperplasia." *Archivos Espanoles De Urolgia* 48, no. 1 (1995): 97–103.

Greca, P., and R. Volpi. "Esperienze sull'uso di un nuovo farmaco nel trattamento medico dell'adenoma prostatico." *Urologia* 52 (1985): 532–5.

Greenway, F. L., and G. A. Bray. "Regional Fat Loss from the Thigh in Obese Women after Adrenergic Modulation." *Clinical Therapeutics* 9, no. 6 (1987).

Greer, F. R., et al. "Bone Mineral Content and Serum 25-hydroxyvitamin D Concentrations in Breast-Fed Infants with and without Supplemental Vitamin D: One-Year Follow-up." *Journal of Pediatrics* 100, no. 6 (1982): 919–22.

Greger, J. L., C. D. Davis, J. W. Suttie, and B. J. Lyle. "Intake, Serum Concentrations, and Urinary Excretion of Manganese by Adult Males." *American Journal of Clinical Nutrition* 51 (1990): 457–61.

Greger, J. L., et al. "Calcium, Magnesium, Phosphorus, Copper, and Manganese Balance in Adolescent Females." *American Journal of Clinical Nutrition* 31 (1978): 117–21.

Grobbee, D. E., and A. Hofman. "Effect of Calcium Supplementation on Diastolic Blood Pressure in Young People with Mild Hypertension." *Lancet* 2 (1986): 703–6.

Gropper, S. S., and P. B. Acosta. "Brief Communicaton: The Therapeutic Effect of Fiber in Treating Obesity." *Journal of the American College of Nutrition* 6, no. 6 (1987): 533–5.

Gruchow, H., K. Sobocinski, and J. Barboriak. "Calcium Intake and the Relationship of Dietary Sodium and Potassium to Blood Pressure." *American Journal of Clinical Nutrition* 48 (1988): 1463–70.

Gupta, S., P. George, V. Gupta, V. R. Tandon, and K. R. Sundaram. "Tylophora Indica in Bronchial Asthma—A Double-Blind Study." *Indian Journal of Medical Research* 69 (1979): 981–9.

Gupta, V., et al. "Effect of Aspartame on Plasma Amino Acid Profiles of Diabetic Patients with Chronic Renal Failure." *American Journal of Clinical Nutrition* 49 (1989): 1302–6.

Gutteridge, J. M. C., et al. "Copper and Iron Complex Catalytic for Oxygen Radical Reactions in Sweat from Human Athletes." *Clinica Chimica Acta* 145 (1985): 267–73.

Haeger, K. "Long-Time Treatment of Intermittent Claudication with Vitamin E." *American Journal of Clinical Nutrition* 27 (1974): 1179–81.

Hale, W. E., et al. "Use of Nutritional Supplements in an Ambulatory Elderly Population." *Journal of the American Geriatrics Society* 30, no. 6 (1982): 401–3.

Hall, J. L., L. A. Gonder-Frederick, W. W. Chewning, J. Silveira, and P. E. Gold. "Glucose Enhancement of Performance on Memory Tests in Young and Aged Humans." *Neuropsychologia* 27, no. 9 (1989): 1129–38.

Hallberg, L., M. Brune, and L. Rossander. "Iron Absorption in Man: Ascorbic Acid and Dose-Dependent Inhibition by Phytate." *American Journal of Clinical Nutrition* 49 (1989): 140–4.

Hallberg, L., M. Brune, and I. Rossander. "Low Bioavailability of Carbony Iron in Man: Studies on Iron Fortification of Wheat Flour." *American Journal of Clinical Nutrition* 43 (1986): 59–67.

Hallberg, L., A. Norrby, and L. Solvell. "Oral Iron with Succinic Acid in the Treatment of Iron Deficiency Anaemia." *Scandinavian Journal of Haematology* 8 (1971): 104–11.

Hallberg, L., L. Rossander-Hulthen, and E. Gramatkovski. "Iron Fortification of Flour with a Complex Ferric Orthophosphate." *American Journal of Clinical Nutrition* 50 (1989): 129–35.

Hallberg, L., et al. "Calcium: Effect of Different Amounts on Nonheme- and Heme-iron Absorption in Humans." *American Journal of Clinical Nutrition* 53 (1991): 112–9.

Hamalainen, E., H. Adlercreutz, P. Puska, and P. Pietinen. "Diet and Serum Sex Hormones in Healthy Men." *Journal of Steroid Biochemistry and Molecular Biology* 20, no. 1 (1984): 459–64.

Hamalainen, E., H. Tikkanen, M. Harkonen, H. Naveri, and H. Adlercreutz. "Serum Lipoproteins, Sex Hormones, and Sex Hormone Binding Globulin in Middle-Aged Men of Different Physical Fitness and Risk of Coronary Heart Disease." *Atherosclerosis* 67 (1987): 155–62.

Hanak, T., and M.-H. Bruckel. "Behandlung von leichten stabilen Formen der Angina pectoris mit Crataegutt novo: Eine placebokontrollierte Doppelblindstudie." *Therapiewoche* 33 (1983): 4331–3.

Hankinson, S. E., et al. "Nutrient Intake and Cataract Extraction in Women: A Prospective Study." *BMJ* 305 (1992): 335–39.

Hansen, C., J. Leklem, and L. Miller. "Changes in Vitamin B-6 Status Indicators of Women Fed a Constant Protein Diet with Varying Levels of Vitamin B-6." *American Journal of Clinical Nutrition* 66 (1997): 1379–87.

Hansgen, K-D., J. Vesper, and M. Ploch. "Multicenter Double-Blind Study Examining the Antidepressant Effectiveness of the Hypercium Extract LI 160." *Journal of Geriatric Psychiatry and Neurology* 7, supplement 1 (1994): S15–8.

Harenberg, J., C. Giese, and R. Zimmermann. "Effect of Dried Garlic on Blood Coagulation, Fibrinolysis, Platelet Aggregation, and Serum Cholesterol Levels in Patients with Hyperlipoproteinemia." *Atherosclerosis* 74 (1988): 247–9.

Harman, D. "Free Radical Involvment in Aging: Pathophysiology and Therapeutic Implications." *Drugs and Aging* 3, no. 1 (1993): 60–80.

Harris, T. B., et al. "Carrying the Burden of

Cardiovascular Risk in Old Age: Associations of Weight and Weight Change with Prevalent Cardiovascular Disease, Risk Factors, and Health Status in the Cardiovascular Health Study." *American Journal of Clinical Nutrition* 66 (1997): 837–44.

Harris, W. S., W. E. Connor, N. Alam, and D. R. Illingworth. "Reduction of Postprandial Triglyceridemia in Humans by Dietary n-3 Fatty Acids." *Journal of Lipid Research* 29 (1988): 1451–60.

Harris, W. S., W. E. Connor, S. B. Inkeles, and D. R. Illingworth. "Dietary Omega-3 Fatty Acids Prevent Carbohydrate-Induced Hypertriglyceridemia." *Metabolism* 33, no. 11 (1984): 1016–9.

Harris, W. S., W. E. Connor, and M. P. McCurry. "The Comparative Reductions of the Plasma Lipids and Lipoproteins by Dietary Polyunsaturated Fats: Salmon Oil Versus Vegetable Oils." *Metabolism* 32, no. 2 (1983): 179–84.

Harris, W. S., C. A. Dujovne, M. Zucker, and B. Johnson. "Effects of a Low Saturated Fat, Low Cholesterol Fish Oil Supplement in Hypertriglyceridemic Patients." *Annals of Internal Medicine* 109 (1988): 465–70.

Hartmann, E., C. Spinweber, and J. Fernstrom. "Tryptophan and Human Sleep: An Analysis of Forty-three Studies." *Progress in Tryptophan and Serotonin Research* (1984): 297–304.

Hartz, S. C., et al. "Nutrient Supplement Use by Healthy Elderly." *Journal of the American College of Nutrition* 7, no. 2 (1988): 119–28.

Harvey, J. A., et al. "Superior Calcium Absorption from Calcium Citrate Than Calcium Carbonate Using External Forearm Counting." *Journal of the American College of Nutrition* 9, no. 6 (1990): 583–7.

Hassan, M. A., et al. "Free Amino Acids, Copper, Iron, and Zinc Composition in Sera of Patients with Thyrometabolic Diseases." *Hormone and Metabolic Research* 22 (1990): 117–20.

Hassig, C., J. Tong, and S. Schreiber. "Fiber-Derived Butyrate and the Prevention of Colon Cancer." *Chemistry and Biology* 4 (1997): 783–9.

Havel, R. J. "Dietary Supplement or Drug? The Case of Cholestin." *American Journal of Clinical Nutrition* 69 (1999): 175–6.

Havel, R. J., et al. "Lovastin (Mevinolin) in the Treatment of Heterozygous Familial Hypercholesterolemia." *Annals of Internal Medicine* 107, no. 5 (1987): 609–15.

Haverkate, F., et al. "Production of C-Reactive Protein and Risk of Coronary Events in Stable and Unstable Angina." *Lancet* 349 (1997): 462–6.

Hayatsu, H., T. Negishi, S. Arimoto, and T. Hayatsu. "Porphyrins as Potential Inhibitors Against Exposure to Carcinogens and Mutagens." *Mutation Research* 290 (1993): 79–85.

Hayes, C., M. M. Werler, W. C. Willett, and A. A. Mitchell. "Case-Control Study of Periconceptional Folic Acid Supplementation and Oral Clefts." *American Journal of Epidemiology* 143, no. 12 (1996): 1229–34.

Heaney, R., and C. M. Weaver. "Oxalate: Effect on Calcium Absorbability." *American Journal of Clinical Nutrition* 50 (1989): 830–2.

Heaney, R., K. M. Davies, R. R. Recker, and P. T. Packard. "Long-Term Consistency of Nutrient Intakes in Humans." *Journal of Nutrition* 120 (1990): 869–75.

Heaney, R., K. T. Smith, R. R. Recker, and S. M. Hinders. "Meal Effects on Calcium Absorption." *American Journal of Clinical Nutrition* 49 (1989): 372–6.

Heaney, R., C. Weaver, and M. Fitzsimmons. "Soybean Phytate Content: Effect on Calcium Absorption." *American Journal of Clinical Nutrition* 53 (1991): 745–7.

Heaney, R., A. J. Yates, and A. C. Santora. "Biphosphonate Effects and the Bone Remodeling Transient." *Journal of Bone and Mineral Research* 12, no. 8 (1997): 1143–51.

Heber, D., et al. "Cholesterol-Lowering Effects of a Proprietary Chinese Red-Yeast-Rice Dietary Supplement." *American Journal of Clinical Nutrition* 69 (1999): 231–6.

Heide, M. "Anderung der Ernahrungsweise bei Ubergewicht und Hyperlipoproteinamie." *Lymphologie* 9 (1985): 90–3.

Hellsten, Y. "Oxidation of Urate in Human Skeletal Muscle During Exercise." *Free Radical Biology and Medicine* 22, nos. 1/2 (1997): 169–74.

Hellstrom, L., S. Rossner, E. Hagstrom-Toft, and S. Reynisdottir. "Lipolytic Catecholamine Resistance Linked to x2-adrenoceptor Sensitivity—A Metabolic Predictor of Weight Loss in Obese Subjects." *International Journal of Obesity* 21 (1997): 314–20.

Hemila, H. "Does Vitamin C Alleviate the Symptoms of the Common Cold? A Review of Current Evidence." *Scandinavian Journal of Infectious Diseases* 26 (1994): 1–6.

Hemminki, E., and U. Rimpela. "A Randomized Comparison of Routine Versus Selective Iron Supplementation During Pregnancy." *Journal of the American College of Nutrition* 10, no. 1 (1991): 3–10.

Henderson, V. W., A. Paganini-Hill, C. K. Emanuel, M. E. Dunn, and J. G. Buckwalter. "Estrogen Replacement Therapy in Older Women." *Archives of Neurology* 51 (1994): 47–51.

Henkin, Y., A. Oberman, D. C. Hurst, and J. P. Segrest. "Niacin Revisited: Clinical Observations on an Important but Underutilized Drug." *American Journal of Medicine* 91 (1991): 239–46.

Hennekens, C. H., and J. M. Gaziano. "Antioxidants and Heart Disease: Epidemiology and Clinical Evidence." *Clinical Cardiology* 16 (1993): 10–5.

Henriksson, K., et al. "Gastrin, Gastric Acid Secretion, Gastric Microflors in Patients with Rheumatoid Arthritis." *Annals of the Rheumatic Diseases* 45 (1986): 475–83.

Henrotte, J. G., and C. Levy-Leboyer. "Le comportement de type A—est il module par des facteurs genetiques régulateurs du metabolisme du magnesium de du zinc?" *Magnesium* 4 (1985): 295–302.

Henrotte, J. G., et al. "Blood and Urinary Magnesium, Zinc, Calcium, Free Fatty Acids, and Catecholamines in Type A and Type B Subjects." *Journal of the American College of Nutrition* 4 (1985): 165–72.

Hense, H. W., M. Stender, W. Bors, and U. Keil. "Lack of an Association Between Serum Vitamin E and Myocardial Infarction in a Population with High Vitamin E Levels." *Atherosclerosis* 103 (1993): 21–8.

Herberg, K.-W. "Fahrtuchtigkeit nach Einnahme von Kava-Spezial-Extrakt WS 1490. Doppelblinde plurebokontrolliente." *Zeitschr. Allemein. Med.* 67 (1991): 842–6.

Herranz, L., A. Megia, C. Grande, P. Gonzales-Gancedo, and F. Pallardo. "Dehydroepiandrosterone Sulphate, Body Fat Distribution, and Insulin in Obese Men." *International Journal of Obesity* 19 (1995): 57–60.

Hertog, M., E. J. M. Feskens, P. C. H. Hollman, M. B. Katan, and D. Kromhout. "Dietary Antioxidant Flavonoids and Risk of Coronary Heart Disease: The Zutphen Elderly Study." *Lancet* 342 (1993): 1007–11.

Hertog, M., P. Hollman, M. Katan, and D. Kromhout. "Intake of Potentially Anticarcinogenic Flavonoids and Their Determinants in Adults in the Netherlands." *Nutrition and Cancer* 20, no. 1 (1993): 21–8.

Heule, F. "An Oral Approach to the Treatment of Photodamaged Skin: a Pilot Study." *Journal of International Medicinal Research* 20 (1992): 273–8.

Heymsfield, S. B., et al. "Garcinia Cambogia (Hydroxycitric Acid) as a Potential Anti-obesity Agent: A Randomized Controlled Trial." *JAMA* 280, no. 18 (1998): 1596–1600.

Hill, P., L. Garbaczewski, H. Koppeschaar, J.H.H. Thijssen, F. de Waard, and E. L. Wynder. "Peptide and Steroid Hormones in Subjects at Different Risk for Diet-Related Diseases." *American Journal of Clinical Nutrition* 48 (1988): 782–6.

Hipkiss, A. R., J. Michaelis, P. Syrris, and M. Dreimanis. "Strategies for the Extension of Human Life Span." *Perspectives in Human Biology* 3 (1995): 59–70.

Hiramatsu, K., and S. Arimori. "Increased Superoxide Production by Mononuclear Cells of Patients with Hypertriglyceridemia and Diabetes." *Diabetes* 37 (1988): 832–7.

Ho, K. Y., et al. "Effects of Sex and Age on the Twenty-four-Hour Profile of Growth Hormone Secretion in Man: Importance of Endogenous Estradiol Concentrations." *Journal of Clinical Endocrinology and Metabolism* 64, no. 1 (1987): 51–6.

Ho, L., D. Chang, M. Chang, S. Kuo, and J. Lai. "Mechanism of Immunosuppression of the Antirheumatic Herb TWHf in Human T Cells." *Journal of Rheumatology* 26, no. 1 (1999): 14–24.

Hobbs, C. J., S. R. Plymate, C. J. Rosen, and R. A. Adler. "Testosterone Administration Increases Insulin-like Growth Factor I Levels in Normal Men." *Journal of Clinical*

Endocrinology and Metabolism 7, no. 8 (1998): 776–9.

Hocman, G. "Prevention of Cancer: Vegetables and Plants." *Comparative Biochemistry and Physiology* 93B, no. 2 (1989): 201–12.

Hodis, H. N., et al. "Serial Coronary Angiographic Evidence That Antioxidant Vitamin Intake Reduces Progression of Coronary Artery Atherosclerosis." *JAMA* 273, no. 23 (1995): 1849–54.

Hollman, P., M. Gaag, M. Mengelers, J. Trup, J. De Vries, and M. Katan. "Absorption and Disposition Kinetics of the Dietary Antioxidant Quercetin in Man." *Free Radical Biology and Medicine* 21, no. 5 (1996): 703–7.

Hollowell, J. G., et al. "Homocystinuria and Organic Aciduria in a Patient with Vitamin B12 Deficiency." *Lancet* 2 (1969): 1428.

Horrobin, D. F. "The Importance of Gamma-Linolenic Acid and Prostaglandin E1 in Human Nutrition and Medicine." *Journal of Holistic Medicine* 5, no. 2 (1981): 118–39.

Horton, T. J., and C. A. Geissler. "Aspirin Potentiates the Effect of Ephedrine on the Thermogenic Response to a Meal in Obese but Not Lean Women." *International Journal of Obesity* 15 (1991): 359–66.

Hotz, W. "Nicotinic Acid and Its Derivatives: A Short Survey." *Advances in Lipid Research* 20 (1983): 195–217.

Howard, B. V., W. G. H. Abbott, and B. A. Swinburn. "Evaluation of Metabolic Effects of Substitution of Complex Carbohydrates for Saturated Fat in Individuals with Obesity and NIDDM." *Diabetes Care* 14, no. 9 (1991): 786–95.

Howat, R.C.L., and G. D. Lewis. "The Effect of Bromelain Therapy on Episiotomy Wounds—A Double-Blind Controlled Clinical Trial." *Journal of Obsterics and Gynecology* 79 (1972): 951–3.

Howell, W. H., D. J. McNamara, M. A. Tosca, B. T. Smith, and J. A. Gaines. "Plasma Lipid and Lipoprotein Responses to Dietary Fat and Cholesterol: A Meta-analysis." *American Journal of Clinical Nutrition* 65 (1997): 1747–64.

Hubner, W-D., S. Lande, and H. Podzuweit. "Hypericum Treatment of Mild Depressions with Somatic Symptoms." *Journal of Geriatric Psychiatry and Neurology* 7, supplement 1 (1994): 12–4.

Hudgins, L. C., and J. Hirsch. "Changes in Abdominal and Gluteal Adipose-Tissue Fatty Compositions in Obese Subjects after Weight Gain and Weight Loss." *American Journal of Clinical Nutrition* 53 (1991): 1372–7.

Hughes-Dawson, B., et al. "A Controlled Trial of the Effect of Calcium Supplementation on Bone Density in Postmenopausal Women." *New England Journal of Medicine* 323, no. 13 (1990): 878–83.

Hulshof, K.F.A.M., et al. "Comparison of Dietary Intake Data with Guidelines: Some Potential Pitfalls (Dutch Nutrition Surveillance System)." *Journal of the American College of Nutrition* 12, no. 2 (1993): 176–85.

Hunt, I. F., et al. "Bone Mineral Content in Postmenopausal Women: Comparison of Omnivores and Vegetarians." *American Journal of Clinical Nutrition* 50 (1989): 517–23.

Hunter, D. J., et al. "A Prospective Study of the Intake of Vitamins C, E, and A and the Risk of Breast Cancer." *New England Journal of Medicine* 329, no. 4 (1993): 234–40.

Hunter, J. O. "Food Allergy—or Enterometabolic Disorder?" *Lancet* 338 (1991): 495–6.

Hurson, M., et al. "Metabolic Effects of Arginine in a Healthy Elderly Population." *Journal of Parenteral and Enteral Nutrition* 19, no. 3 (1995): 227–30.

Hustead, V. A., J. L. Greger, and G. R. Gutcher. "Zinc Supplementation and Plasma Concentration of Vitamin A in Preterm Infants." *American Journal of Clinical Nutrition* 47 (1988): 1017–21.

Imai, K., and K. Nakachi. "Cross-Sectional Study of Effects of Drinking Green Tea on Cardiovascular and Liver Diseases." *BMJ* 310 (1995): 693–6.

Innis, S. M., and D. B. Allardyce. "Possible Biotin Deficiency in Adults Receiving Long-Term Total Parental Nutrition." *American Journal of Clinical Nutrition* 37 (1983): 185–7.

Iost, C., et al. "Repleting Hemoglobin in Iron Deficiency Anemia in Young Children Through Liquid Milk Fortification with Bioavailable Iron Amino Acid Chelate." *Journal of the American College of Nutrition* 17, no. 2 (1998): 187–94.

Iseri, L. T., P. Chung, and J. Tobis. "Magnesium Therapy for Intractable Ventricular Tachyarrhythmias in Normomagnesemic Patients." *Western Journal of Medicine* 138, no. 6 (1983): 8238.

Itoh, R., N. Nishiyama, and Y. Suyama. "Dietary Protein Intake and Urinary Excretion of Calcium: A Cross-Sectional Study in a Healthy Japanese Population." *American Journal of Clinical Nutrition* 67 (1998): 438–44.

Ivanovich, P., H. Fellows, and C. Rich. "The Absorption of Calcium Carbonate." *Annals of Internal Medicine* 66, no. 5 (1967): 917–23.

Iwamoto, M., T. Sato, and T. Ishizak. "The Clinical Effect of Crataegutt in Heart Disease of Ischemic or Hypertensive Origin. A Multicenter Double-Blind Study." *Planta Medica* 42, no. 1 (1981): 1–16.

Jacobsen, S., B. Danneskiold-Samsoe, and R. B. Andersen. "Oral S-adenosylmethionine in Primary Fibromyalgia: Double-Blind Clinical Evaluation." *Scandinavian Journal of Rheumatology* 20 (1991): 294–302.

Jacques, P. F., et al. "Long-Term Vitamin C Supplement Use and Prevalence of Early Age-Related Lens Opacities." *American Journal of Clinical Nutrition* 66 (1997): 911–16.

Jacques, P. F., et al. "Relation Between Folate Status, a Common Mutation in Methylenetetrahydrofolate Reductase, and Plasma Homocysteine Concentrations." *Circulation* 93 (1996): 7–9.

Jain, A. K., R. Vargas, S. Gotzkowsky, and F. G. McMahon. "Can Garlic Reduce Levels of Serum Lipids? A Controlled Clinical

Study." *American Journal of Medicine* 94 (1993): 632–5.

Jain, R. C., and C. R. Vyas. "Onion and Garlic in Atherosclerotic Heart Disease." *Medikon* 6, no. 5 (1977): 12–8.

Jain, S. K., et al. "Effect of Modest Vitamin E Supplementation on Blood Glycated Hemoglobin and Triglyceride Levels and Red Cell Indices in Type I Diabetic Patients." *Journal of the American College of Nutrition* 15, no. 5 (1996): 458–61.

Jandak, J., M. Steiner, and P. D. Richardson. "Alpha-tocopherol, an Effective Inhibitor of Platelet Adhesion." *Blood* 73, no. 1 (1989): 141–9.

Jandak, J., M. Steiner, and P. D. Richardson. "Reduction of Platelet Adhesiveness by Vitamin E Supplementation in Humans." *Thrombosis Research* 49 (1988): 393–404.

Jang, M., L. Cai, G. O. Udeani, K. V. Slowing, C. F. Thomas, C.W.W. Beecher, H.H.S. Fong, N. R. Farnsworth, A. D. Kinghorn, R. G. Mehta, R. C. Moon, and J. M. Pezzuto. "Cancer Chemopreventive Activity of Resveratrol, a Natural Product Derived from Grapes." *Science* 275 (1997): 218–20.

Janowsky, J. S., S. K. Oviatt, and E. S. Orwoll. "Testosterone Influences Spatial Cognition in Older Men." *Behavioral Neuroscience* 106 (1994): 325–32.

Jantzky, K., and A. Morreale. "Probable Interaction Between Warfarin and Ginseng." *American Journal of Health-System Pharmacy* 54, 692–3.

Jeng, K.-C., et al. "Supplementation with Vitamins C and E Enhances Cytokine Production by Peripheral Blood Mononuclear Cells in Healthy Adults." *American Journal of Clinical Nutrition* 64 (1996): 960–5.

Jenkins, D.J.A., A. I. Jenkins, T.M.S. Wolever, V. Vuksan, A. V. Rao, L. U. Thompson, and R. G. Josse. "Low Glycemic Index: Lente Carbohydrates and Physiological Effects of Altered Food Frequency." *American Journal of Clinical Nutrition* 59 (1994): 706s–9s

Jenkins, J. A., et al. "Glycemic Index of Foods: A Physiological Basis for Carbohydrate Exchange." *American Journal of Clinical Nutrition* 34 (1981): 362–6.

Jensen, C. A., C. M. Weaver, and D. A. Sedlock. "Iron Supplementation and Iron in Exercising Young Women." *J. Nutr. Biochem.* 2 (1991): 368–73.

Jeppensen, J., et al. "Effects of Low-Fat, High-Carbohydrate Diets on Risk Factors for Ischemic Heart Disease in Postmenopausal Women." *American Journal of Clinical Nutrition* 65 (1997): 1027–33.

Jeukendrup, A., et al. "Effect of Medium-Chain Triacylglycerol and Carbohydrate Ingestion During Exercise on Substrate Utilization and Subsequent Cycling Performance." *American Journal of Clinical Nutrition* 67 (1998): 397–404.

Johannson, I., P. Tidehag, V. Lundberg, and G. Hallmans. "Dental Status, Diet, and Cardiovascular Risk Factors in Middle-Aged People in Northern Sweden." *Community Dentistry and Oral Epidemiology* 22 (1994): 431–6.

Johnson, A., N. Jiang, and E. John Staba. "Whole Ginseng Effects on Human

Response to Demands for Performance." Proceedings of the Third International Ginseng Symposium, Seoul, Korea, 1980.

Johnson, D., H. Ksciuk, H. Woelk, E. Sauerwein-Giese, and A. Frauendorf. "Effects of Hypericum Extract LI 160 Compared with Maprotiline on Resting EEG and Evoked Potentials in Twenty-four Volunteers." *Journal of Geriatric Psychiatry and Neurology* 7, supplement 1 (1994): 44–6.

Johnson, E., N. P. Kadam, D. M. Hylands, and P. J. Hylands. "Efficacy of Feverfew as Prophylactic Treatment of Migraine." *BMJ* 291 (1985): 569–73.

Johnsonton, C. C., et al. "Calcium Supplementation and Increases in Bone Mineral Density in Children." *New England Journal of Medicine* 327 (1992): 82–7.

Johnston, L., L. Vaughan, and H. M. Fox. "Pantothenic Acid Content of Human Milk." *American Journal of Clinical Nutrition* 34 (1981): 2205–9.

Johri, R. K., and U. Zutshi. "An Ayurvedic Formulation 'Trikatu' and Its Constituents." *Journal of Ethnopharmacology* 37 (1992): 85–91.

Joosten, E., et al. "Metabolic Evidence that Deficiencies of Vitamin B12 (Cobalamin), Folate, and Vitamin B6 Occur Commonly in Elderly People." *American Journal of Clinical Nutrition* 58 (1993): 468–76.

Jung, F., C. Mrowietz, H. Kiesewetter, and E. Wenzei. "Effect of Ginkgo Biloba on Fluidity of Blood and Peripheral Microcirculation in Volunteers." *Arzneimittel-Forschung/Drug Research* 40, no. 5 (1990): 589–93.

Jurcic, K., D. Melchart, M. Holzmaan, P. Martin, R. Bauer, A. Doenecke, and H. Wagner. "Zwei Probandenstudien zur Stiumlierung der Granulozyten-phagozytose durch Echinacea-Extrakt-haltige Präparate." *Zeitschrift fur Phytotherapie* 10 (1989): 67–70.

Kaats, G. R., S. C. Keith, D. Pullin, W. G. Squires, J. A. Wise, R. Hesslink, and R. J. Morin. "Safety and Efficacy Evaluation of a Fitness Club Weight-Loss Program." *Advances in Natural Therapy* 15, no. 6 (1998).

Kaats, G. R., et al. "The Short-Term Therapeutic Efficacy of Treating Obesity with a Plan of Improved Nutrition and Moderate Caloric Restriction." *Curr. Ther. Res.* 51, no. 2 (1992): 261–74.

Kagan, B. L., D. L. Sultzer, N. Rosenlicht, and R. H. Gerner. "Oral S-adenosylmethionine in Depression: A Randomized, Double-Blind, Placebo-Controlled Trial." *American Journal of Psychiatry* 147, no. 5 (1990): 591–5.

Kalbfleisch, W., and H. Pfalzgraf. "Odemprotektiva: Aquipotente Dosierung: Robkastaniensamenextrakt und O-B-hydroxyethyl-rutosideim Vergleich." *Therapiewoche* 39 (1989): 3703–7.

Kales, A., E. O. Bixler, J. D. Kales, and M. B. Scharf. "Comparative Effectiness of Nine Hypnotic Drugs: Sleep Laboratory Studies." *Journal of Clinical Pharmacology* (1977): 207–13.

Kallner, A., D. Hartmann, and D. H. Horning. "On the Requirements of Ascorbic Acid in Man: Steady-State Turnover and Body

Pool in Smokers." *American Journal of Clinical Nutrition* 34 (1981): 1347–55.

Kallner, A., D. Horning, and R. Pellikka. "Formation of Carbon Dioxide from Ascorbate in Man." *American Journal of Clinical Nutrition* 41 (1985): 609–13.

Kaltwasser, J. P., E. Werner, and M. Niechzial. "Bioavailability and Therapeutic Efficacy of Bivalent and Trivalent Iron Preparations." *Arzneimittel-Forschung* 37 (1987): 122–8.

Kamanna, V. S., and N. Chandrasekhara. "Biochemical and Physiological Effects of Garlic (Allium Sativum Linn.)." *Journal of Scientific and Industrial Research* 42 (1983): 353–7.

Kampen, D. L., and B. B. Sherwin. "Estrogen Use and Verbal Memory in Healthy Postmenopausal Women." *Obstetrics and Gynecology* 83, no. 6 (1994): 979–83.

Kanarek, R. B., and D. Swinney. "Effects of Food Snacks on Cognitive Performance in Male College Students" *Appetite* 14 (1990): 15–27.

Kang, S-S., P.W.K. Wong, and M. Norusis. "Homocysteinemia Due to Folate Deficiency." *Metabolism* 36 (1987): 458–62.

Kant, A. K., and G. Block. "Dietary Vitamin B6 Intake and Food Sources in the U.S. Population: NHANES II, 1976–1980." *American Journal of Clinical Nutrition* 52 (1990): 707–16.

Kasai, K., M. Kobayashi, and S. Shimoda. "Stimulatory Effect of Glycine on Human Growth Hormone Secretion." *Metabolism* 27, no. 2 (1978): 201–9.

Kaul, L., and J. Nidiry. "High-Fiber Diet in the Treatment of Obesity and Hypercholesterolemia." *Journal of the National Medical Association* 85 (1993): 231–2.

Kaye, G. L., J. C. Blake, and A. K. Burroughs. "Metabolism of Exogenous S-adenosyl-l-methionine in Patients with Liver Disease." *Drugs* 40, no. 3 (1990): 124–8.

Keen, H., J. Payan, J. Allawi, J. Walker, G. A. Jamal, A. I. Weir, L. M. Henderson, E. A. Bissessar, P. J. Watkins, M. Sampson, E.A.M. Gale, J. Scarfello, H. G. Boddie, K. J. Hardy, P. K. Thomas, P. Misra, and J. Halonen. "Treatment of Diabetic Neuropathy with Gamma-linolenic Acid." *Diabetes Care* 16, no. 1 (1993): 8–15.

Kelly, G. S. "Sports Nutrition: A Review of Selected Nutritional Supplements For Bodybuilders and Strength Athletes." *Alternative Medicine Review* 2, no. 3 (1997): 184–201.

Kelly, S. E., et al. "Effect of Meal Composition on Calcium Absorption: Enhancing Effect of Carbohydrate Polymers." *Gastroenterology* 87 (1984): 596–600.

Keltikangas-Jarvinen, L., et al. "Relationships Between the Pituitary-Adrenal Hormones, Insulin, and Glucose in Middle-Aged Men: Moderating Influence of Psychosocial Stress." *Metabolism* 47, no. 12 (1998): 1440–9.

Kendler, B. S. "Garlic (Allium Sativum) and Onion (Allium Cepa): A Review of Their Relationships to Cardiovascular Disease." *Preventive Medicine* 16 (1987): 670–85.

Kern, W., C. Dodt, J. Born, and H. L. Fehm. "Changes in Cortisol and Growth Hormone Secretion During Nocturnal Sleep in the Course of Aging." *Journal of Gerontology* (1996): M3–9.

Kerzberg, E. M., E.J.A. Roldan, G. Castelli, and E. D. Huberman. "Combination of Glycosaminoglycans and Acetylsalicylic Acid in Knee Osteoarthrosis." *Scandinavian Journal of Rheumatology* 16 (1987): 377–80.

Khaw, K.-T., and E. Barrett-Connor. "Dietary Potassium and Stroke-Associated Mortality." *New England Journal of Medicine* 316, no. 3 (1987): 235–40.

Kiesewetter, H., et al. "Effects of Garlic on Blood Fluidity and Fibrinolytic Activity: A Randomised, Placebo-Controlled, Double-Blind Study." *British Journal of Clinical Practice* 44 (1990): 24–9.

Kimm, S.Y.S. "The Role of Dietary Fiber in the Development and Treatment of Childhood Obesity." *Pediatrics* 96 (1996): 1010–4.

Kingsbury, K. J., D. M. Morgan, C. Aylott, and R. Emmerson. "Effect of Ethyl Arachidonate, Cod-Liver Oil, and Corn Oil on the Plasma-Cholesterol Level." *Lancet* (1961): 739–41.

Kinsell, L. W., G. D. Michaels, G. Walker, and R. E. Visintine. "The Effect of a Fish-Oil Fraction on Plasma Lipids." *Diabetes* 10, no. 4 (1961): 316–9.

Kinzler, E., J. Kromer, and E. Lehmann. "Wirksamkeit eines Kava-Spezial-Extraktes bei Patienten mit Angst-, Spannungs-, und Erregungszustanden nicht-psychotischer Genese: Doppelblind-Studie gegen Plazebo uber 4 Wochen." *Arzneimittel-Forschung* 41 (1991): 584–8.

Kirt, S. J., et al. "Arginine Stimulates Wound Healing and Immune Function in Elderly Human Beings." *Surgery* 114 (1993): 155–60.

Kiyose, C., et al. "Biodiscrimination of Alpha-tocopherol Stereoisomers in Humans After Oral Administration." *American Journal of Clinical Nutrition* 65 (1997): 785–9.

Kleijnen, J., and P. Knipschild. "Ginkgo Biloba." *Lancet* 340 (1992): 1136–9.

Kleine, M., G. M. Stauder, and E. W. Beese. "The Intestinal Absorption of Orally Administered Hydrolytic Enzymes and Their Effects in the Treatment of Acute Herpes Zoster as Compared with Those of Oral Acylovir Therapy." *Phytomedicine* 2, no. 1 (1995): 7–15.

Knekt, P., et al. "Antioxidant Vitamin Intake and Coronary Mortality in a Longitudinal Population Study." *American Journal of Epidemiology* 139, no. 12 (1994): 1180–9.

Knekt, P., et al. "Dietary Antioxidants and the Risk of Lung Cancer." *American Journal of Epidemiology* 134, no. 5 (1991): 471–9.

Knipschild, P., M. van Dongen, E. van Rossum, and J. Kleijnen. "Clinical Experience with Ginkgo in Patients with Cerebral Insufficiency." *Revista Brasileira de Neurologia* 30 (1994): 18–25S

Knox, T. A., et al. "Calcium Absorption in Elderly Subjects on High- and Low-Fiber

Diets: Effect of Gastric Acidity." *American Journal of Clinical Nutrition* 53 (1991): 1480–6.

Knuiman, J. T., A. C. Beynen, and M. B. Katan. "Lecithin Intake and Serum Cholesterol." *American Journal of Clinical Nutrition* 49 (1989): 266–8.

Kohlmeier, L., and S. B. Hastings. "Epidemiologic Evidence of a Role of Carotenoids in Cardiovascular Disease Prevention." *American Journal of Clinical Nutrition* 62, supplement 65 (1995): 1370–6.

Kok, F. J., et al. "Serum Selenium, Vitamin Antioxidants, and Cardiovascular Mortality: A Nine-Year Follow-up Study in the Netherlands." *American Journal of Clinical Nutrition* 45 (1987): 462–8.

Kok, F. J., J. Schrijver, A. Hofman, J.C.M. Witteman, D.A.C.M. Kruyssen, W. J. Remme, and H. A. Valkenburg. "Low Vitamin B6 Status in Patients with Acute Myocardial Infarction." *American Journal of Cardiology* 63 (1989): 513–6.

Konig, B. "A Long-Term (Two Years) Clinical Trial with S-adenosylmethionine for the Treatment of Osteoarthritis." *American Journal of Medicine* 83, no. 5A (1997): 89–94.

Konig, G. M., and A. D. Wright. "Marine Natural Products Research: Current Directions and Future Potential." *Planta Medica* 62 (1996): 193–211.

Kono, S., K. Shinchi, N. Ikeda, F. Yanai, and K. Imanishi. "Green Tea Consumption and Serum Lipid Profiles: A Cross-Sectional Study in Northern Kyushu, Japan." *Preventive Medicine* 21 (1992): 526–31.

Koppeschaar, H.P.F., C. D. ten Horn, J.H.H. Thijssen, M. D. Page, C. Dieguez, and M. F. Scanlon. "Differential Effects of Arginine on Growth Hormone Releasing Hormone and Insulin Induced Growth Hormone Secretion." *Clinical Endocrinology* 35 (1992): 487–90.

Korpela, H., et al. "Effect of Selenium Supplementation After Acute Myocardial Infarction." *Res Comm in Chem Path and Pharma* 65, no. 2 (1989): 249–52.

Kovacs, A. B. "Efficacy of Ipriflavone in the Prevention and Treatment of Postmenopausal Osteoporosis." *Agents and Actions* 41 (1994): 86–7.

Kraft, K. "Artichoke Leaf Extract—Recent Findings Reflecting Effects on Lipid Metabolism, Liver, and Gastrointestinal Tracts." *Phytomedicine* 4, no. 4 (1997): 369–78.

Kramer, T. R., and B. J. Burri. "Modulated Mitogenic Proliferative Responsiveness of Lymphocytes in Whole-Blood Cultures After a Low-Carotene Diet and Mixed-Carotenoid Supplementation in Women." *American Journal of Clinical Nutrition* 65 (1997): 871–5.

Krassowski, J., J. Rousselle, E. Maeder, and J. Felber. "The Effect of Ornithine Alpha-ketoglutarate on Growth Hormone (GH) and Prolactin (PRL) Release in Normal Subjects." *Endokrynologia Polska* 37, no. 1 (1986): 11–5.

Kremer, J. "Effects of Modulation of Inflammatory and Immune Parameters in Patients with Rheumatic and Inflammatory Disease Receiving Dietary Supplementation of n-3 and n-6 Fatty Acids." *Lipids* 31 (1996): S243–7.

Krinsky, N. "Effects of Carotenoids in Cellular and Animal Systems." *American Journal of Clinical Nutrition* 53 (1991): 238–46.

Krotkiewski, M., et al. "Zinc and Muscle Strength and Endurance." *Acta Physiologica Scandinavica* 116 (1982): 309–11.

Kubo, M., K. Namba, N. Nagamoto, T. Nagao, J. Nakanishi, H. Uno, and H. Nishimura. "A New Phenolic Glucoside, Curculigoside from Rhizomes of Curculigo Orchioides." *Journal of Medicinal Plant Research* 47 (1983): 52–5.

Kulkarni, R. R., et al. "Treatment of Osteoarthritis with a Herbomineral Formulation: A Double-Blind, Placebo-Controlled, Crossover Study." *Journal of Ethnopharmacology* 33 (1991): 91–5.

Kumpulainen, J., et al. "Selenium Status of Exclusively Breast-Fed Infants as Influenced by Maternal Organic or Inorganic Selenium Supplementation." *American Journal of Clinical Nutrition* 42 (1985): 829–35.

Kupfer, S. R., L. E. Underwood, R. C. Bexter, and D. R. Clemmons. "Enhancement of the Anabolic Effects of Growth Hormone and Insulin-like Growth Factor I by Use of Both Agents Simultaneously." *Journal of Clinical Investigation* 91 (1993): 391–6.

Kuppurajan, K., K. Srinivasan, and K. Janaki. "A Double-Blind Study of the Effect of Mandookaparni on the General Mental Ability of Normal Children." *Jour Res. Ind. Med. Yoga & Homeo* 13, no. 1 (1978): 37–41.

Kuratsune, H., et al. "Acylcarnitine Deficiency in Chronic Fatigue Sydrome." *Clinical Infectious Diseases* 18 (1994): S62–7.

Kushi, L. H., A. R. Folsom, R. J. Prineas, P. J. Mink, Y. Wu, and R. M. Bostick. "Dietary Antioxidant Vitamins and Death from Coronary Heart Disease in Postmenopausal Women." *New England Journal of Medicine* 334, no. 18 (1996): 1156–62.

Laakmann, G., C. Schule, T. Baghai, and M. Kieser. "St. John's Wort in Mild to Moderate Depression: The Relevance of Hyperforin for the Clinical Efficacy." *Pharmacopsychiatry* 31, supplement 1 (1998): 54–9.

Laine, L. A., E. Bentley, and P. Chandrasoma. "Effect of Oral Iron Therapy on the Upper Gastrointestinal Tract: A Prospective Evaluation." *Digestive Diseases and Sciences* 33, no. 2 (1988): 172–7.

Lakshmanan, F. L., et al. "Magnesium Intakes, Balances, and Blood Levels of Adults Consuming Self-Selected Diets." *American Journal of Clinical Nutrition* 40 (1984): 1380–9.

Lalor, B. C., D. Bhatnagar, P. H. Winocour, M. Ishola, S. Arrol, M. Brading, and P. N. Durrington. "Placebo-Controlled Trial of the Effects of Guar Gum and Metformin on Fasting Blood Glucose and Serum Lipids in Obese, Type 2 Diabetic Patients." *Diabetic Medicine* 7 (1990): 242–5.

Lambert, M. I., J. A. Hefer, R. P. Millar, and P. W. Macfarlane. "Failure of Commercial Oral Amino Acid Supplements to Increase Serum Growth Hormone Concentrations in Male Body-Builders." *International Journal of Sport Nutrition* 3 (1993): 298–305.

Landgren, F., B. Israelsson, A. Lindgren, B. Hultberg, A. Andersson, and L. Brattstrom. "Plasma Homocysteine in Acute Myocardial Infarction: Homocysteine-Lowering Effect of Folic Acid." *Journal of Internal Medicine* 237 (1995): 381–8.

Landin, K., et al. "Decreased Skeletal Muscle Potassium in Obesity." *Acta Medica Scandinavica* 223 (1988): 507–13.

Landsberg, L., and J. B. Young. "Sympathoadrenal Activity and Obesity: Physiological Rationale for the Use of Adrenergic Thermogenic Drugs." *International Journal of Obesity* 17 (1993): S29–34.

Lane, I. W., and E. Contreras. "High Rate of Bioactivity (Reduction in Gross Tumor Size) Observed in Advanced Cancer Patients Treated with Shark Cartilage Material." *Journal of Naturopathic Medicine* 3, no. 1 (1992): 86–8.

Langv, E. "Einmalige i.v. Gabe eines Crataegus-Extraktes beichronischer Herzinsuffizienz NYHA II. Welche hamodynamische Akutwirkungen?" *Therapiewoche* 38 (1991): 2448–54.

Langner, E., S. Greifenberg, and J. Gruenwald. "Ginger: History and Use." *Advances in Therapy* 15, no. 1 (1998): 25–44.

Lanza, E., Y. Jones, G. Block, and L. Kessler. "Dietary Fiber Intake in the U.S. Population." *American Journal of Clinical Nutrition* 46 (1987): 790–7.

La Rue, A., et al. "Nutritional Status and Cognitive Functioning in a Normally Aging Sample: A Six-Year Reassessment." *American Journal of Clinical Nutrition* 65 (1997): 20–9.

Lassus, A., L. Jeskanen, H. P. Happonen, and J. Santalahti. "Imedeen for the Treatment of Degenerated Skin in Females." *Journal of International Medical Research* 19 (1991): 147–52.

Lau, B.H.S., F. Lam, and R. Wang-Cheng. "Effect of an Odor-Modified Garlic Preparation on Blood Lipids." *Nutrition Research* 7 (1987): 139–49.

Laughlin, G. A., and S.S.C. Yen. "Nutritional and Endocrine-Metabolic Aberrations in Amenorrheic Athletes." *Journal of Clinical Endocrinology and Metabolism* 81 (1996): 4301–9.

Layer, P. and G. Groger. "Fate of Pancreatic Enzymes in the Human Intestinal Lumen in Health and Pancreatic Insufficiency." *Digestion* 54, supplement 2 (1993): 10–4.

Lazarou, J., B. H. Pomeranz, and P. N. Corey. "Incidence of Adverse Drug Reactions in Hospitalized Patients." *JAMA* 279, no. 15 (1998): 1200–4.

Leaf, A., and P. C. Weber. "Cardiovascular Effects of n-3 Fatty Acids." *New England Journal of Medicine* 318, no. 9 (1988): 549–57.

Leathwood, P., and F. Chauffard. "Aqueous Extract of Valerian Reduces Latency to Fall Asleep in Man." *Planta Medica* (1985): 144–8.

Leathwood, P., F. Chauffard, E. Heck, and R. Munoz-Box. "Aqueous Extract of Valerian Root (Valeriana Officinalis L.) Improves

Sleep Quality in Man." *Pharmacology, Biochemistry and Behavior* 17 (1982): 65–71.

Le Bars, P., et al. "A Placebo-Controlled, Double-Blind, Ramdomized Trial of an Extract of Ginkgo Biloba for Dementia." *JAMA* 278, no. 16 (1997): 1327–32.

Lecomte, A. "A Double-Blind Study Confirms the Effects on Weight of Bean Husk Arkocaps." *Association Mondiale de Phototherapie* no. 1 (June 1985): 41–4.

Lees, A. M., H.Y.I. Mok, R. S. Lees, M. A. McCluskey, and S. M. Grundy. "Plant Sterols as Cholesterol-Lowering Agents: Clinical Trials in Patients with Hypercholesterolemia and Studies of Sterol Balance." *Atherosclerosis* 28 (1977): 325–38.

Lefavi, R. G., R. A. Anderson, R. E. Keith, G. D. Wilson, J. L. McMillan, and M. H. Stone. "Efficacy of Chromium Supplementation in Athletes: Emphasis on Anabolism." *International Journal of Sport Nutrition* 2 (1992): 111–22.

Lefavi, R. G., et al. "Lipid-Lowering Effect of a Dietary Chromium (III)–Nicotinic Acid Complex in Male Athletes." *Nutrition Research* 13 (1993): 239–49.

Le Gal, M., P. Cathebras, and K. Struby. "Pharmaton Capsules in the Treatment of Functional Fatigue: A Double-Blind Study Versus Placebo Evaluated by a New Methodology." *Phytotherapy Research* 10 (1996): 49–53.

Lehmann, E., E. Kinzler, and J. Friedemann. "Efficacy of Special Kava Extract in Patients with States of Anxiety, Tension, and Excitedness of Non-mental Origin—A Double-Blind Placebo-Controlled Study of Four Weeks' Treatment." *Phytomedicine* 3, no. 2 (1996): 113–9.

Lehmann, E., E. Klieser, A. Klimke, H. Krach, and R. Sparz. "The Efficacy of Cavain in Patients Suffering from Anxiety." *Pharmacopsychiatry* 22 (1989): 258–62.

Lei, X., and G.C.Y. Chiou. "Cardiovascular Pharmacology of Panax Notoginseng (Burk) F. H. Chen and Salvia Miltiorrhiza." *American Journal of Chinese Medicine* 14, nos. 3–4 (1986): 145–52.

Lei, X., and G.C.Y. Chiou. "Studies on Cardiovascular Actions in Salvia Miltiorrhiza." *American Journal of Chinese Medicine* 14, nos. 1–2 (1986): 26–32.

Leon, A. S. "Physiological Interactions Between Diet and Exercise in the Etiology and Prevention of Ischaemic Heart Disease." *Annals of Clinical Research* 20 (1988): 114–20.

Leslie, J. "A Comparative Trial of a New Controlled-Release Iron Tablet (Ferrocontin) and a Slow-Release Ferrous Sulphate Preparation (Feospan Spansule Capsules)." *Clinical Trials Journal* 16, no. 1 (1979): 2–4.

Leuchtgens, V. H. "Crataegus-Spezialextrakt WS 1442 bei Herzinsuffizienz NYHA II: Eine palzebokontrollierte randomisierte Doppelblindstudie." *Fortschritte der Medizin* 111 (1993): 352–4.

Levine, M., et al. "Vitamin C Pharmacokinetics in Healthy Volunteers: Evidence for a Recommended Dietary Allowance." *Proceedings of the National Academy of Science of the United States of America* 93 (1996): 3704–9.

Lewis, N., M. Marcus, A. Behling, and J. Greger. Calcium Supplements and Milk: Effects on Acid-Base Balance and on Retention of Calcium, Magnesium, and Phosphorus." *American Journal of Clinical Nutrition* 49 (1989): 527–33.

Liangzheng, Z., et al. "Clinical and Experimental Studies on Tong Yu Ling in the Treatment of Diabetic Hyperlipemia." *Journal of Traditional Chinese Medicine* 12, no. 3 (1992): 163–8.

Lichton, I. J. "Dietary Intake Levels and Requirements of Mg and Ca for Different Segments of the U.S. Population." *Magnesium* 8 (1988): 117–23.

Lieber, C. S. "The Influence of Alcohol on Nutritional Status." *Nutrition Reviews* 46, no. 7 (1988): 241–54.

Lieberman, H. R., B. J. Spring, and G. S. Garfield. "The Behavioral Effects of Food Constituents: Strategies used in Studies of Amino Acids, Protein, Carbohydrate, and Caffeine." *Nutritional Reviews* (May 1986): 61–70.

Lijnen, P., et al. "Erythrocyte, Plasma, and Urinary Magnesium in Men Before and After a Marathon." *European Journal of Applied Physiology and Occupational Physiology* 58 (1988): 252–6.

Liljeberg, H.G.M., and I.M.E. Bjorck. "Delayed Gastric Emptying Rate as a Potential Mechanism for Lowered Glyce-mia After Eating Sourdough Bread: Studies in Humans and Rats Using Test Products with Added Organic Acids or an Organic Salt." *American Journal of Clinical Nutrition* 64 (1996): 886–93.

Lindberg, J. S., et al. "Magnesium Bioavailability from Magnesium Citrate and Magnesium Oxide." *Journal of the American College of Nutrition* 9, no. 1 (1990): 48–55.

Linde, K., et al. "St. John's Wort for Depression—An Overview and Meta-analysis of Randomised Clinical Trials." *BMJ* 313 (1996): 253–8.

Lindeberg, S., et al. "Age Relations of Cardiovascular Risk Factors in a Traditional Melanesian Society: The Kitava Study." *American Journal of Clinical Nutrition* 66 (1997): 845–52.

Lindenberg, V. D., and H. Pitule-Schodel. "D,L-Kavain im Vergleich zu Oxazepam bei Angstzustanden: Doppelblindstudie zur klinischen Wirksamkeit." *Fortschritte der Medizin* 108, no. 2 (1990): 31–4.

Lippman, S. M., and F. L. Meyskens. "Vitamin A Derivatives in the Prevention and Treatment of Human Cancer." *Journal of the American College of Nutrition* 7, no. 4 (1988): 269–84.

Lipsky, P. E., and X. Tao. "A Potential New Treatment for Rheumatoid Arthritis: Thunder God Vine." *Seminars in Arthritis and Rheumatism* 26, no. 5 (1997): 712–23.

Liske, E. "Therapeutic Efficacy and Safety of Cimicifuga Racemosa for Gynecologic

Disorders." *Advances in Therapy* 15, no. 1 (1998): 58–65.

Lisper, H-O., and B. Eriksson. "Effects of the Length of a Rest Break and Food Intake on Subsidiary Reaction-Time Performance in an Eight-Hour Driving Task." *Journal of Applied Psychology* 65, no. 1 (1980): 117–22.

Liu, Jia-Sen, and Yuan-Long Zhu. "The Structures of Huperzine A and B, Two New Alkaloids Exhibiting Marked Anti-cholinesterase Activity." *Canada Journal of Chemistry* 64 (1986): 837–9.

Liviero, L., P. P. Puglisi, P. Morazzoni, and E. Bombardelli. "Antimutagenic Activity of Procyanidins from Vitis Vinifera Fitoter-apia." 65, no. 3 (1994): 203–9.

Livingstone, P. D., and C. Jones. "Treatment of Intermittent Claudication with Vitamin E." *Lancet* (1958): 602–4.

Lloyd, T., et al. "Calcium Supplementa-tion and Bone Mineral Density in Ado-lescent Girls." *JAMA* 270, no. 7 (1983): 841–4.

Lloyd, T., et al. "Dietary Caffeine Intake and Bone Status of Postmenopausal Women." *American Journal of Clinical Nutrition* 65 (1997): 1826–30.

Lobelenz, J. "Extractum Sabal fructus bei Benigner Prostatahyperplasie (BPH): Klin-ische Prufung im Stadium I und II." *Thera-peutikon* 6 (1992): 34–7.

Loehrer, F.M.T., R. Schwab, C. P. Angst, W. E. Haefeli, and B. Fowler. "Influence of Oral S-adenosylmethionine on Plasma 5-methyltetrahydrofolate, S-adenosylhomo-cysteine, Homocysteine, and Methionine in Healthy Humans." *Journal of Pharmacology and Experimental Therapeutics* 262, no. 2 (1997): 345–50.

Longnecker, M., et al. "Selenium in Diet, Blood, and Toenails in Relation to Human Health in a Seleniferous Area." *American Journal of Clinical Nutrition* 53 (1991): 1288–94.

Longobardi, S., et al. "Reevaluation of Growth Hormone (GH) Secretion in Sixty-nine Adults Diagnosed as GH-Deficient Patients During Childhood." *Journal of Clinical Endocrinology and Metabolism* 81 (1996): 1244–7.

Lonnerdal, B., A. Cederblad, L. Davidsson, and B. Sandstrom. "The Effect of Individ-ual Components of Soy Forumla and Cows' Milk Formula on Zinc Bioavailability." *American Journal of Clinical Nutrition* 40 (1984): 1064–70.

Looker, A., et al. "Vitamin-Mineral Supple-ment Use: Association with Dietary Intake and Iron Status of Adults." *Journal of the American Dietetic Association* 88 (1988): 808–14.

Losonczy, K. G., T. B. Harris, and R. J. Havlik. "Vitamin E and Vitamin C Supplement Use and Risk of All-Cause and Coronary Heart Disease Mortality in Older Persons: The Established Populations for Epidemiologic Studies of the Elderly." *American Journal of Clinical Nutrition* 64 (1996): 190–6.

Loughead, J. L., et al. "A Role for Magnesium in Neonatal Parathyroid Gland Function?" *Journal of the American College of Nutrition* 10, no. 2 (1991): 123–6.

Lovejoy, J., and M. DiGirolamo. "Habitual Dietary Intake and Insulin Sensitivity in Lean and Obese Adults." *American Journal of Clinical Nutrition* 55 (1992): 1174–9.

Lowik, M.R.H., et al. "Dose-Response Relationships Regarding Vitamin B-6 in Elderly People: A Nationwide Nutritional Survey (Dutch Nutritional Surveillance System)." *American Journal of Clinical Nutrition* 50 (1989): 391–9.

Lowik, M.R.H., et al. "Nutrition and Aging: Nutritional Status of 'Apparently Healthy' Elderly (Dutch Nutrition Surveillance System)." *Journal of the American College of Nutrition* 9, no. 1 (1990): 18–27.

Luft, F. C., et al. "The Effect of Dietary Interventions to Reduce Blood Pressure in Normal Humans." *Journal of the American College of Nutrition* 8, no. 6 (1989): 495–503.

Luley, C., et al. "Lack of Efficacy of Dried Garlic in Patients with Hyperlipoproteinemia." *Arzneimittel-Forschung* 36 (1986): 766–8.

Lundeberg, S., et al. "Growth Hormone Improves Muscle Protein Metabolsim and Whole Body Nitrogen Economy in Man During a Hyponitrogenous Diet." *Metabolism* 40, no. 3 (1991): 315–22.

Luoma, P. V., H. Korpela, E. A. Sotaniemi, and J. Kumpulainen. "Serum Selenium, Glutathione Peroxidase, Lipids, and Human Liver Microsomal Enzyme Activity." *Biological Trace Element Research* 8 (1985): 113–21.

Luoma, P. V., S. Nayha, K. Sikkila, and J. Hassi. "High Serum Alpha-tocopherol, Albumin, Selenium, and Cholesterol, and Low Mortality from Coronary Heart Disease in Northern Finland." *Journal of Internal Medicine* 237 (1995): 49–54.

Luostarinen, R., R. Wallin, L. Wibell, and T. Saldeen. "Vitamin E Supplementation Counteracts the Fish Oil–Induced Increase of Blood Glucose in Humans." *Nutrition Research* 15, no. 7 (1995): 953–68.

Lupton, J. R., J. L. Morin, and M. C. Robinson. "Barley Bran Flour Accelerates Gastrointestinal Transit Time." *Journal of the American Dietetic Association* 93 (1993): 881–5.

Lupton, J. R., M. C. Robinson, and J. L. Morin. "Cholesterol-Lowering Effect of Barley Bran Flour and Oil." *Journal of the American Dietetic Association* 94 (1994): 65–70.

Lyle, R. M., C. L. Melby, and G. C. Hyner. "Metabolic Differences Between Subjects Whose Blood Pressure Did or Did Not Respond to Oral Calcium Supplementation." *American Journal of Clinical Nutrition* 47 (1988): 1030–5.

Lyle, R. M., et al. "Blood Pressure and Metabolic Effects of Calcium Supplementation in Normotensive White and Black Men." *JAMA* 257, no. 13 (1987): 1772–6.

Ma, J., A. R. Folsom, L. Lewis, and J. H. Eckfeldt. "Relation of Plasma Phosopholipid and Cholesterol Ester Fatty Acid Composition to Carotid Artery Intima-media Thickness: The Atherosclerosis Risk in Communities (ARIC) Study." *American Journal of Clinical Nutrition* 65 (1997): 551–9.

Maccario, M., et al. "Effect of Bromocriptine on Insulin, Growth Hormone, and Prolactin Responses to Arginine in Obesity." *Journal of Endocrinological Investigation* 19 (1996): 219–23.

Maccario, M., et al. "In Obesity the Somatotrope Response to Either Growth Hormone–Releasing Hormone or Arginine Is Inhibited by Somatostatin or Pirenzepine but Not by Glucose." *Journal of Clinical Endocrinology and Metabolism* 80 (1995): 3774–8.

Macfarlane, B. J., et al. "Effect of Traditional Oriental Soy Products on Iron Absorption." *American Journal of Clinical Nutrition* 51 (1990): 873–80.

MacGregor, J. T., et al. "Spontaneous Genetic Damage in Man: Evaluation of Interindividual Variability, Relationship Among Markers of Damage, and Influence of Nutritional Status." *Mutation Research* 377 (1997): 125–35.

Maezaki, Y., et al. "Hypocholesterolemic Effect of Chitosan in Adult Males." *Bioscience, Biotechnology, and Biochemistry* 57, no. 9 (1993): 1439–44.

Malaise, M., R. Marcolongo, D. Uebelhart, and E. Vignon. "Efficacy and Tolerability of 800 mg Oral Chondroitin 4 and 6 Sulfate in the Treatment of Knee Osteoarthritis: A Randomized, Double-Blind, Multicentre Study Versus Placebo." Proceedings European League Against Rheumatism (EULAR) Symposium, Geneva, 1998.

Malinow, M. R., et al. "The Effects of Folic Acid Supplementation on Plasma Total Homocysteine Are Modulated by Multivitamin Use and Methylenetetrahydrofolate Reductase Genotypes." *Arteriosclerosis, Thrombosis, and Vascular Biology* 17, no. 6 (1997): 1157–62.

Malinow, M. R., et al. "Reduction of Plasma Homocysteine Levels by Breakfast Cereal Fortified with Folic Acid in Patients with Coronary Heart Disease." *New England Journal of Medicine* 338, no. 15 (1998): 1009–15.

Malone, W. F. "Studies Evaluating Antioxidants and B-carotene as Chemopreventives." *American Journal of Clinical Nutrition* 53 (1991): 305–13S

Mandressi, A., et al. "Terapia medica dell'adenoma prostatico: Confronto della efficacia dell'estratto di Serenoa repens (Permixon) versus l'estratto di pigeum Africanum e placebo." *Urologia* 50 (1983): 752–8.

Mani, U. V., et al. "Glycemic Index of Traditional Indian Carbohydrate Foods." *Journal of the American College of Nutrition* 9, no. 6 (1990): 573–7.

Manku, M. S., D. F. Horrobin, N. L. Morse, S. Wright, and J. L. Burton. "Essential Fatty Acids in the Plasma Phospholipids of

Patients with Atopic Eczema." *British Journal of Dertmatology* 100 (1984): 643–8.

Manning, C. A., J. L. Hall, and P. E. Gold. "Glucose Effects on Memory and Other Neuropsychological Tests in Elderly Humans." *Psychological Science* 1, no. 5 (1990): 307–11.

Mantzioris, E., M. J. James, R. A. Gibson, and L. G. Cleland. "Dietary Substitution with an Alpha-linolenic Acid-Rich Vegetable Oil Increases Elcosapentaenoic Acid Concentrations in Tissues." *American Journal of Clinical Nutrition* 59 (1994): 1304–9.

Marchand, L. L., J. H. Hanking, L. N. Kolonel, and L. R. Wilkens. "Vegetable and Fruit Consumption in Relation to Prostate Cancer Risk in Hawaii: A Reevaluation of Effect of Dietary B-carotene." *American Journal of Epidemiology* 133 (1991): 215–9.

Marin, P., M. Krotkiewski, B. Andersson, and P. Bjorntorp. "Muscle Fiber Composition and Capillary Density in Women and Men with NIDDM." *Diabetes Care* 17, no. 5 (1994): 382–6.

Markus, R. A., W. J. Mack, S. P. Azen, and H. N. Hodis. "Influence of Lifestyle Modification on Atherosclerotic Progression Determined by Ultrasonographic Change in the Common Cartoid Intima-media Thickness." *American Journal of Clinical Nutrition* 65 (1997): 1000–4.

Marshall, J. D., C. B. Hazlett, D. W. Spady, and H. A. Quinney. "Comparison of Convenient Indicators of Obesity." *American Journal of Clinical Nutrition* 51 (1990): 22–8.

Martin, R. F., M. Janghorbani, and V. R. Young. "Experimental Selenium Restriction in Healthy Adult Humans: Change in Selenium Metabolism Studied with Stable-Istope Methodology." *American Journal of Clinical Nutrition* 49 (1989): 854–61.

Martin, R. F., et al. "Ascorbic Acid–Selenite Interactions in Humans Studied with an Oral Dose of SeO3." *American Journal of Clinical Nutrition* 49 (1989): 862–9.

Martinez, B., S. Kasper, S. Ruhrmann, and H-J. Moller. "Hypericum in the Treatment of Seasonal Affective Disorders." *Journal of Geriatric Psychiatry and Neurology* 7, supplement 1 (1994): S29–32.

Mathur, N. B., A. M. Dwarkadas, V. K. Sharma, K. Saha, and N. Jain. "Anti-Infective Factors in Preterm Human Colostrum." *Acta Pediatrica Scandinavica* 79 (1990): 1039–44.

Matkovic, V. "Calcium Metabolism and Calcium Requirements During Skeletal Modeling and Consolidation of Bone Mass." *American Journal of Clinical Nutrition* 54 (1991): 245–60.

Mato, J. M., L. Alvarez, P. Ortiz, and M. A. Pajares. "S-adenosylmethionine Synthesis: Molecular Mechanisms and Clinical Implications." *Pharmacology and Therapeutics* 73, no. 3 (1997): 265–80.

Matteini, M., et al. "GH Secretion by Arginine Stimulus: The Effect of Both Low Doses and Oral Arginine Administered Before Standard Test." *Bollettino—Societa Italiana Biologia Sperimentale* 56 (1980): 2254–60.

Mattes, R. D., et al. "Dietary Evaluation of Patients with Smell and/or Taste Disorders." *American Journal of Clinical Nutrition* 51 (1990): 233–40.

Mattson, F. H., B. A. Erickson, and A. M. Kligman. "Effect of Dietary Cholesterol on Serum Cholesterol in Man." *American Journal of Clinical Nutrition* 25 (1972): 589–94.

Mattson, F. H., S. M. Grundy, and J. R. Crouse. "Optimizing the Effect of Plant Sterols on Cholesterol Absorption in Man." *American Journal of Clinical Nutrition* 35 (1982): 697–700.

Mauriege, P., et al. "Regional Differences in Adipose Tissue Metabolism Between Sedentary and Endurance-Trained Women." *Journal of Clinical Endocrinology and Metabolism* 273 (1997): 497–506.

Maver, A. "Terapia medica dell'ipertrofia fibro-adenomatosa della prostata mediante una nuova sostanza vegetale." *Urologia* 63 (1972): 2126–36.

May, B., H.-D. Kuntz, M. Kieser, and S. Kohler. "Efficacy of a Fixed Peppermint Oil/Caraway Oil Combination in Non-ulcer Dyspepsia." *Arneimittel-Forschung* 46 (1996): 1149–53.

May, J. M., Z.-C. Qu, and C. E. Cobb. "Accessibility and Reactivity of Ascorbate 6-palmitate Bound to Erythrocyte Membranes." *Free Radical Biology and Medicine* 21, no. 4 (1996): 471–80.

Mazess, R., and H. Barden. "Bone Density in Premenopausal Women: Effects of Age, Dietary Intake, Physical Activity, Smoking, and Birth-Control Pills." *American Journal of Clinical Nutrition* 53 (1991): 132–42.

Mazieres, B., et al. "Le Chondrotine sulfate dans le traitement de la gonarthrose et de la coxarthrose: Resultats a 5 mois, d'une etude prospective multicentrique, controlee, en double aveugle, versus placebo." *Rev. Rhum. Mal. Osteoartic.* 59, nos. 7–8 (1992): 466–72.

Mazzuoli, G., et al. "Effects of Ipriflavone on Bone Remodeling in Primary Hyperparathyroidism." *Bone and Mineral* 19, supplement 1 (1992): S27–33.

McCarron, D. A., and C. D. Morris. "Blood Pressure Response to Oral Calcium in Persons with Mild to Moderate Hypertension." *Annals of Internal Medicine* 103 (1985): 825–31.

McCrindle, B. W., E. Helden, and W. T. Conner. "Garlic Extract Therapy in Children with Hypercholesterolemia." *Archives of Pediatrics and Adolescent Medicine* 152 (1998): 1089–94.

McCune, M. A., H. O. Perry, S. A. Muller, and W. M. O'Fallon. "Treatment of Recurrent Herpes Simplex Infections with L-lysine Monohydrochloride." *Cutis* 34 (1984): 366–73.

McDougall, J., K. Litzau, E. Haver, V. Saunders, and G. A. Spiller. "Rapid Reduction of Serum Cholesterol and Blood Pressure by a Twelve-Day, Very Low Fat, Strictly Vegetarian Diet." *Journal of the American College of Nutrition* 14, no. 5 (1995): 491–6.

McGregor, N. R., et al. "Preliminary Determination of a Molecular Basis to Chronic

Fatigue Syndrome." *Biochemical and Molecular Medicine* 57 (1996): 73–80.

McIntosh, G. H., J. Whyte, R. McArthur, and P. J. Nestel. "Barley and Wheat Foods: Influence on Plasma Cholesterol Concentrations in Hypercholesterolemic Men." *American Journal of Clinical Nutrition* 53 (1991): 1205–9.

McLeod, M. N., B. N. Gaynes, and R. N. Golden. "Chromium Potentiation of Antidepressant Pharmacotherapy for Dysthymic Disorder in Five Patients." *Journal of Clinical Psychiatry* 60 (1999): 237–40.

McMahon, B., S. Yen, D. Trichopoulos, K. Warren, and G. Nardi. "Coffee and Cancer of the Pancreas." *New England Journal of Medicine* 304, no. 11 (1981): 630–3.

McMahon, F. G., and R. Vargas. "Can Garlic Lower Blood Pressure? A Pilot Study." *Pharmacotherapy* 13, no. 4 (1993): 406–7.

McNaugton, L., G. Egan, and G. Caelli. "A Comparison of Chinese and Russian Ginseng as Ergogenic Aids to Improve Various Facets of Physical Fitness." *International Clinical Nutrition Review* 9, no. 1 (1989): 31–4.

Meacham, S. L., L. J. Taper, and S. L. Volpe. "Effect of Boron Supplementation on Blood and Urinary Calcium, Magnesium, and Phosphorus, and Urinary Boron in Athletic and Sedentary Women." *American Journal of Clinical Nutrition* 61 (1995): 341–5.

Meadows, N. J., et al. "Oral Iron and the Bioavailability of Zinc." *BMJ* 287 (1983): 1013–4.

Mei, M., Q. Zhuang, G. Liu, and W. Xie. "Rapid Screening Method for Hypocholesterolemic Agents." *Acta Pharmaceutica Sinica* 14, no. 1 (1979): 24–6.

Meier, C. R., L. E. Derby, S. S. Jick, C. Vasilakis, and H. Jick. "Antibiotics and Risk of Subsequent First-time Acute Myocardial Infarction." *JAMA* 281, no. 5 (1999): 427–31.

Meiselman, H. L., and B. P. Halpern. "Human Judgments of Gymnema Sylvestre and Sucrose Mixtures." *Physiology and Behavior* 5 (1970): 945–8.

Mejia, L. A., and F. Chew. "Hematological Effect of Supplementing Anemic Children with Vitamin A Alone and in Combination with Iron." *American Journal of Clinical Nutrition* 48 (1988): 595–600.

Mekki, N., et al. "Effects of Lowering Fat and Increasing Dietary Fiber on Fasting and Postprandial Plasma Lipids in Hypercholesterolemic Subjects Consuming a Mixed Mediterranean-Western Diet." *American Journal of Clinical Nutrition* 66 (1997): 1443–51.

Melchart, D., K. Linde, F. Worku, R. Bauer, and H. Wagner. "Immunomodulation with Echinacea—A Systematic Review of Controlled Clinical Trials." *Phytomedicine* 1 (1994): 245–54.

Melchior, J., S. Palm, and G. Wikman. "Controlled Clinical Study of Standardized Andrographis Paniculata Extract in Common Cold—A Pilot Trial." *Phytomedicine* 3, no. 4 (1996/97): 315–8.

Melhus, H., et al. "Excessive Dietary Intake of Vitamin A Is Associated with Reduced Bone Mineral Density and Increased Risk for Hip Fracture." *Annals of Internal Medicine* 129, no. 10 (1998): 770–8.

Melis, G. B., et al. "Ipriflavone and Low Doses of Estrogens in the Prevention of Bone Mineral Loss in Climacterium." *Bone and Mineral* 19 (1992): S49–56.

Mendelson, W. B., R. A. Lantigua, R. J. Wyatt, J. C. Gillin, and L. S. Jacobs. "Piperidine Enhances Sleep-Related and Insulin-Induced Growth Hormone Secretion: Further Evidence for a Cholinergic Secretory Mechanism." *Journal of Clinical Endocrinology and Metabolism* 52, no. 3 (1981): 409–15.

Mennen, L. I., et al. "The Association of Dietary Fat and Fiber with Coagulation Factor VII in the Elderly: The Rotterdam Study." *American Journal of Clinical Nutrition* 65 (1997): 732–6.

Merry, P., M. Grootveld, J. Lunec, and D. R. Blake. "Oxidative Damage to Lipids Within the Inflamed Human Joint Provides Evidence of Radical-Mediated Hypoxic-Reperfusion Injury." *American Journal of Clinical Nutrition* 53 (1991): 362–9.

Metcoff, J. "Intracellular Amino Acid Levels as Predictors of Protein Synthesis." *Journal of the American College of Nutrition* 5 (1986): 107–20.

Metzker, H., M. Kieser, and U. Holscher. "Wirksamkeit eines Sabal-Urtica-Kombinationspräparats bei der Behandlung der benigen Prostatahyperplasie (BPH)." *Urolge B* 36 (1996): 292–300.

Meydani, S. N., et al. "Vitamin B-6 Deficiency Impairs Interleukin 2 Production and Lymphocyte Proliferation in Elderly Adults." *American Journal of Clinical Nutrition* 53 (1991): 1275–80.

Meyer, F., I. Bairati, and G. R. Dagenais. "Lower Ischemic Heart Disease Incidence and Mortality Among Vitamin Supplement Users." *Canadian Journal of Cardiology* 12, no. 10 (1996): 930–4.

Meyer, J. S., et al. "Neurotransmitter Precursor Amino Acids in the Treatment of Multi-Infarct Dementia and Alzheimer's Disease." *Journal of the American Geriatrics Society* 25, no. 7 (1977): 289–98.

Meyskens, F. Jr., and A. Manetta. "Prevention of Cervical Intraepithelial Neoplasia and Cervical Cancer." *American Journal of Clinical Nutrition* 62 (1995): 1417–9.

Mezzetti, A., et al. "Vitamins E, C, and Lipid Peroxidation in Plasma and Arterial Tissue of Smokers and Non-smokers." *Atherosclerosis* 112 (1995): 91–9.

Michaelsson, G., L. Juhlin, and K. Ljunghall. "A Double-Blind Study of the Effect of Zinc and Oxytetracycline in Acne Vulgaris." *Swedish Journal of Dermatology* 97 (1977): 561–5.

Michaelsson, G., L. Juhlin, and A. Vahlquist. "Effects of Oral Zinc and Vitamin A in Acne." *Archives of Dermatology* 113 (1977): 31–6.

Michnovicz, J. J., H. Adlercreutz, and H. L. Bradlow. "Changes in Levels of Urinary Estrogen Metabolites After Oral Indole-3-carbinol Treatment in Humans." *Journal of the National Cancer Institute* 89, no. 10 (1997): 718–23.

Micozzi, M. S., et al. "Plasma Carotenoid Response to Chronic Intake of Selected Foods and B-carotene Supplements in Men." *American Journal of Clinical Nutrition* 55 (1992): 1120–5.

Miettinen, T. A., and Y. A. Kesaniemi. "Cholesterol Absorption: Regulation of Cholesterol Synthesis and Elimination and Within-Population Variations of Serum Cholesterol Levels." *American Journal of Clinical Nutrition* 49 (1989): 629–35.

Miller, F., A. Svardal, P. Aukrust, R. Berge, P. Ueland, and S. Froland. "Elevated Plasma Concentration of Reduced Homocysteine in Patients with Human Immunodeficiency Virus Infection." *American Journal of Clinical Nutrition* 63 (1996): 242–8.

Miller, J., D. Smith, L. Flora, M. Peacock, and C. Johnston Jr. "Calcium Absorption in Children Estimated from Single and Double Stable Calcium Isotope Techniques." *Clinica Chimica Acta* 183 (1989): 107–14.

Miller, L. G. "Herbal Medicinals: Selected Interactions; Considerations Focusing on Known or Potential Drug-Herb Interactions." *Archives of Internal Medicine* 158 (1998): 2200–11.

Miller, W. C., M. G. Niederpruem, J. P. Wallace, and A. K. Lindeman. "Dietary Fat, Sugar, and Fiber Predict Body Fat Content." *Journal of the American Dietetic Association* 94, no. 6 (1994): 612–5.

Milne, D. B., et al. "Folate Status of Adult Males Living in a Metabolic Unit: Possible Relationships with Iron Nutriture." *American Journal of Clinical Nutrition* 37 (1983): 768–73.

Miskolczi, P., K. Kozma, M. Polgar, and L. Vereczkey. "Pharmacokinetics of Vinpocetine and Its Main Metabolite Apovincaminic Acid Before and After the Chronic Oral Administration of Vinpocetine to Humans." *European Journal of Drug Metabolism and Pharmacokinetics* 15, no. 1 (1990): 1–5.

Misra, D. N., and G. D. Shukla. "Mustong in Sexual Inadequacy—A Clinical Trial." *Indian Medical Gazette* (1984): 322–3.

Mitcheva, M., H. Astroug, D. Drenska, A. Popov, and M. Kassarova. "Biochemical and Morphological Studies on the Effects of Anthocyans and Vitamin E on Carbon Tetrachloride Induced Liver Injury." *Cellular and Molecular Biology* 39, no. 4 (1993): 443–8.

Miyazaki, Manabu. "The Effect of a Cerebral Vasodilator, Vinpocetine, on Cerebral Vascular Resistance Evaluated by the Doppler Ultrasonic Technique in Patients with Cerebrovascular Diseases." *Journal of Vascular Diseases* 46, no. 1 (1995): 53–8.

Mock, D. M., and D. D. Stadler. "Conflicting Indicators of Biotin Status from a Cross-sectional Study of Normal Pregnancy."

Journal of the American College of Nutrition 16, no. 3 (1997): 252–7.

Mohan, J. C., R. Arora, and M. Khaliullah. "Preliminary Observations on Effect of Lactobacillus Sporogenes on Serum Lipid Levels in Hypercholesterolemic Patients." *Indian Journal of Medical Research* 92 (1990): 431–2.

Monnier, V. M., D. R. Sell, H. N. Ramanakoppa, and S. Miyata. "Mechanism of Protection Against Damage Mediated by the Maillard Reaction in Aging." *Gerontology* 37 (1991): 152–65.

Moore, T. J. "The Role of Dietary Electrolytes in Hypertension." *Journal of the American College of Nutrition* 8 (1989): 68S–80S.

Morales, A. J., J. J. Nolan, J. C. Nelson, and S. S. C. Yen. "Effects of Replacement Dose of Dehydroepiandrosterone in Men and Women of Advancing Age." *Journal of Clinical Endocrinology and Metabolism* 76, no. 6 (1994): 1360–7.

Morck, T. A., et al. "Iron Availability from Infant Food Supplements." *American Journal of Clinical Nutrition* 34 (1981): 2630–4.

Morita, H., and H. Itokawa. "Cytotoxic and Antifungal Diterpenes from the Seeds of Alpinia Galanda." *Planta Medica* (1988): 117–20.

Morrison, H. I., D. Schaubel, M. Desmeules, and D. T. Wigle. "Serum Folate and Risk of Fatal Coronary Heart Disease." *JAMA* 24 (1996): 1893–6.

Mortensen, L., and P. Charles. "Bioavailability of Calcium Supplements and the Effect of Vitamin D: Comparisons Between Milk, Calcium Carbonate, and Calcium Carbonate plus Vitamin D." *American Journal of Clinical Nutrition* 63 (1996): 354–7.

Mortola, J., and S. Yen. "The Effects of Oral DHEA on Endocrine-Metabolic Parameters in Postmenopausal Women." *Journal of Clinical Endrocrinology and Metabolism* 71 (1990): 696–704.

Mossad, S. B., M. L. Macknin, S. V. Medendorp, and P. Mason. "Zinc Gluconate Lozenges for Treating the Common Cold: A Randomized, Double-Blind, Placebo-Controlled Study." *Annals of Internal Medicine* 125, no. 2 (1996): 81–8.

Motulsky, H. J., and P. A. Insel. "Adrenergic Receptors in Man: Direct Identification, Physiologic Regulation, and Clinical Alterations." *New England Journal of Medicine* 307, no. 1 (1982): 18–27.

Mudd, S. H., et al. "The Natural History of Homocystinuria Due to Cytathionine B-synthase Deficiency." *American Journal of Human Genetics* 37 (1985): 1–31.

Mueller, B. M. "Effects of Hypericum Extract HYP 811 in Patients with Psychovegetative Disorders." *Advances in Therapy* 15, no. 4 (1998): 23–8.

Mueller, B. M. "St. John's Wort for Depressive Disorders: Results of an Outpatient Study with the Hypericum Preparation HYP 811." *Advances in Therapy* 15, no. 2 (1998): 109–16.

Murphy, J. J., S. Hepinstall, and J. R. A. Mitchell. "Randomised Double-Blind Placebo-

Controlled Trial of Feverfew in Migraine Prevention." *Lancet* (1988): 189–92.

Murray, R., W. P. Bartoli, D. E. Eddy, and M. K. Horn. "Physiological and Performance Responses to Nicotinic-Acid Ingestion During Exercise." *Medicine and Science in Sports and Exercise* (1995): 1057–62.

Nagaya, T., et al. "Serum Lipid Profile in Relation to Milk Consumption in a Japanese Population." *Journal of the American College of Nutrition* 15, no. 6 (1996): 625–9.

Nair, P. P., et al. "Diet, Nutrition Intake, and Metabolism in Populations at High and Low Risk for Colon Cancer: Dietary Cholesterol, B-sitosterol, and Stigmasterol." *American Journal of Clinical Nutrition* 40 (1984): 927–30.

Nakamura, S., et al. "Effect of Ipriflavone on Bone Mineral Density and Calcium-Related Factors in Elderly Females." *Calcified Tissue International* 51, supplement 1 (1992): S30–4.

Natali, A., et al. "Effects of Acute Hypercarnitinemia During Increased Fatty Substrate Oxidation in Man." *Metabolism* 42, no. 5 (1993): 594–600.

Naurath, H. J., E. Joosten, R. Riezler, S. P. Stabler, R. H. Allen, and J. Lindenbaum. "Effects of Vitamin B12, Folate, and Vitamin B6 Supplements in Elderly People with Normal Serum Vitamin Concentrations." *Lancet* 346 (1995): 85–9.

Naylor, S., F. J. Hanke, L. V. Manes, and P. Crews. "Chemical and Biological Aspects of Marine Monoterpenes." *Progress in the Chemistry of Organic Natural Products* 44 (1983): 190–241.

Nelson, L. H., and L. A. Tucker. "Diet Composition Related to Body Fat in Multivariate Study of 203 Men." *Journal of the American Dietetic Association* 96, no. 3 (1996): 771–7.

Nelson, M., E. Fisher, F. Dilmanian, G. Dallal, and W. Evans. A One-Year Walking Program and Increased Dietary Calcium in Postmenopausal Women: Effects on Bone." *American Journal of Clinical Nutrition* 53 (1991): 1304–11.

Nestel, P. J. "Fish Oil Attenutates the Cholesterol-Induced Rise in Lipoprotein Cholesterol." *American Journal of Clinical Nutrition* 43 (1986): 752–7.

Nestel, P. J., W. E. Connor, M. F. Reardon, S. Connor, S. Wong, and R. Boston. "Suppression by Diets Rich in Fish Oil of Very Low Density Lipoprotein Production in Man." *Journal of Clinical Investigation* 74 (1984): 82–9.

Nestler, J., C. O. Barlascini, J. N. Clore, and W. G. Blackard. "Dehydroepiandrosterone Reduces Serum Low Density Lipoprotein Levels and Body Fat but Does Not Alter Insulin Sensitivity in Normal Man." *Journal of Clinical Endocrinology and Metabolism* 66, no. 1 (1988): 57–61.

Nestler, J., N. A. Beer, D. J. Jakubowicz, and R. M. Beer. "Effects of a Reduction in Circulating Insulin by Metformin on Serum

Dehydroepiandrosterone Sulfate in Nondiabetic Men." *Journal of Clinical Endocrinology and Metabolism* 78, no. 3 (1994): 549–554.

Neve, J., F. Vertongen, and P. Capel. "Selenium Supplementation in Healthy Belgian Adults: Response in Platelet Glutathione Peroxidase Activity and Other Blood Indices." *American Journal of Clinical Nutrition* 48 (1988): 139–43.

Newcomer, A. D., H. S. Park, P. C. O'Brien, and D. B. McGill. "Response of Patients with Irritable Bowel Syndrome and Lactase Deficiency Using Unfermented Acidophilus Milk." *American Journal of Clinical Nutrition* 38 (1983): 257–63.

Newsome, D. A., et al. "Macular Degeneration and Elevated Serum Ceruloplasmin." *Investigative Ophthalmology and Visual Science* 27 (1986): 1675–80.

Nicar, M. J., and C. Y. C. Pak. "Calcium Bioavailability from Calcium Carbonate and Calcium Citrate." *Journal of Clinical Endocrinology and Metabolism* 61 (1985): 391–3.

Nielsen, F. H., C. D. Hunt, L. M. Mullen, and J. R. Hunt. "Effect of Dietary Boron on Mineral, Estrogen, and Testosterone Metabolism in Postmenopausal Women." *FASEB* 1 (1987): 394–7.

Nirenberg, D. W., et al. "Determinants of Increase in Plasma Concentration of B-carotene after Chronic Oral Supplementation." *American Journal of Clinical Nutrition* 53 (1991): 1443–9.

Nishi, Y., et al. "Transient Partial Growth Hormone Deficiency Due to Zinc Deficiency." *Journal of the American College of Nutrition* 8, no. 2 (1989): 93–7.

Niwa, Y., Y. Miyachi, K. Ishimoto, and T. Kanoh. "Why Are Natural Plant Medicinal Products Effective in Some Patients and Not in Others with the Same Disease?" *Planta Medica* 57 (1991): 299–304.

Noakes, M., et al. "Effect of High-Amylose Starch and Oat Bran on Metabolic Variables and Bowel Function in Subjects with Hypertriglyceridemia." *American Journal of Clinical Nutrition* 64 (1996): 944–51.

Nord, J., et al. "Treatment with Bovine Hyperimmune Colostrum of Cryptosporidial Diarrhea in AIDS Patients." *AIDS* 4 (1990): 581–4.

Nowson, C. A., et al. "A Co-twin Study of the Effect of Calcium Supplementation on Bone Density During Adolescence." *Osteoporosis International* 7 (1997): 219–25.

O'Conolly, V. M., W. Jansen, G. Bernhoft, and G. Bartsch. "Behandlung der nachlassenden Herzleistung: Therapie mit standardisiertem Crataegus-Extrakt im hoheren Lebensalter." *Fortschritte der Medizin* 104 (1986): 805–8.

O'Dea, K. "Westernization and Non-insulin-dependent Diabetes in Australian Aborigines." *Ethnicity and Disease* 1 (1991): 171–87.

Oh, M. S., et al. "D-lactic Acidosis in a Man with the Short-Bowel Sydrome." *New England Journal of Medicine* 301, no. 5 (1979): 249–52.

Oka, H., S. Yamamoto, T. Kuroki, S. Harihara, T. Marumo, S. Kim, T. Monna, K. Kobayashi, and T. Tango. "Prospective Study of Chemoprevention of Hepatocellular Carcinoma with Sho-saiko-to (TJ-9)." *Cancer* 76, no. 5 (1995): 743–9.

Olszewski, A. J., and MuCully, K. S. "Homocysteine Metabolism and the Oxidative Modification of Proteins and Lipids." *Free Radical Biology and Medicine* 14 (1993): 683–93.

Omaye, S. T., et al. "Blood Antioxidants Changes in Young Women Following B-carotene Depletion and Repletion." *Journal of the American College of Nutrition* 15, no. 5 (1996): 469–74.

Omdahl, J. L., et al. "Nutritional Status in a Healthy Elderly Population: Vitamin D." *American Journal of Clinical Nutrition* 36 (1982): 1225–33.

Orwoll, E., R. Weigel, S. Oviatt, M. McClung, and L. Deftos. "Calcium and Cholecalciferol: Effects of Small Supplements in Normal Men." *American Journal of Clinical Nutrition* 48 (1988): 127–30.

Osterheider, M., A. Schmidtke, and H. Beckmann. "Behandlung depressiver Syndrome mit Hypericum (Johanniskraut)—eine placeboknotrollierte Doppelblindstudie." *Fortschritte der Neurologie-Psychiatrie* 60, no. 2 (1992): 210–1.

Pace-Asciak, C. R., O. Rounova, S. E. Hahn, E. P. Diamandis, and D. M. Goldberg. "Wines and Grape Juices as Modulators of Platelet Aggregation in Healthy Human Subjects." *Clinica Chimica Acta* 246 (1996): 163–82.

Packer, L., H. J. Tritschler, and K. Wessel. "Neuroprotection by the Metabolic Antioxidant Alpha-lipoic Acid." *Free Radical Biology and Medicine* 20, nos. 1–2 (1997): 359–78.

Pak, C. Y. C., A. Stewart, and S. D. S. Haynes. "Effect of Added Citrate or Malate on Calcium Absorption from Calcium-Fortified Orange Juice." *Journal of the American College of Nutrition* 13, no. 6 (1994): 575–7.

Palareti, G., et al. "Blood Coagulation Changes in Homocystinuria: Effects of Pyridoxine and Other Specific Therapy." *Journal of Pediatrics* 109, no. 6 (1986): 1001–6.

Palasciano, G., et al. "The Effect of Silymarin on Plasma Levels of Malon-Dialdehyde in Patients Receiving Long-Term Treatment with Psychotropic Drugs." *Curr. Therap. Res.* 55, no. 5 (1994): 537–45.

Palozza, P., and N. Krinsky. "Astaxanthin and Canthaxanthin Are Potent Antioxidants in a Membrane Model." *Archives of Biochemistry and Biophysics* 297, no. 2 (1992): 291–5.

Pancharuniti, N., et al. "Plasma Homocysteine, Folate, and Vitamin B12 Concentrations and Risk for Early Onset Coronary Artery Disease." *American Journal of Clinical Nutrition* 59 (1994): 940–8.

Pannunzio, E., et al. "Serenoa repens vs. gestonorone caproato nel trattamento dell' ipertrofia prostatica benigna." *Urologica* 53 (1986): 696–705.

Paolisso, G., M. R. Tagliamonte, M. Rosaria, D. Manzella, A. Gambardella, and M. Varricchio. "Oxidative Stress and Advancing Age: Results in Healthy Centenarians." *Journal of the American Geriatrics Society* 46 (1998): 833–8.

Paolisso, G., et al. "Daily Magnesium Supplements Improve Glucose Handling in Elderly Subjects." *American Journal of Clinical Nutrition* 55 (1992): 1161–7.

Paolisso, G., et al. "Improved Insulin Response and Action by Chronic Magnesium Administration in Aged NIDDM Subjects." *Diabetes Care* 12, no. 4 (1989): 265–9.

Paolisso, G., et al. "Metabolic Benefits Deriving from Chronic Vitamin C Supplementation in Aged Non-insulin-dependent Diabetics." *Journal of the American College of Nutrition* 14, no. 4 (1995): 387–92.

Paranjpe, P., P. Patki, and B. Patwardhan. "Ayurvedic Treatment of Obesity: A Randomised Double-Blind, Placebo-Controlled Clinical Trial." *Journal of Ethnopharmacology* 29 (1990): 1–11.

Parfitt, V. J., P. Rubba, C. Boloton, G. Marotta, M. Hartog, and M. Mancini. "A Comparison of Antioxidant Status and Free Radical Peroxidation of Plasma Lipoproteins in Healthy Young Persons from Naples and Bristol." *European Heart Journal* 15 (1994): 871–6.

Parnham, M. J. "Benefit-Risk Assessment of the Squeezed Sap of the Purple Coneflower (Echinacea Purpurea) for Long-Term Oral Immunostimulation." *Phytomedicine* 3, no. 1 (1996): 95–102.

Parry, G. J., and D. E. Bredesen. "Sensory Neuropathy with Low-Dose Pyridoxine." *Neurology* 35 (1985): 1466–8.

Passeri, M., et al. "Acetyl-l-carnitine in the Treatment of Mildly Demented Elderly Patients." *International Journal of Clinical Pharmacological Research* 10, nos. 1–2 (1990): 75–9.

Passeri, M., et al. "Effect of Ipriflavone on Bone Mass in Elderly Osteoporotic Women." *Bone and Mineral* 19 (1992): S57–62.

Paulev, P.-E., R. Jordal, and N. S. Pedersen. "Dermal Excretion of Iron in Intensely Training Athletes." *Clinica Chimica Acta* 127 (1983): 19–27.

Pavelka, K., R. Manopulo, and L. Busci. "Double-Blind, Dose-Effect Study of Oral Chondroitin 4 & 6 Sulfate 1200 mg, 800 mg, 200 mg, and Placebo in the Treatment of Knee Osteoarthritis." Proceedings, European League Against Rheumatism (EULAR) Symposium, Geneva, 1998.

Peacock, M. "Calcium Absorption Efficiency and Calcium Requirements in Children and Adolescents." *American Journal of Clinical Nutrition* 54 (1991): 261S–5S

Pelletier, V., L. Marks, D. A. Wagner, R. A. Hoerr, and V. R. Young. "Branched-Chain Amino Acid Interactions with Reference to Amino Acid Requirements in Adult Men: Leucine Metabolism at Different Valine and Isoleucine Intakes." *American Journal of Clinical Nutrition* 54 (1991): 402–7.

Peretz, A., J. Neve, J. Desmedt, J. Duchateau, M. Dramaix, and J-P. Famaey. "Lymphocyte Response Is Enhanced by Supplementation of Elderly Subjects with Selenium-Enriched Yeast." *American Journal of Clinical Nutrition* 53 (1991): 1323–8.

Perez-Campo, R., M. Lopez-Torres, S. Cadenas, C. Rojas, and G. Barja. "The Rate of Free Radical Production as a Determinant of the Rate of Aging: Evidence from the Comparative Approach." *Journal of Comparative Physiology. B* 168 (1998): 149–58.

Perry, A., et al. "Relation Between Anthropometric Measures of Fat Distribution and Cardiovascular Risk Factors in Overweight Pre- and Postmenopausal Women." *American Journal of Clinical Nutrition* 66 (1997): 829–36.

Perticone, F., D. Borelli, R. Ceravolo, and P. L. Mattioli. "Antiarrhythmic Short-term Protective Magnesium Treatment in Ischemic Dilated Cardiomyopathy." *Journal of the American College of Nutrition* 9, no. 5 (1990): 492–9.

Pessah-Rasmussen, H., et al. "Eighty-year-old Men without Cardiovascular Disease in the Community of Malmo: Smoking Characteristics and Ultrasound Findings, with Special Reference to Glutathione Transferase and Pyridoxal-5-phosphate." *Journal of Internal Medicine* 228 (1990): 17–22.

Petkov, V. "Pharmakologische Untersuchungen der Droge Panax Ginseng C. A. Meyer." *Arzneimittel-Forschung* 9 (1959): 305–11.

Petkov, V. W. "Pharmakologische und klinische Untersuchungen des Knoblauchs." *Deutsche Apotheker-Zeitung* 106 (1966): 1861–7.

Petkov, V. "Plants with Hypotensive, Antiatheromatous, and Coronarodilatating Action." *American Journal of Chinese Medicine* 7, no. 3 (1979): 197–236.

Petkov, V., and A. H. Mosharrof. "Effects of Standardized Ginseng Extract on Learning, Memory, and Physical Capabilities." *American Journal of Chinese Medicine* 15, nos. 1–2 (1987): 19–29.

Philippi, A. F., et al. "Glucosamine, Chondroitin, and Manganese Ascorbate for Degenerative Joint Disease of the Knee or Low Back: A Randomized, Double-Blind, Placebo-Controlled Pilot Study." *Military Medicine* 164 (1999): 85–91.

Phillips, J. D., et al. "Magnesium Absorption in Human Ileum." *Journal of the American College of Nutrition* 10, no. 3 (1991): 200–4.

Phillipson, B. E., D. W. Rothrock, W. E. Connor, W. S. Harris, and D. R. Illingworth. "Reduction of Plasma Lipids, Lipoproteins, and Apoproteins by Dietary Fish Oils in Patients with Hypertriglyceridemia." *New England Journal of Medicine* 312, no. 19 (1985): 1210–6.

Piatti, P. M., et al. "Insulin Sensitivity and Lipid Levels in Obese Subjects After Slimming Diets with Different Complex and Simple Carbohydrate Content." *International Journal of Obesity* 17 (1993): 375–81.

Pineda, O., H. D. Ashmead, J. M. Perez, and C. P. Lemus. "Effectiveness of Iron Amino Acid Chelate on the Treatment of Iron Deficiency Anemia in Adolescents." *Journal of Applied Nutrition* 46, nos. 1–2 (1994): 1–13.

Pines, A., H. Raafat, A. H. Lynn, and J. Whittington. "Clinical Trial of Microcrystalline Hydroxyapatite Compound ('Ossopan') in the Prevention of Osteoporosis Due to Corticosteroid Therapy." *Current Medical Research and Opinion* 8, no. 10 (1984): 734–42.

Pinsky, M. J. "Treatment of Intermittent Claudication with Alpha-tocopherol." *Journal of the American Podiatry Association* 70, no. 9 (1980): 454–8.

Pittler, M. H., and E. Ernst. "Horse-Chesnut Seed Extract for Chronic Venous Insufficiency." *Archives of Dermatology* 134 (1998): 1258–60.

Plioplys, A. V., and S. Plioplys. "Amantadine and L-carnitine Treatment of Chronic Fatigue Syndrome." *Neuropsychobiology* 35 (1997): 16–23.

Plioplys, A. V., and S. Plioplys. "Serum Levels of Carnitine in Chronic Fatigue Syndrome: Clinical Correlates." *Neuropsychobiology* 32 (1995): 132–8.

Pochart, P., et al. "Survival of Bifidobacteria Ingested via Fermented Milk During Their Passage Through the Human Small Intestine: An In Vivo Study Using Intestinal Perfusion." *American Journal of Clinical Nutrition* 55 (1992): 78–80.

Pollak, O. J. "Reduction of Blood Cholesterol in Man." *Circulation* 7 (1953): 702–6.

Pollitt, E., R. L. Leibel, and D. Greenfield. "Brief Fasting, Stress, and Cognition in Children." *American Journal of Clinical Nutrition* 34 (1981): 1526–33.

Pollitt, E., N. L. Lewis, G. Garza, and R. L. Shulman. "Fasting and Cognitive Function." *Journal of Psychiatric Research* 17, no. 2 (1983): 169–74.

Posner, B. M., L. A. Cupples, D. Gagnon, P. W. F. Wilson, K. Chetwynd, and D. Felix. "The Rationale and Potential Efficacy of Preventive Nutrition in Heart Disease: The Framingham Offspring-Spouse Study." *Archives of Internal Medicine* 153 (1993): 1549–56.

Poulsen, H. E., S. Loft, and K. Vistisen. "Extreme Exercise and Oxidative DNA Modification." *Journal of Sports Sciences* 14 (1996): 343–6.

Power, S. K., and S. Dodd. "Caffeine and Endurance Performance." *Sports Medicine* 2 (1985): 165–74.

Powers, J. S., et al. "Assessment of Nutritional Status in Noninstitutionalized Elderly." *Southern Medical Journal* 82, no. 8 (1989): 990–4.

Prasa, K., and J. Kalra. "Oxygen Free Radicals and Hypercholesterolemic Atherosclerosis: Effect of Vitamin E." *American Heart Journal* 125 (1993): 958–73.

Prasad, A. S. "Discovery of Human Zinc Deficiency and Studies in an Experimental Human Model." *American Journal of Clinical Nutrition* 53 (1991): 403–12.

Prchal, J. T., M. E. Conrad, and H. W. Skalka. "Association of Presenile Cataracts with Heterozygosity for Galactosaemic States and with Riboflavin Deficiency." *Lancet* (1978): 982–4.

Princen, H. M. G., et al. "Supplementation with Vitamin E but Not B-carotene In Vivo Protects Low Density Lipoprotein from Lipid Peroxidation In Vitro; Effect of Cigarette Smoking." *Arteriosclerosis and Thrombosis* 12 (1992): 554–62.

Princen, H. M. G., et al. "Supplementation with Low Doses of Vitamin E Protects LDL from Lipid Peroxidation in Men and Women." *Arteriosclerosis, Thrombosis, and Vascular Biology* 15, no. 3 (1995): 325–33.

Prinz, R. J., W. A. Roberts, and E. Hantman. "Dietary Correlates of Hyperactive Behavior in Children." *Journal of Consulting and Clinical Psychology* 48, no. 6 (1980): 760–9.

Prudden, J. F. "The Clinical Acceleration of Healing with a Cartilage Preparation." *JAMA* 192, no. 5 (1965): 92–6.

Prudden, J. F. "The Treatment of Human Cancer with Agents Prepared from Bovine Cartilage." *Journal of Biological Response Modifiers* 4 (1985): 551–84.

Pujalte, J. M., et al. "Double-Blind Clinical Evaluation of Oral Glucosamine Sulphate in the Basic Treatment of Osteoarthrosis." *Current Medical Research and Opinion* 7, no. 2 (1980): 110–4.

Qureshi, Asaf, et al. "Lowering of Serum Cholesterol in Hypercholesterolemic Humans by Tocotrienols (Palmvitee)." *American Journal of Clinical Nutrition* 53, supplement 45 (1991): 1021–6.

Racette, S. B., W. M. Kohrt, M. Landt, and J. O. Holloszy. "Response of Serum Leptin Concentrations to 7 d of Energy Restriction in Centrally Obese African Americans with Impaired or Diabetic Glucose Tolerance." *American Journal of Clinical Nutrition* 66 (1997): 33–7.

Ragan, M. A., and K.-W. Glombitza. "Phlorotannins, Brown Algal Polyphenols." *Progress in Phycological Research* 4 (1986): 130–241.

Raman, A., and C. Lau. "Anti-diabetic Properties and Phytochemistry of Momordica Charantia L. (Cucurbitaceae)." *Phytomedicine* 2, no. 4 (1996): 349–62.

Ramaswamy, A. S., S. M. Periyasamy, and N. Basu. "Pharmacological Studies on Centella Asiatica Linn (Brahma Manduki) (N. O. Umbelliferae)." *Jour Res. Ind. Med.* 4, no. 2 (1970): 160–75.

Ranno, S., G. Minaldi, G. Viscusi, G. Di Marco, and C. Consoli. "Efficacia e tollerabilita del trattamento dell'adenoma prostatico con Tadenan 50." *Il Progresso Medico* 42 (1986): 165–9.

Rao, M. V. R. A., K. Srinivasan, and T. Koteswara Rao. "The Effect of Centella Asiatica on the General Mental Ability of Mentally Retarded Children." *Indian Journal of Psychiatry* 19, no. 4 (1977): 54–9.

Rao, M. V. R. A., S. P. Usha, S. S. Rajagopalan, and R. Sarangan. "Six Months' Results of a Double-Blind Trial to Study the Effect of Mandookaparni and Punarnava on Normal Adults." *Jour. Res. Ind. Med* 2, no. 1 (1967): 79–85.

Rapoport, J. L., et al. "Behavioral and Cognitive Effects of Caffeine in Boys and Adult Males." *Journal of Nervous and Mental Disease* 169, no. 11 (1981): 726–32.

Rasic, J. L. "The Role of Dairy Food Containing Bifido- and Acidophilus Bacteria in Nutrition and Health?" *North European Dairy Journal* (1983): 80–8.

Rasmussen, K., J. Moller, M. Lyngbak, A. M. Pedersen, and L. Dybkjaer. "Age- and Gender-Specific Reference Intervals for Total Homocysteine and Methylmalonic Acid in Plasma Before and After Vitamin Supplementation." *Clinical Chemistry* 42, no. 4 (1996): 630–6.

Reddy, M. B., and J. D. Cook. "Assessment of Dietary Determinants of Nonheme-Iron Absorption in Humans and Rats." *American Journal of Clinical Nutrition* 54 (1991): 723–8.

Regnstrom, J., et al. "Inverse Relation Between the Concentration of Low-density-lipoprotein Vitamin E and Severity of Artery Disease." *American Journal of Clinical Nutrition* 63 (1996): 377–85.

Reh, C., P. Laux, and N. Schenk. "Hypericum-Extrakt bei Depressionen—Eine Wirksame." *Alternative Therapiewoche* 42 (1992): 1576–81.

Rehn, D., M. Unkauf, P. Klein, V. Jost, and P. W. Luckner. "Comparative Clinical Efficacy and Tolerability of Oxerutins and Horse Chestnut Extract in Patients with Chronic Venous Insufficiency." *Arzneimittel-Forschung* 46, no. 5 (1996): 483–7.

Reichelt, J. "Antimicrobial Activity from Marine Algae: Results of a Large-Scale Screening Programme." *Hydrobiologia* 116/117 (1984): 158–67.

Reid, I. R., D. J. A. Gallagher, and J. Bosworth. "Prophylaxis Against Vitamin D Deficiency in the Elderly by Regular Sunlight Exposure." *Age and Ageing* 15 (1986): 35–40.

Remes, K., K. Kuoppasalmi, and H. Aldereutz. "Effect of Physical Exercise and Sleep Deprivation on Plasma Androgen Levels: Modifying Effect of Physical Fitness." *International Journal of Sports Medicine* 6 (1985): 131–5.

Reuter, H. D. "Garlic (Allium Sativum L.) in the Prevention and Treatment of Atherosclerosis." *British Journal of Phytotherapy* 3. no. 1 (1993/4): 3–9.

Reynolds, E. H., M. W. P. Carney, and B. K. Toone. "Methylation and Mood." *Lancet* (July 1984): 196–8.

Rhode, B. M., P. Arseneau, B. A. Cooper, M. Katz, B. M. Filfix, and L. D. MacLean. "Vitamin B12 Deficiency After Gastric Surgery for Obesity." *American Journal of Clinical Nutrition* 63, no. 1 (1996): 103–9.

Riella, M. C., J. W. Broviac, M. Wells, and B. H. Scribner. "Essential Fatty Acid Deficiency in Human Adults During Total Parenteral Nutrition." *Annals of Internal Medicine* 83 (1975): 786–9.

Riemersma, R. A., D. A. Wood, C. C. A. Macintryre, R. A. Elton, K. F. Gey, and M. F. Oliver. "Risk of Angina Pectoris and Plasma Concentrations of Vitamins A, C, and E and Carotene." *Lancet* 337 (1991): 1–5.

Riemersma, R. A., et al. "Plasma Antioxidants and Coronary Heart Disease: Vitamins C, and E, and Selenium." *European Journal of Clinical Nutrition* 44 (1990): 143–50.

Rigaud, D., K. R. Ryttig, L. A. Angel, and M. Apfelbaum. "Overweight Treated with Energy Restriction and a Dietary Fibre Supplement:

A Six-Month Randomized, Double-Blind, Placebo-Controlled Trial." *International Journal of Obesity* 14 (1990): 763–9.

Riggs, K., A. Spiro III, K. Tucker, and D. Rush. "Relations of Vitamin B-12, Vitamin B-6, Folate, and Homocysteine to Cognitive Performance in the Normative Aging Study." *American Journal of Clinical Nutrition* 63 (1996): 306–14.

Rimm, E., et al. "Vegetable, Fruit, and Cereal Fiber Intake and Risk of Coronary Heart Disease Among Men." *JAMA* 275, no. 6 (1996): 447–51.

Ringbom, T., L. Segura, Y. Noreen, P. Perera, and L. Bohlin. "Ursolic Acid from Plantago Major, a Selective Inhibitor of Cycloxygenase-2 Catalyzed Prostaglandin Biosynthesis." *J. Nut. Prod.* 61 (1998): 1212–5.

Ringer, T. V., et al. "Beta-carotene's Effects on Serum Lipoproteins and Immunologic Indices in Humans." *American Journal of Clinical Nutrition* 53 (1991): 688–94.

Ripsin, C. M., et al. "Oat Products and Lipid Lowering: A Meta-analysis." *Journal of the American Medical Association* 267 (1992): 3317–25.

Risser, W. L., et al. "Iron Deficiency in Female Athletes: Its Prevalence and Impact on Performance." *Medicine and Science in Sports and Exercise* 20, no. 2 (1987): 116–21.

Roberts, C. C., et al. "Adequate Bone Mineralization in Breast-Fed Infants." *Journal of Pediatrics* 99, no. 2 (1981): 192–6.

Roberts, H. J. "Reactions Attributed to Aspartame-Containing Products: 551 Cases." *Journal of Applied Nutrition* 40, no. 2 (1988): 85–94.

Robertson, D., J. Frolich, K. Carr, J. Watson, J. Hollifield, D. Shand, and J. Oates. "Effects of Caffeine on Plasma Renin Activity, Catecholamines, and Blood Pressure." *New England Journal of Medicine* 298 (1978): 181–6.

Robinson, K., et al. "Hyperhomocysteinemia and Low Pyridoxal Phosphate: Common and Independent Reversible Risk Factors for Coronary Artery Disease." *Circulation* 92 (1995): 2825–30.

Rock, C. L., et al. "Racial Group Differences in Plasma Concentrations of Antioxidant Vitamins and Carotenoids in Hemodialysis Patients." *American Journal of Clinical Nutrition* 65 (1997): 844–50.

Roesler, J., et al. "Application of Purified Polysaccharides from Cell Cultures of the Plant Echinacea Purpurea to Test Subject Mediates Activation of the Phagocyte System." *International Journal of Immunopharmacology* 13, no. 7 (1991): 931–41.

Rolls, B. J. "Carbohydrates, Fats, and Satiety." *American Journal of Clinical Nutrition* 61 (1995): 960–7S.

Romics, I., H. Schmitz, and D. Frang. "Experience in Treating Benign Prostatic Hypertrophy with Sabal Serrulata for One Year." *International Urology and Nephrology* 25, no. 6 (1993): 565–69.

Rosen, L. A., M. E. Bender, S. Sorrell, S. R. Booth, M. L. McGarth, and R. S. Drabman. "Effects of Sugar (Sucrose) on Children's Behavior." *Journal of Consulting and Clinical Psychology* 56, no. 4 (1988): 583–9.

Rosenbaum, J. F., M. Fava, W. E. Felk, M. H. Pollack, L. S. Cohen, B. M. Cohen, and G. S. Zubenko. "The Antidepressant Potential of Oral S-adeno-l-methionine." *Acta Psychiatrica Scandinavica* 81 (1990): 432–6.

Rossander-Hulten, L., et al. "Competitive Inhibition of Iron Absorption by Manganese and Zinc in Humans." *American Journal of Clinical Nutrition* 54 (1991): 152–6.

Rossner, S., D. Von Zweigbergk, A. Ohlin, and K. Ryttig. "Weight Reduction with Dietary Fibre Supplements." *Acta Medica Scandinavica* 222 (1987): 83–8.

Roth-Mathews, Micheline. "Carotenoids and Cancer Prevention—Experimental and Epidemiological Studies." *Pure and Applied Chemistry* 57, no. 5 (1985): 717–22.

Roveda, S., and P. Colombo. "Sperimentazione clinica controllata sulla bioequivalenza terapeutica e sulla tollerabilita dei prodotti a base di Serenoa repens in capsule da 160 mg o capsule rettali da 640 mg." *Arch. Med. Interna.* 46 (1994): 61–75.

Rudofsky, G., A. Neib, K. Otto, and K. Seibel. "Odemprotektive Wirkung und klinische Wirsamkeit von Robkastaniensamenextrakt im Doppeltblindversuch." *Phlebologie und Proktologie* 15 (1986): 47–54.

Rumessen, J. J., S. Bode, O. Hamberg, and E. Gudmand-Hoyer. "Fructans of Jerusalem Artichokes: Intestinal Transport, Absorption, Fermentation, and Influence on Blood Glucose, Insulin, and C-peptide Responses in Healthy Subjects." *American Journal of Clinical Nutrition* 52 (1990): 675–81.

Russel, M. G., et al. "'Modern Life' in the Epidemiology of Inflammatory Bowel Disease: A Case-Control Study with Special Emphasis on Nutritional Factors." *European Journal of Gastroenterology and Hepatology* 10 (1996): 243–9.

Russell, R. M. "Nutrition." *JAMA* 275, no. 23 (1996): 1828–9.

Russell, R. M., S. K. Dutta, E. V. Oaks, I. H. Rosenberg, and A. C. Giovetti. "Impairment of Folic Acid Absorption by Oral Pancreatic Extracts." *Digestive Diseases and Sciences* 25, no. 5 (1980): 369–73.

Ruz, M., et al. "Development of Dietary Model for the Study of Mild Zinc Deficiency in Humans and Evalution of Some Biochemical and Functional Indices of Zinc Status." *American Journal of Clinical Nutrition* 43 (1991): 1294–1303.

Rytter, E., C. Erlanson-Albertsson, L. Lindahl, U. Viberg, B. Akesson, and R. Oste. "Changes in Plasma Insulin, Enterostatin, and Lipoprotein Levels During an Energy-Restricted Dietary Regimen Including a New Oat-Based Liquid Food." *Annals of Nutritional Metabolism* 40 (1996): 212–20.

Ryttig, K. R., G. Tellnes, L. Hiegh, E. Boe, and H. Fagerthun. "A Dietary Fibre Supplement and Weight Maintenance After

Weight Reduction: A Randomized, Double-Blind, Placebo-Controlled Long-Term Trial." *International Journal of Obesity* 13 (1989): 165–71.

Sacks, F. M. "Dietary Fats and Blood Pressure: A Critical Review of the Evidence." *Nutrition Reviews* 47, no. 10 (1989): 291–300.

Sainani, G. S., D. B. Desai, N. H. Gorhe, S. M. Natu, D. V. Pise, and P. G. Sainani. "Effect of Dietary Garlic and Onion on Serum Lipid Profile in Jain Community." *Indian Journal of Medical Research* 69 (1979): 776–80.

Saku, K., et al. "Effects of Chinese Herbal Drugs on Serum Lipids, Lipoproteins and Apolipoproteins in Mild to Moderate Essential Hypertensive Patients." *Journal of Human Hypertension* 6 (1992): 393–5.

Salim, A. S. "Sulfhydryl-Containing Agents in the Treatment of Gastric Bleeding Induced by Nonsteroidal Anti-inflammatory drugs." *Can J Surg* 36, no. 1 (1993): 53–8.

Salmenpera, L. "Vitamin C Nutrition During Prolonged Lactation: Optimal in Infants While Marginal in Some Mothers." *American Journal of Clinical Nutrition* 40 (1984): 1050–6.

Salonen, J., et al. "Effects of Antioxidant Supplementation on Platelet Function: A Randomized Pair-Matched, Placebo-Controlled, Double-Blind Trial in Men with Low Antioxidant Status." *American Journal of Clinical Nutrition* 53 (1991): 1222–9.

Salonen, J. T., et al. "Serum Fatty Acids, Apolipoproteins, Selenium, and Vitamin Antioxidants and the Risk of Death from Coronary Artery Disease." *American Journal of Cardiology* 56 (1985): 226–31.

Sanders, T.A.B., D. R. Sullivan, J. Reeve, and G. R. Thompson. "Triglyceride-Lowering Effect of Marine Polyunsaturates in Patients with Hypertriglyceridemia." *Arteriosclerosis* 5 (1985): 459–65.

Sanders, T.A.B., and K. M. Younger. "The Effect of Dietary Supplements of w-3 Polyunsaturated Fatty Acids on the Fatty Acid Composition of Platelets and Plasma Choline Phosphoglycerides." *British Journal of Nutrition* 45 (1981): 613–6.

Sandstrom, B., A. Cederblad, and B. Lonnderdal. "Zinc Absorption from Human Milk, Cow's Milk, and Infant Formulas." *Am. J. Dis. Child* 137 (1983): 726–9.

Santos, M. S., et al. "Natural Killer Cell Activity in Elderly Men Is Enhanced by B-carotene Supplementation." *American Journal of Clinical Nutrition* 64 (1996): 772–7.

Saradeth, T., et al. "Does Garlic Alter the Lipid Pattern in Normal Volunteers?" *Phytomedicine* 1 (1994): 183–5.

Sathyanathan, T. J. "Effect of Mustong on Sexual Dysfunction in Male Diabetes." *Indian Medical Gazette* (1985): 196–7.

Sato, T., N. Igarashi, K. Miyagawa, M. Shimizu, T. Nishikawa, and T. Hashimoto. "Mutual Priming Effects of GHRH and Arginine on GH Secretion: Informative

Procedure for Evaluating GH Secretory Dynamics." *Endocrinol. Japon.* 37, no. 4 (1990): 501–9.

Sauberlich, H. E., et al. "Ascorbic Acid and Erythorbic Acid Metabolism in Pregnant Women." *American Journal of Clinical Nutrition* 50 (1989): 1039–49.

Savage, D. G., J. Lindenbaum, S. P. Stabler, and R. H. Allen. "Sensitivity of Serum Methylamalonic Acid and Total Homocysteine Determinations for Diagnosing Cobalamin and Folate Deficiencies." *American Journal of Medicine* 96 (1994): 239–45.

Saynor, R., and D. Verel. "Effect of a Marine Oil High in Eicosapentaenoic Acid on Blood Lipids and Coagulation." *Clinical Pharmacology and Therapeutics* 8 (1980): 378–9.

Saynor, R., D. Verel, and T. Gillott. "The Long-Term Effect of Dietary Supplementation with Fish Lipid Concentrate on Serum Lipids, Bleeding Time, Platelets, and Angina." *Atherosclerosis* 50 (1984): 3–10.

Scarpignato, C., and P. Rampal. "Prevention and Treatment of Traveler's Diarrhea: A Clinical Pharmacological Approach." *Chemotherapy* 41, supplement 1 (1995): 48–81.

Schauss, A. G. "Lactobacillus Acidophilus: Method of Action, Clinical Application, and Toxicity Data." *Journal of Advancement in Medicine* 3, no. 3 (1990): 163–78.

Schellenberg, R., S. Sauer, and W. Dimpfel. "Pharmacodynamic Effects of Two Different Hypericum Extracts in Healthy Volunteers Measured by Quantitative EEG." *Pharmacopsychiatry* 31, supplement 1 (1998): 44–53.

Scherer, J. "Kava-Kava Extract in Anxiety Disorders: An Outpatient Observation Study." *Advances in Therapy* 15, no. 4 (1998): 29–37.

Schmidt, J. M., and J. S. Greenspoon. "Aloe Vera Dermal Wound Gel Is Associated with a Delay in Wound Healing." *Obsterics and Gynecology* 78, no. 1 (1991): 115–7.

Schmidt, U., U. Kuhn, M. Ploch, and W.-D. Hubner. "Efficacy of the Hawthorn (Crataegus) Preparation LI 132 in Seventy-eight Patients with Chronic Congestive Heart Failure Defined as NYHA Functional Class II." *Phytomedicine* 1 (1994): 17–24.

Schmidt, U., et al. "Psychomotorische Leistungverbesserung: Antidepressive Therapie mit Johanniskraut." *Therapiewoche* 2 (1995): 106–12.

Schneider, C. L., and D. J. Nordlund. "Prevalence of Vitamin and Mineral Supplement Use in the Elderly." *Journal of Family Practice* 17, no. 2 (1983): 243–7.

Scholmerich, J., et al. "Bioavailability of Zinc from Zinc-Histidine Complexes: I Comparison with Zinc Sulfate in Healthy Men." *American Journal of Clinical Nutrition* 45 (1987): 1480–6.

Scholmerich, J., et al. "Bioavailability of Zinc from Zinc-Histidine Complexes: II. Studies on Patients with Liver Cirrhosis and the Influence of the Time of Application." *American Journal of Clinical Nutrition* 45 (1987): 1487–91.

Schorah, C. J., et al. "Total Vitamin C, Ascorbic Acid, and Dehydroascorbic Acid Concentrations in Plasma of Critically Ill Patients." *American Journal of Clinical Nutrition* 63 (1996): 760–5.

Schuette, S. A., and J. B. Knowles. "Intestinal Absorption of Ca(H2PO4)2 and Ca Citrate Compared by Two Methods." *American Journal of Clinical Nutrition* 47 (1988): 884–8.

Schuette, S., J. Knowles, and H. Ford. "Effect of Lactose or its Component Sugars on Jejunal Calcium Absorption in Adult Man." *American Journal of Clinical Nutrition* 50 (1989): 1084–7.

Schuette, S. A., N. J. Yasillo, and C. M. Thompson. "The Effect of Carbohydrates in Milk on the Absorption of Calcium by Postmenopausal Women." *Journal of the American College of Nutrition* 10, no. 2 (1991): 132–9.

Schulz, H., C. Stolz, and J. Muller. "The Effect of Valerian Extract on Sleep Polygraphy in Poor Sleepers: A Pilot Study." *Pharmacopsychiatry* 27 (1994): 147–51.

Schulz, V., W. Hubner, and M. Ploch. "Clinical Trials with Phyto-psychopharmacological Agents." *Phytomedicine* 4, no. 4 (1997): 379–387.

Schwartz, J., and S. T. Weiss. "Relationship Between Dietary Vitamin C Intake and Pulmonary Function in the First National Health and Nutrition Examination Survey (NHANES I)." *American Journal of Clinical Nutrition* 59 (1994) 110–4.

Schwartz, R., H. Spencer, and J. J. Welsh. "Magnesium Absorption in Human Subjects from Leafy Vegetables, Intrinsically Labeled with Stable Mg." *American Journal of Clinical Nutrition* 39 (1984): 571–6.

Schwartz, R., H. Spencer, and R. A. Wentworth. "Measurement of Magnesium in Man Using Stable Mg as a Tracer." *Clinica Chimica Acta* 87 (1978): 265–73.

Seddon, J. M., et al. "Dietary Carotenoids, Vitamins A, C, and E, and Advanced Age-Related Macular Degeneration." *JAMA* 272 (1994): 1413–20.

Seim, H. C., and K. B. Holtmeier. "Effects of a Six-Week, Low-Fat Diet on Serum Cholesterol, Body Weight, and Body Measurements." *Family Practice Research Journal* 12, no. 4 (1992): 411–9.

Seim, H. C., et al. "Effects of Six-Week, Low-Fat Diet on Serum Cholesterol, Body Weight, and Body Measurements." *Family Practice Research Journal* 12, no. 4 (1992): 411–9.

Selhub, J., F. P. Jacques, P. W. F. Wilson, D. Rush, and I. H. Rosenberg. "Vitamin Status and Intake as Primary Determinants of Homocysteinemia in an Elderly Population." *JAMA* 270 (1993): 2693–8.

Selhub, J., et al. "Association between Plasma Homocysteine Concentrations and Extracranial Carotid-Artery Stenosis." *New England Journal of Medicine* 332, no. 5 (1995): 286–91.

Seligman, P. A., et al. "Measurements of Iron Absorption from Prenatal Multivitamin-

Mineral Supplements." *Obstetrics and Gynecology* 61, no. 3 (1983): 356–61.

Sentipal, J., G. Wardlaw, J. Mahan, and V. Matkovic. "Influence of Calcium Intake and Growth Indexes on Vertebral Bone Mineral Density in Young Females." *American Journal of Clinical Nutrition* 54 (1991): 425–8.

Shanmugasundaram, E. R. B., et al. "Use of Gymnema Sylvestre Leaf Extract in the Control of Blood Glucose in Insulin-Dependent Diabetes Mellitus." *Journal of Ethnopharmacology* 30 (1990): 281–94.

Sharma, H. M., B. D. Triguna, and D. Chopra. "Maharishi Ayur-Veda: Modern Insights into Ancient Medicine." *JAMA* 265, no. 20 (1991): 2633–7.

Sharma, K. K., A. L. Sharma, K. K. Dwivedi, and P. K. Sharma. "Effect of Raw and Boiled Garlic on Blood Cholesterol in Butter Fat Lipaemia." *Indian Journal of Nutrition and Dietetics* 13 (1976): 7–10.

Shead, A., et al. "Effects of Phyllanthus Plant Extracts on Duck Hepatitis B Virus In Vitro and In Vivo." *Antiviral Research* 18 (1992): 127–38.

Sheehan, M. P., and D. J. Atherton. "A Controlled Trial of Traditional Chinese Medicinal Plants in Widespread Non-exudative Atopic Eczema." *British Journal of Dermatology* 136 (1993): 179–84.

Sheehan, M. P., et al. "Efficacy of Traditional Chinese Herbal Therapy in Adult Atopic Dermatitis." *Lancet* 340 (1992): 13–7.

Sherman, V. L., et al. "Do Patients Receiving Regular Haemodialysis Need Folic Acid Supplements?" *BMJ* 285 (1982): 96–7.

Shickikawa, K., M. Igarashi, S. Sugawara, and Y. Iwasaki. "Clinical Evaluation of High Molecular Weight Sodium Hyaluronate (SPH) on Osteoarthritis of the Knee— Multi-center Well-Controlled Comparative Study." 14, no. 3 (1983): 545–58.

Shivpuri, D. N., M. P. S. Menon, and D. Prakash. "A Crossover Double-Blind Study on Tylophora Indica in the Treatment of Asthma and Allergic Rhinitis." *Journal of Allergy* 43, no. 3 (1969): 145–50.

Shivpuri, D. N., S. C. Singhal, and D. Prakash. "Treatment of Asthma with an Alcoholic Extract of Tylophora Indica: A Cross-over Double-Blind Study." *Annals of Allergy* 30 (1972): 407–12.

Siegenberg, D., et al. "Ascorbic Acid Prevents the Dose-Dependent Inhibitory Effects of Polyphenols and Phytates on Nonheme-Iron Absorption." *American Journal of Clinical Nutrition* 53 (1991): 537–41.

Sies, H., and N. I. Krinsky. "The Present Status of Antioxidant Vitamins and B-carotene." *American Journal of Clinical Nutrition* 62 (1996): 1299S–3000S.

Siliprandi, N., et al. "Metabolic Changes Induced by Maximal Exercise in Human Subjects Following L-carnitine Administration." *Biochimica et Biophysica Acta* 1034 (1990): 17–21.

Silverstone, B. Z., L. Landau, D. Berson, and J. Sternbuch. "Zinc and Copper Metabolism in Patients with Senile Macular Degeneration." *Annals of Ophthalmology* 17 (1985): 419–22.

Simeon, D. T., and S. Grantham-McGregor. "Effects of Missing Breakfast on the Cognitive Functions of School Children of Differing Nutritional Status." *American Journal of Clinical Nutrition* 49 (1989): 646–53.

Simkin, P. A. "Oral Zinc Sulphate in Rheumatoid Arthritis." *Lancet* (1976): 539–42.

Simon, J. A. "Vitamin C and Cardiovascular Disease: A Review." *Journal of the American College of Nutrition* 11, no. 2 (1992): 107–25.

Simons, L. A., et al. "On the Effect of Garlic on Plasma Lipids and Lipoproteins in Mild Hypercholesterolaemia." *Atherosclerosis* 113 (1995): 219–25.

Simopoulos, A. "Evolutionary Aspects of Diets: Fatty Acids, Insulin Resistance, and Obesity." In T.B. VanItallie and A.P. Simopoulos, eds., *Obesity: New Directions in Assessment and Management.* Philadelphia: Charles Press, 1995.

Singh, A., et al. "Dietary Intakes and Biochemical Markers of Selected Minerals: Comparison of Highly Trained Runners and Untrained Women." *Journal of the American College of Nutrition* 9 (1990): 65–75.

Singh, A., et al. "Magnesium, Zinc, and Copper Status of U.S. Navy SEAL Trainees." *American Journal of Clinical Nutrition* 49 (1989): 695–700.

Singh, R. B., and D. Downing. "Antioxidants and Coronary Artery Disease." *Journal of Nutritional and Environmental Medicine* 5 (1995): 219–24.

Singh, R. B., S. Ghosh, M. A. Niaz, R. Singh, R. Beegum, H. Chibo, Z. Shoumin, and A. Postiglione. "Dietary Intake, Plasma Levels of Antioxidant Vitamins, and Oxidative Stress in Relation to Coronary Artery Disease in Elderly Subjects." *American Journal of Cardiology* 76 (1995): 1233–8.

Singh, R. B., M. A. Niaz, S. Ghosh, R. Beegum, I. Bishnoi, P. Agarwal, and A. Agarwal. "Dietary Intake and Plasma Levels of Antioxidant Vitamins in Health and Disease: A Hospital-Based Case-Control Study." *Journal of Nutritional and Environmental Medicine* 5 (1995): 235–42.

Singhal, P. C., and L. D. Joshi. "Glycemic and Cholesterolemic Role of Ginger and Til." *Jour. Sci. Res. Pl. & Med.* 4, no. 3 (1983): 18–20.

Sjogren, A., C.-H. Floren, and A. Nilsson. "Evaluation of Magnesium Status in Crohn's Disease as Assessed by Intracellular Analysis and Intravenous Magnesium Infusion." *Scandinavian Journal of Gastroenterology* 23 (1988): 555–61.

Sklodowska, M., et al. "Selenium and Vitamin E Concentrations in Plasma and Erythrocytes of Angina Pectoris Patients." *Trace Elements in Medicine* 8, no. 3 (1991): 113–7.

Skoryna, S. C. "Effect of Oral Supplementation with Stable Strontium." *CMA* 125 (1981): 703–12.

Slota, T., N. A. Kozlov, and H. V. Ammon. "Comparison of Cholesterol and Beta-sitosterol: Effects on Jejunal Fluid Secretion Induced by Oleate, and Absorption from Micellar Solutions." *Gut* 24 (1983): 653–8.

Smirnov, V. V., and S. R. Reznick. "Modern Views of Mechanism of Healing Action of Probiotics from Bacterium of Bacillus Family." *Microbiological Journal* 55, no. 4 (1993): 92–104.

Smith, A., S. Leekam, A. Ralph, and G. McNeill. "The Influence of Meal Composition on Post-lunch Changes in Performance Efficiency and Mood." *Appetite* 10 (1988): 195–203.

Smith, A., and C. Miles. "Acute Effects of Meals, Noise, and Nightwork." *British Journal of Psychology* 77 (1986): 377–87.

Smith, H. R., A. Memom, C. J. Smart, and K. Dewbury. "The Value of Permixon in Benign Prostatic Hypertrophy." *British Journal of Urology* 58 (1986): 36–40.

Smith, K., R. Heaney, L. Flora, and S. Hinders. "Calcium Absorption from a New Calcium Delivery System (CCM)." *Calcified Tissue International* 41 (1987): 351–2.

Smith, U. "Dietary Fibre, Diabetes, and Obesity." *International Journal of Obesity* 11, supplement 1 (1987): 27–31.

Sneed, S. M., C. Zane, and M. R. Thomas. "The Effects of Ascorbic Acid, Vitamin B6, Vitamin B12, and Folic Acid Supplementation on the Breast Milk and Maternal Nutritional Status of Low Socieconomic Lactating Women." *American Journal of Clinical Nutrition* 34 (1981): 1338–46.

Sobota, A. E. "Inhibition of Bacterial Adherence by Cranberry Juice: Potential Use for the Treament of Urinary Tract Infections." *Journal of Urology* 131 (1984): 1013–6.

Soholm, B. "Clinical Improvement of Memory and Other Cognitive Functions by Ginkgo Biloba: Review of Relevant Literature." *Advances in Therapy* 15, no. 1 (1998): 66–77.

Solum, T. T., K. R. Ryttig, E. Solum, and S. Larsen. "The Influence of a High-Fibre Diet on Body Weight, Serum Lipids, and Blood Pressure in Slightly Overweight Persons." *International Journal of Obesity* 11, no. 1 (1987): 67–71.

Sorensen, G., et al. "Work-Site Nutrition Intervention and Employees' Dietary Habits: The Treatwell Program." *American Journal of Public Health* 82, no. 6 (1992): 877–80.

Sowers, M. R., and R. B. Wallace. "Retinol, Supplemental Vitamin A and Bone Status." *Journal of Clinical Epidemiology* 43, no. 7 (1990): 693–9.

Spencer, H., et al. "Effect of Zinc Supplements on the Intestinal Absorption of Calcium." *Journal of the American College of Nutrition* 6, no. 1 (1987): 47–51.

Spiers, P., D. Myers, G. S. Hochanadel, H. R. Lieberman, and P. J. Wurtman. "Citicoline Improves Verbal Memory in Aging." *Archives of Neurology* 53 (1996): 441–8.

Spring, B., J. Chiodo, and D. J. Bowen. "Carbohydrates, Tryptophan, and Behavior: A Methodological Review." *Psychological Bulletin* 102, no. 2 (1987): 234–56.

Spring, B., H. R. Lieberman, G. Swope, and G. S. Garfield. "Effects of Carbohydrates on Mood and Behavior." *Nutrition Reviews* (May 1986): 51–60.

Spring, B., O. Maller, J. Wurtman, L. Digman, and L. Cozolino. "Effects of Protein and Carbohydrate Meals on Mood and Performance: Interactions with Sex and Age." *Journal of Psychiatric Research* 17, no. 2 (1982): 155–67.

Spring, B., et al. "Psychobiological Effects of Carbohydrates." *Journal of Clinical Psychiatry* 50, supplement 5 (1989): 27–33.

Srinivasan, V., et al. "Pantothenic Acid Nutritional Status in the Elderly—Institutionalized and Noninstitutionalized." *American Journal of Clinical Nutrition* 34 (1981): 1736–42.

Stamler, J., A. W. Caggiula, and G. A. Grandits. "Relation of Body Mass and Alcohol, Nutrient, Fiber, and Caffeine Intakes to Blood Pressure in the Special Intervention and Usual Care Groups in the Multiple Risk Factor Intervention Trial." *American Journal of Clinical Nutrition* 65 (1997): 338–65.

Standord, J. L., et al. "Combined Estrogen and Progestin Hormone Replacement Therapy in Relation to Risk of Breast Cancer in Middle-Aged Women." *JAMA* 274, no. 4 (1995): 139–42.

Staniforth, D. H., I. M. Baird, J. Fowler, and R. E. Lister. "The Effects of Dietary Fibre on Upper and Lower Gastro-intestinal Transit Times and Faecal Bulking." *Journal of International Medical Research* 18 (1991): 228–33.

Stanko, R. T., D. L. Tietze, and J. E. Arch. "Body Composition, Energy Utilization, and Nitrogen Metabolism with a 4.25-MJ/d Low-Energy Diet Supplemented with Pyruvate." *American Journal of Clinical Nutrition* 56 (1992): 30–5.

Stanton, C. and R. Gray. "Effects of Caffeine Consumption on Delayed Conception." *American Journal of Epidemiology* 142, no. 12 (1995): 1322–9.

Starling, R. D., T. A. Trappe, K. R. Short, M. Sheffield-Moore, A. C. Jozsi, W. J. Fink, and D. L. Costill. "Effect of Inosine Supplementation on Aerobic and Anaerobic Cycling Performance." *Official Journal of the American College of Sports Medicine* (1996): 1993–8.

Steben, R. E., and P. Boudreaux. "The Effects of Pollen and Protein Extracts on Selected Blood Factors and Performance of Athletes." *Journal of Sports Medicine* 18 (1978): 221–6.

Steichen, J. J., et al. "Elevated Serum 1,25-dihydroxy Vitamin D Concentrations in Rickets of Very Low-Birth-Weight Infants." *Journal of Pediatrics* 99, no. 2 (1981): 293–8.

Stein, J., and C. A. Borden. "Causative and Beneficial Algae in Human Disease Conditions: A Review." *Phycologia* 23, no. 4 (1984): 485–501.

Steinberg, D., et al. "The Anticarcinogenic Activity of Clycrrhizin: Preliminary Clinical Trials." *Israel Journal of Dental Sciences* 2 (1989): 153–7.

Steiner, M. "Untersuchungen zur odemvermindernden und odemprotektiven Wirkung von Robkastaniensamenextrakt." *Phlebologie und Proktologie* 19 (1990): 239–42.

Steiner, M., and J. Anastasi. "Vitamin E: An Inhibitor of the Platelet Release Reaction." *Journal of Clinical Investigation* 57 (1976): 732–7.

Steiner, M., H. Khan, D. Holbert, and R. I. Lin. "A Double-Blind Crossover Study in Moderately Hypercholesterolemic Men That Compared the Effect of Aged Garlic Extract and Placebo Administration on Blood Lipids." *American Journal of Clinical Nutrition* 64 (1996): 866–70.

Stekel, A., et al. "Prevention of Iron Deficiency by Milk Fortification: II. A Field Trial with a Full-Fat Acidified Milk." *American Journal of Clinical Nutrition* 47 (1988): 265–9.

Stellon, A., A. Davies, A. Webb, and R. Williams. "Microcrystalline Hydroxyapatite Compound in Prevention of Bone Loss in Corticosteroid-Treated Patients with Chronic Active Hepatitis." *Postgraduate Medicine Journal* 61 (1985): 791–6.

Stendig-Lindberg, G., et al. "Changes in Serum Magnesium Concentration After Strenuous Exercise." *Journal of the American College of Nutrition* 6, no. 1 (1987): 35–40.

Stensvold, I., A. Tverdal, K. Solvoll, and O. P. Foss. "Tea Consumption, Relation to Cholesterol, Blood Pressure, and Coronary and Total Mortality." *Preventive Medicine* 21 (1992): 546–53.

Stephens, N., et al. "Randomised Controlled Trial of Vitamin E in Patients with Coronary Disease: Cambridge Heart Antioxidant Study (CHAOS)." *Lancet* 347 (1996): 781–6.

Stoa-Birketvedt, G. "Effect of Cimetidine Suspension on Appetite and Weight in Overweight Subjects." *BMJ* 306 (1993): 1091–2.

Stolzenberg-Solomon, R. Z., et al. "Pancreatic Cancer Risk and Nutrition-Related Methyl-Group Availability Indicators in Male Smokers." *Journal of the National Cancer Institute* 91, no. 6 (1999): 535–41.

Strain, E., G. Mumford, K. Silverman, and R. Griffiths. "Caffeine Dependence Syndrome: Evidence from Case Histories and Experimental Evaluations." *JAMA* 272, no. 13 (1994): 1043–8.

Strauch, G., et al. "Comparison of Finasteride and Serenoa Repens in the Inhibition of 5-alpha Reductase in Healthy Male Volunteers." *European Urology* 26 (1994): 247–52.

Strazzullo, P., et al. "Abnormalities of Calcium Metabolism in Essential Hypertension." *Clinical Science* 65 (1983): 137–41.

Street, D. A., G. W. Comstock, R. H. Salkeld, W. Schuep, and M. J. Klag. "Serum Antioxidants and Myocardial Infarction. Are Low Levels of Carotenoids and Alpha-tocopherol Risk Factors for Myocardial Infarction?" *Circulation* 90, no. 3 (1994): 1154–61.

Sturniolo, G. C., M. M. Molokhia, R. Shields, and L. A. Turnberg. "Zinc Absorption in Crohn's Disease." *Gut* 21 (1980): 387–91.

Subhan, Z., and I. Hindmarch. "Psychopharmacological Effects of Vinpocetine in Normal Healthy Volunteers." *European Journal of Clinical Pharmacology* 28 (1985): 567–71.

Sullivan, D. R., T. A. B. Sanders, I. M. Trayner, and G. R. Thompson. "Paradoxical Elevation of LDL Apoprotein B Levels in Hypertriglyceridaemic Patients and Normal Subjects Ingesting Fish Oil." *Atherosclerosis* 61 (1986): 129–34.

Suminski, R. R., et al. "Acute Effect of Amino Acid Ingestion and Resistance Exercise on Plasma Growth Hormone Concentration in Young Men." *International Journal of Sport Nutrition* 7 (1997): 48–60.

Summer, A. E., et al. "Elevated Methylmalonic Acid and Total Homocysteine Levels Show High Prevalence of Vitamin B12 Deficiency After Gastric Surgery." *Annals of Internal Medicine* 124 (1996): 469–76.

Sundaram, G. S., R. London, S. Manimekalai, P. P. Nair, and P. Goldstein. "Alpha-tocopherol and Serum Lipoproteins." *Lipids* 16, no. 4 (1981): 223–7.

Sundberg, B., et al. "Mixed-Linked B-glucan from Breads of Different Cereals Is Partly Degraded in the Human Ileostomy Model." *American Journal of Clinical Nutrition* 65 (1996): 878–85.

Sundstrom, H., et al. "Serum Selenium and Glutathione Peroxidase, and Plasma Lipid Peroxides in Uterine, Ovarian, or Vulvar Cancer, and Their Responses to Antioxidants in Patients with Ovarian Cancer." *Cancer Letters* 24 (1984): 1–10.

Superko, H. R., W. Bortz, P. T. Williams, J. J. Albers, and P. D. Wood. "Caffeinated and Decaffeinated Coffee Effects on Plasma Lipoprotein Cholesterol, Apolipoproteins, and Lipase Activity: A Controlled, Randomized Trial." *American Journal of Clinical Nutrition* 54 (1991): 599–605.

Svenson, K. L. G., R. Hallgren, E. Johansson, and U. Lindh. "Reduced Zinc in Peripheral Blood Cells from Patients with Inflammatory Connective Tissue Diseases." *Inflammation* 9, no. 2 (1985): 189–97.

Swift, L., et al. "Medium-Chain Fatty Acids: Evidence for Incorporation into Chylomicron Triglycerides in Humans." *American Journal of Clinical Nutrition* 52 (1990): 834–6.

Takahara, J., et al. "Stimulatory Effects of Gamma-hydroxybutyric Acid on Growth Hormone and Prolactin Release in Humans." *Journal of Clinical Endocrinology and Metabolism* 44 (1977): 1014–7.

Tang, G., C. Serfaty-Lacrosniere, M. E. Camilo, and R. M. Russell. "Gastric Acidity Influences the Blood Response to a B-carotene Dose In Humans." *American Journal of Clinical Nutrition* 64 (1996): 622–6.

Tao, X., L. S. Davis, K. Hashimoto, and P. E. Lipsky. "The Chinese Herbal Remedy T2 Inhibits Mitogen-Induced Cytokine Gene Transcription by T Cells, but Not Initial Signal Transduction." *Journal of Pharmacology and Experimental Therapeutics* 276, no. 1 (1996): 316–25.

Tao, X., H. Schulze-Koops, L. Ma, J. Cai, Y. Mao, and P. E. Lipsky. "Effects of Tripterygium Wilfordii Hook F Extracts on Induction of Cyclooxygenase 2 Activity and Prostaglandin E2 Production." *Arthritis and Rheumatism* 41, no. 1 (1998): 130–8.

Tapadinhas, M., I. Rivera, and A. Bignamini. "Oral Glucosamine Sulphate in the Management of Arthrosis: Report on a Multicentre Open Investigation in Portugal." *Pharmatherapeutica* 3 (1982): 157–68.

Tarr, J. B., T. Tamura, and E. L. R. Stokstad. "Availability of Vitamin B6 and Pantothenate in an Average American Diet in Man." *American Journal of Clinical Nutrition* 34 (1981): 1328–37.

Tatami, R., et al. "Regression of Coronary Atherosclerosis by Combined LDL-apheresis and Lipid-Lowering Drug Therapy in Patients with Familial Hypercholesterolemia: A Multicenter Study." *Atherosclerosis* 95 (1992): 1–13.

Tauchert, M., M. Ploch, and W.-D. Hubner. "Wirksamkeit des Weißdorn-Extraktes LI 132 im Vergleich mit Captopril: Multizentrische Doppelblindstudie bei 132 Patienten mit Herzinsuffizienz im Stadium II nach NYHA." *Munch. med. Wochenschrift* 136 (1994): S27–33.

Tauchert, M., G. Siegel, and V. Schulz. "Weißdorn-Extrakt als pflanzliches Cariacum: Neubewertung der therapeutischen Wirksamkeit." *Munch. med. Wochenschrift* 136 (1994): S3–5.

Tavoni, A., C. Vitali, S. Bombardieri, and G. Pasero. "Evaluation of S-adenosylmethionine in Primary Fibromyalgia." *American Journal*

of Medicine 83, supplement 5A (1987): 107–10.

Teas, J. "The Dietary Intake of Laminaria, a Brown Seaweed, and Breast Cancer Prevention." *Nutrition and Cancer* 4, no. 3 (1983): 217–20.

Teresi, M. E., and D. E. Morgan. "Attitudes of Healthcare Professionals Toward Patient Counseling on Drug-Nutrient Interactions." *Annals of Pharmacotherapy* 28 (1994): 576–9.

Tesch, P. A., H. Johansson, and P. Kaiser. "The Effect of Ginseng, Vitamins, and Minerals on the Physical Work Capacity of Middle-aged Men." *Lakartidningen* 84 (1987): 4326–8.

Thayer, R. E. "Energy, Tiredness, and Tension Effects of a Sugar Snack Versus Moderate Exercise." *Journal of Personality and Social Psychology* 52, no. 1 (1987): 119–25.

Thruvengadam, K. V., et al. "Tylophora Indica in Bronchial Asthma." *Journal of Indian Medicine* 71, no. 7 (1977): 172–6.

Tikkanen, H. O., E. Hamalainen, S. Sarna, H. Adlercreutz, and M. Harkonen. "Associations Between Skeletal Muscle Properties, Physical Fitness, Physical Activity, and Coronary Heart Disease Risk Factors in Men." *Atherosclerosis* 137, no. 3 (1998): 77–89.

Tikkanen, H. O., H. Naveri, and M. Harkonen. "Skeletal Muscle Fiber Distribution Influences Serum High-Density Lipoprotein Cholesterol Levels." *Atherosclerosis* 120 (1996): 1–5.

Tirosh, O., Y. Katzhendler, Y. Barenholz, I. Ginsburg, and R. Kohen. "Antioxidant Properties of Amidothionophosphates: Novel Antioxidant Molecules." *Free Radical Biology and Medicine* 20, no. 3 (1996): 421–32.

Tisserand, R. "Aromatherapy: Clinical Use of Essential Oils to Affect Positive Mental and Physical States." *International Journal of Aromatherapy* 6, no. 3 (1995): 14–9.

Toborek, M., and B. Hennig. "Is Methionine an Atherogenic Amino Acid?" *Journal of Optimal Nutrition* 3, no. 2 (1994): 80–3.

Todd, S., M. Woodward, C. Bolton-Smith, and H. Tunstall-Pedoe. "An Investigation of the Relationship Between Antioxidant Vitamin Intake and Coronary Heart Disease in Men and Women Using Discriminant Analysis." *Journal of Clinical Epidemiology* 48, no. 2 (1995): 297–305.

Toft, I., K. H. Bonaa, O. C. Ingebretsen, A. Nordoy, and T. Jonseen. "Effects of n-3 Polyunsaturated Fatty Acids on Glucose Homeostasis and Blood Pressure in Essential Hypertension: A Randomized, Controlled Trial." *Annals of Internal Medicine* 123 (1995): 911–8.

Toner, M. M., et al. "Metabolic and Cardiovascular Responses to Exercise with Caffeine." *Ergonomics* 25, no. 12 (1982): 1175–83.

Tordoff, M. G., and A. M. Alleva. "Effect of Drinking Soda Sweetened with Aspartame or High-Fructose Corn Syrup on Food Intake and Body Weight." *American Journal of Clinical Nutrition* 51 (1990): 963–9.

Tremblay, A., G. Plourde, J.-P. Despres, and C. Bouchard. "Impact of Dietary Fat Content and Fat Oxidation on Energy Intake in Humans." *American Journal of Clinical Nutrition* 49 (1989): 799–805.

Tremblay, A., et al. "Effect of Intensity of Physical Activity on Body Fatness and Fat Distribution." *American Journal of Clinical Nutrition* 51 (1990): 153–7.

Trent, L. K., and T. L. Conway. "Dietary Factors Related to Physical Fitness Among Navy Shipboard Men." *American Journal of Health Promotion* 3, no. 2 (1988): 12–25.

Tuntawiroon, M., et al. "Dose-Dependent Inhibitory Effect of Phenolic Compounds in Foods on Nonheme-Iron Absorption in Men." *American Journal of Clinical Nutrition* 53 (1991): 554–7.

Turnlund, J. R., W. R. Keyes, H. L. Anderson, and L. L. Acord. "Copper Absorption and Retention in Young Men at Three Levels of Dietary Copper by Use of Stable Isotope Cu1–4." *American Journal of Clinical Nutrition* 49 (1989): 870–8.

Tuttle, W. W., K. Daum, L. Myers, and C. Martin. "Effect of Omitting Breakfast on the Physiologic Response in Men." *Journal of the American Dietetic Association* 26 (1950): 332–5.

Tuttle, W. W., M. Wilson, and K. Daum. "Effect of Altered Breakfast Habits on Physiologic Response." *Journal of Applied Physiology* 1, no. 8 (1949): 545–59.

Ubbink, J. B., W.J.H. Vermaak, A. van der Merwe, and P. J. Becker. "Vitamin B12, Vitamin B6, and Folate Nutritional Status in Men with Hyperhomocysteinemia." *American Journal of Clinical Nutrition* 57 (1993): 47–53.

Ubbink. J. B., W.J.H. Vermaak, A. van der Merwe, P. J. Becker, R. Delport, and H. C. Potgieter. "Vitamin Requirements for the Treatment of Hyperhomocysteinemia in Humans." *Journal of Nutrition* 124 (1994): 1927–33.

Umegaki, K., et al. "Beta-carotene Prevents X-ray Induction of Micronuclei in Human Lymphocytes." *American Journal of Clinical Nutrition* 59 (1994): 409–12.

Urberg, M., J. Benyi, and R. John. "Hypocholesterolemic Effects of Nicotinic Acid and Chromium Supplementation." *Journal of Family Practice* 27, no. 6 (1988): 603–6.

Urberg, M., and M. B. Zemel. "Evidence for Synergism Between Chromium and Nicotinic Acid in the Control of Glucose Tolerance in Elderly Humans." *Metabolism* 36, no. 9 (1987): 896–9.

Urgert, R., N. Essed, G. van der Weg, T. Kosmeijer-Schuil, and M. Katan. "Separate Effects of the Coffee Diterpenes Cafestol and Kahweol on Serum Lipids and Liver Aminotransferases." *American Journal of Clinical Nutrition* 65 (1997): 519–24.

Ushiroyama, T., S. Okamura, A. Ikeda, and M. Ueki. "Efficacy of Ipriflavone and 1alpha Vitamin D Therapy for the Cessation of Vertebral Bone Loss." *International Journal of Gynecology and Obstetrics* 48 (1995): 283–88.

Vajaradul, Y. "Double-Blind Clinical Evaluation of Intra-Articular Glucosamine in Outpatients with Gonarthrosis." *Clinical Therapy* 3 (1981): 336–43.

Valberg, L. S., P. R. Flanagan, A. Kertesz, and D. C. Bondy. "Zinc Absorption in Inflammatory Bowel Disease." *Digestive Diseases and Sciences* 31, no. 7 (1986): 724–31.

Valente, M., et al. "Effects of One-Year Treatment with Ipriflavone on Bone in Postmenopausal Women with Low Bone Mass." *Calcified Tissue International* 54 (1994): 377–80.

Van Beresteijn, E., J. Brussaard, and M. van Schaik. "Relationship Between the Calcium-to-Protein Ratio in Milk and Urinary Calcium Excretion in Healthy Adults—A Controlled Crossover Study." *American Journal of Clinical Nutrition* 52 (1990): 142–6.

Van Dau, N., et al. "The Effects of a Traditional Drug, Turmeric (Curcuma Longa), and Placebo on the Healing of Duodenal Ulcer." *Phytomedicine* 5, no. 1 (1998): 29–34.

Van den Berg, M., et al. "Hyperhomocysteinaemia and Endothelial Dysfunction in Young Patients with Peripheral Arterial Occlusive Disease." *European Journal of Clinical Investigation* 25 (1995): 176–81.

Van de Ven, M.L.H.M., M. S. Westerterp-Plantenga, L. Wouters, and W.H.M. Saris. "Effects of Liquid Preloads with Different Fructose/Fibre Concentrations on Subsequent Food Intake and Ratings of Hunger in Women." *Appetite* 23 (1994): 139–46.

Van Duyn, M.A.S., T. A. Leo, M. E. McIvor, K. M. Behali, J. E. Michnowski, and

A. L. Mendeloff. "Nutritional Risk of High-Carbohydrate, Guar Gum Dietary Supplementation in Non-insulin-dependent Diabetes Mellites." *Diabetes Care* 9, no. 5 (1986): 497–503.

Van Gent, C. M., J. B. Luten, H. C. Bronsgeest-Schoute, and A. Ruiter. "Effect, on Serum Lipid Levels of w-3 Fatty Acids, of Ingesting Fish-Oil Concentrate." *Lancet* (1979): 1249–50.

Van Lente, F., R. Daher, and J. A. Waletzky. "Vitamin E Compared with Other Potential Risk Factor Concentrations in Patients with and without Coronary Artery Disease: A Case-Matched Study." *Eur. J. Clin. Chem. Clin Biochem.* 32 (1994): 583–7.

Van Rooij, J., G. Van der Stegen, R. Schoemaker, C. Kroon, J. Burggraaf, L. Hollaar, T. Vroon, A. Smelt, and A. Cohen. "A Placebo-Controlled Parallel Study of the Effect of Two Types of Coffee Oil on Serum Lipids and Transaminases: Identification of Chemical Substances Involved in the Cholesterol-Raising Effect of Coffee." *American Journal of Clinical Nutrition* 61 (1995): 1277–83.

Vannucchi, H., and F. S. Moreno. "Interaction of Niacin and Zinc Metabolism in Patients with Alcoholic Pellagra." *American Journal of Clinical Nutrition* 50 (1989): 364–9.

Varma, S. D. "Scientific Basis for Medical Therapy of Cataracts by Antioxidants." *American Journal of Clinical Nutrition* 53 (1991): 335–45.

Vido, L., P. Facchin, L. Antonello, D. Gobber, and F. Rigon. "Childhood Obesity Treatment: Double-Blinded Trial on Dietary Fibres (Glucomannan) Versus Placebo." *Paediatr. Puedol.* 28 (1993): 133–6.

Vinson, J. A., and P. Bose. "Comparative Bioavailability to Humans of Ascorbic Acid Alone or in a Citrus Extract." *American Journal of Clinical Nutrition* 48 (1988): 601–4.

Vita, A. J., R. B. Terry, H. B. Hubert, and J. F. Fries. "Aging, Health Risks, and Cumulative Disability." *New England Journal of Medicine* 338 (1998): 1035–41.

Volz, H.-P., and M. Kieser. "Kava-kava Extract WS 1490 Versus Placebo in Anxiety Disorders—A Randomized Placebo-Controlled Twenty-five-Week Outpatient Trial." *Pharmacopsychiatry* 30 (1997): 1–5.

Von Lossonczy, T. O., A. Ruiter, H. C. Bronsgeest-Schoute, C. M. van Gent, and R.J.J. Hermus. "The Effect of a Fish Diet on Serum Lipids in Healthy Human Subjects." *American Journal of Clinical Nutrition* 31 (1978): 1340–6.

Vorbach, E. U., and K. H. Arnold. "Wirksamkeit und Vertraglichkeit von Baldrianextrakt (LI 156) versus Placebo bei behandlungbedurftigen Insomnien." *Z. Phytother. Abstractband.* S11 (1995).

Vorbach, E. U., et al. "Efficacy and Tolerability of St. John's Wort Extract LI 160 Versus Imipramine in Patients with Severe Depressive Episodes According to ICD-10." *Pharmacopsychiatry* 30 (1997): 81–5.

Vorberg, G. "Ginkgo Biloba (GBE): A Long-Term Study of Chronic Cerebral Insufficiency in Geriatric Patients." *Clinical Trials Journal* 22, no. 2 (1985): 149–57.

Wagner, H. "Search for New Plant Constituents with Potential Antiphlogistic and Antiallergic Activity." *Planta Medica* 55 (1989): 235–41.

Wahlqvist, M. L., N. Wattanapenpaiboon, F. A. Macrae, J. R. Lambert, R. Maclennon, B. H. Hsu-Hage, and Australian Prevention Project Investigators. "Changes in Serum Carotenoids in Subjects with Colorectal Adenomas After Twenty-four Months of B-carotene Supplementation." *American Journal of Clinical Nutrition* 60 (1994): 936–43.

Walker, K. Z., et al. "Body Fat Distribution and Non-insulin-dependent Diabetes: Comparison of a Fiber-Rich, High-Carbohydrate, Low-Fat (23%) and a 35% Fat Diet High in Monounsaturated Fat." *American Journal of Clinical Nutrition* 63 (1996): 254–60.

Wander, R. C., S.-H. Du, S. O. Ketchum, and K. E. Rowe. "Effects of Interaction of RRR-alpha-tocopheryl Acetate and Fish Oil on Low-Density-Lipoprotein Oxidation in Postmenopausal Women with and without Hormone-Replacement Therapy." *American Journal of Clinical Nutrition* 63 (1996): 184–93.

Wang, J., et al. "Multicenter Clinical Trial of the Serum Lipid-Lowering Effects of a Monascus Purpureus (Red Yeast) Rice Preparation from Traditional Chinese Medicine." *Current Therapeutic Research* 58, no. 12 (1997): 964–78.

Wannmacher, L., et al. "Plants Employed in the Treatment of Anxiety and Insomnia: II. Effect of Infusions of Aloysia Triphylla on Experimental Anxiety in Normal Volunteers." *Fitoterapia* 61, no. 5 (1990): 449–53.

Warnecke, G., H. Pfaender, G. Gerster, and E. Gracza. "Wirksamkeit von Kawa-Kawa-Extrakt beim klimakterischen Syndrom: Eine Doppelblindstudie mit einem neuen Monopraparat." *Zeitschrift fur Phytotherapie* 11 (1990): 81–6.

Warnecke, V. G. "Psychosomatische Dysfunktionen im weiblichen Klimakterium." *Fortschritte der Medizin* 109, no. 4 (1991): 119–22.

Wastney, M. E., and R. I. Henkin. "Calculation of Zinc Absorption in Humans Using Tracers by Fecal Monitoring and a Compartmental Approach." *Journal of Nutrition* 119 (1989): 1438–43.

Watanabe, J., F. Umeda, H. Wakasugi, and H. Ibayashi. "Effect of Vitamin E on Platelet Aggregation in Diabetes Mellitus." *Thrombosis and Haemostasis* 51, no. 3 (1984): 313–6.

Watanabe, S., et al. "Effects of L- and DL-carnitine on Patients with Impaired Exercise Tolerance." *Japanese Heart Journal* 36 (1995): 319–31.

Watson, R. R., R. H. Prabhala, P. M. Plezia, and D. S. Alberts. "Effect of B-carotene on Lymphocyte Subpopulations in Elderly Humans: Evidence for a Dose-Response Relationship." *American Journal of Clinical Nutrition* 53 (1991): 90–4.

Watson, W. S., et al. "A Simple Blood Sample Method for Measuring Oral Zinc Absorption in Clinical Practice." *Clin. Phys. Physiol. Meas.* 8 (1987): 173–8.

Weber, J., J. M. Were, H. W. Julius, and J. J. M. Marx. "Decreased Iron Absorption in Patients with Active Rheumatoid Arthritis, with and without Iron Deficiency." *Annals of the Rheumatic Diseases* 47 (1988): 404–9.

Weikl, A., and H.-S. Noh. "Der Einfluß von Crataegus bei globaler Herzinsuffizienz" (The Influence of Crataegus in Global Cardiac Insufficiency). *Herz Gefaße* 11 (1992): 516–24.

Weikl, A., et al. "Crataegus Special Extract WS 1442: Objective Proof of Efficacy in Patients with Cardiac Insufficiency (NYHA II)." *Fortschritte der Medizin* 114 (1996): 291–6.

Weiliang, W., X. Mingyu, B. Xiaofeng, and W. Xiufeng. "The Treatment of Forty-four Cases of Simple Obesity with TCM." *Journal of Traditional Chinese Medicine* 9, no. 4 (1989): 283–4.

Weisburger, J. H. "Nutritional Approach to Cancer Prevention with Emphasis on Vitamins, Antioxidants, and Carotenoids." *American Journal of Clinical Nutrition* 53 (1991): 226–37S

Welbourne, T. C. "Increased Plasma Bicarbonate and Growth Hormone After an Oral Glutamine Load." *American Journal of Clinical Nutrition* 61 (1995): 1058–61.

Wene, J. D., W. E. Connor, and L. DenBesten. "The Development of Essential Fatty Acid Deficiency in Healthy Men Fed Fat-Free Diets Intravenously and Orally." *Journal of Clinical Investigation* 36 (1975): 127–34.

Werner, E., and J. P. Kaltwasser. "Judgement of Measured Values of Intestinal Iron Absorption." *Arzneimittel-Forschung* 37 (1987): 116–21.

Wesnes, K. A., et al. "The Cognitive, Subjective, and Physical Effects of a Ginkgo Biloba/Panax Ginseng Combination in Healthy Volunteers with Neurasthenic Complaints." *Psychopharmacology Bulletin* 33, no. 4 (1997): 677–83.

Westphal, J., M. Horning, and K. Leonhardt. "Phytotherapy in Functional Upper Abdominal Complaints." *Phytomedicine* 2, no. 4 (1996): 285–91.

Wheatley, D. "LI 160, an Extract of St. John's Wort, Versus Amitriptyline in Mildly to Moderately Depressed Outpatients—A Controlled Six-Week Clinical Trial." *Pharmacopsychiatry* 30 (1997): 77–80.

Whyte, K. F., G. J. Addis, R. Whitesmith, and J. L. Reid. "Adrenergic Control of Plasma Magnesium in Man." *Clinical Science* 72 (1987): 135–8.

Wiesenauer, M. "Comparison of Solid and Liquid Forms of Homeopathic Remedies for Tonsillitis." *Advances in Therapy* (November/December 1998): 362–71.

Wiklund, I., J. Karlberg, and B. Lund. "A Double-Blind Comparison of the Effect on Quality of Life of a Combination of Vital

Substances Including Standardized Ginseng G115 and Placebo." *Current Therapeutic Research* 55, no. 1 (1994): 32–42.

Wilcken, D.E.L., N.P.B. Dudman, P. A. Tyrell, and M. R. Robertson. "Folic Acid Lowers Elevated Plasma Homocysteine in Chronic Renal Insufficiency: Possible Implication for Prevention of Vascular Disease." *Metabolism* 34 (1988): 1073–7.

Wilcken, D.E.L., V. J. Gupta, and A. K. Betts. "Homocysteine in the Plasma of Renal Transplant Recipients: Effects of Cofactors of Methionine Metabolism." *Clinical Science* 61 (1981): 743–9.

Williams, C. H., S. A. Witherly, and R. K. Buddington. "Influence of Dietary Neosugar on Selected Bacterial Groups of the Human Faecal Microbiota." *Microbial Ecology in Health and Disease* 7 (1994): 91–7.

Williams, C. L. "Importance of Dietary Fibre in Childhood." *Journal of the American Dietetic Association* 95, no. 10 (1995): 1140–9.

Williams, H.T.G., D. Fenna, and R. A. Macbeth. "Alpha Tocopherol in the Treatment of Intermittent Claudication." *Surgery, Gynecology, and Obstetrics* (April 1971): 662–6.

Winters, W. D., R. Benavides, and W. J. Clouse. "Effects of Aloe Extracts on Human Normal and Tumor Cells In Vitro." *Economic Botany* 35, no. 1 (1981): 89–95.

Wisker, E., R. Nagel, T. K. Tanudjaja, and W. Feldheim. "Calcium, Magnesium, Zinc, and Iron Balances in Young Women: Effects of a Low-Phytate Barley-Fiber Concentrate." *American Journal of Clinical Nutrition* 54 (1991): 553–9.

Woelk, H., et al. "Behandlung von Angst-Patienten: Doppelblindstudie; Kava-Spezialextrakt WS 1490 versus Benzodiazepine." *Z. Allg. Med.* 69 (1993): 271–7.

Wolever, T.M.S., D.J.A. Jenkins, V. Vuksan, A. I. Jenkins, G. S. Wong, and R. G. Josse. "Beneficial Effect of Low-Glycemic Index Diet in Overweight NIDDM Subjects." *Diabetes Care* 15, no. 4 (1997): 562–4.

Wong, A.H.C., M. Smith, and H. S. Boon. "Herbal Remedies in Psychiatric Practice." *Arch. Gen. Psychiatry* 55 (1998): 1033–44.

Wood, R. J., and J. J. Zheng. "High Dietary Calcium Intakes Reduce Zinc Absorption and Balance in Humans." *American Journal of Clinical Nutrition* 65 (1997): 1803–9.

Worthington-Roberts, B. S., M. W. Breskin, and E. R. Monsen. "Iron Status of Premenopausal Women in a University Community and Its Relationship to Habitual Dietary Sources of Protein." *American Journal of Clinical Nutrition* 47 (1988): 275–9.

Wu, A. H., M. C. Pike, and D. O. Stram. "Meta-analysis: Dietary Fat Intake, Serum Estrogen Levels, and the Risk of Breast Cancer." *Journal of the National Cancer Institute* 91, no. 6 (1999): 529–34.

Wurtman, J. J., A. Brzeizinski, R. J. Wurtman, and B. Laferrere. "Effect of Nutrient Intake on Premenstrual Depression." *American Journal of Obstetrics and Gynecology* 161 (1989): 1128–34.

Yetiv, J. Z. "Clinical Applications of Fish Oils." *JAMA* 260, no. 5 (1988): 665–70.

Yeum, K.-J., et al. "Human Plasma Carotenoid Response to the Ingestion of Controlled Diets High in Fruits and Vegetables." *American Journal of Clinical Nutrition* 64 (1996): 594–602.

Yim, T. K., W. K. Wu, D. H. F. Mak, and K. M. Ko. "Myocardial Protective Effect of an Anthraquinone-Containing Extract of Polygonum Multiflorum Ex Vivo." *Planta Medica* 64 (1998): 607–11.

Yingming, G., and A. Shufen. "Yishou-Jianghzi (De-blood-lipid) Tablets in the Treatment of Hyperlipemia." *Journal of Traditional Chinese Medicine* 15, no. 3 (1996): 178–9.

Yongchaiyudha, S., et al. "Antidiabetic Activity of Aloe Vera L. Juice: II. Clinical Trial in Diabetes Mellitus Patients in Combination with Glibenclamide." *Phytomedicine* 3, no. 3 (1996): 245–8.

Yost, T. J., and R. H. Eckel. "Hypocaloric Feeding in Obese Women: Metabolic Effects of Medium-Chain Triglyceride Substitution." *American Journal of Clinical Nutrition* 49 (1989): 326–30.

Yu, B. P. "Aging and Oxidative Stress: Modulation by Dietary Restriction." *Free Radical Biology and Medicine* 21, no. 5 (1996): 651–68.

Zahafonetis, C.J.D. "Preliminary and Short Reports: Darkening of Gray Hair During Para-amino-benzoic-acid Therapy." *Journal of Investigative Dermatology* (1950): 399–401.

Zarkadas, M., et al. "Sodium Chloride Supplementation and Urinary Clacium Excretion in Postmenopausal Women." *American Journal of Clinical Nutrition* 50 (1989): 1088–94.

Zavaroni, I., et al. "Risk Factors for Coronary Artery Disease in Healthy Persons with Hyperinsulnemia and Normal Glucose Tolerance." *New England Journal of Medicine* 320, no. 11 (1989): 702–6.

Zemel, P. C., et al. "Metabolic and Hemodynamic Effects of Magnesium Supplementation in Patients with Essential Hypertension." *American Journal of Clinical Nutrition* 51 (1990): 665–9.

Zhang, Y. H., et al. "Possible Immunologic Involvement of Antioxidants in Cancer Prevention." *American Journal of Clinical Nutrition* 62 (1995): 1477–82.

Zhdanova, I. V., et al. "Sleep-Inducing Effects of Low Doses of Melatonin Ingested in the Evening." *Clinical Pharmacology and Therapeutics* 57 (1995): 552–8.

Zheng, W., et al. "Retinol, Antioxidant Vitamins, and Cancers of the Upper Digestive Tract in a Prospective Cohort Study of Postmenopausal Women." *American Journal of Epidemiology* 142, no. 9 (1995): 955–60.

Zhi-Xu, G., et al. "Efficacy of Tablet Huperzine A on Memory, Cognition, and Behavior in Alzheimer's Disease." *Acta Pharmacologica Sinica* 16, no. 5 (1995): 391–5.

Ziegler, R. G. "Vegetables, Fruits, and Carotenoids and the Risk of Cancer." *American*

Journal of Clinical Nutrition 53 (1991): 251–9S

Zorgniottie, A. W., and E. F. Lizza. "Effect of Large Doses of the Nitric Oxide Precursor, L-arginine, on Erectile Dysfunction." *International Journal of Impotence Research* 6 (1994): 33–6.

Zuin, M., et al. "Effects of a Preparation Containing a Standardized Ginseng Extract Combined with Trace Elements and Multivitamins Against Hepatotoxin-Induced Chronic Liver Disease in the Elderly." *Journal of International Medical Research* 15 (1987): 276–81.

INDEX

ABOUT THE AUTHOR

Daniel Gastelu, M.S., M.F.S., is founder of Supplementfacts™ International, a company devoted to providing reliable information about nutrition and dietary supplements. He serves as director of nutritional sciences for the International Sports Sciences Association and is actively involved in many facets of the dietary supplement industry, including product development, manufacturing, and regulatory affairs. Daniel Gastelu developed and coauthored the ISSA's Specialist in Performance Nutrition certification program and course book, which is used to certify doctors, physical therapists, fitness trainers, strength coaches, and nutritionists. Daniel Gastelu is a graduate of Rutgers University, where he taught science courses. He is a Master Fitness Trainer, and Specialist in Performance Nutrition. He also creates and teaches continuing education courses about nutrition and dietary supplements for pharmacists. During the past two decades Daniel Gastelu has developed hundreds of health care products, including dietary supplements, sports nutritionals, nutraceutical foods, and OTC drugs. He directed innovative research programs examining the effects of different nutrition programs on body composition, health, and physical performance. In recent years Daniel Gastelu has worked on numerous projects with prominent health experts, such as Shari Lieberman, Ph.D., Cherie Calbom, M.S., C.N., Stephen Gullo, Ph.D., Ann Louise Gittleman, M.S., Varro Tyler, Ph.D., Frederick J. Vagnini, M.D., Frederick C. Hatfield, Ph.D., Richard Simmons, Jack La Lanne, Denise Austin, and Tony Little. Recent books include *Dynamic Nutrition for Maximum Performance, All About Sports Nutrition, All About Bioflavonoids, All About Carnitine, Avery's Sports Nutrition Almanac,* and *Performance Nutrition: The Complete Guide.*

SUPPLEMENTFACTS.COM

As a purchaser of *The Complete Nutritional Supplements Buyer's Guide,* you are invited to visit my special SUPPLEMENTFACTS™ Web site. I created the SUPPLEMENTFACTS Web site as a means to offer my readers periodic updates to this book.

Just go on-line to access the http://www.supplementfacts.com™ Web site and follow the simple instructions to register for your use. To get access to the site, you will be asked to enter your special password, which is contained in this book.

The Complete Nutritional Supplement Buyer's Guide is part of Daniel Gastelu's SUPPLEMENTFACTS™ health book series.